the complete **superfoods** cookbook

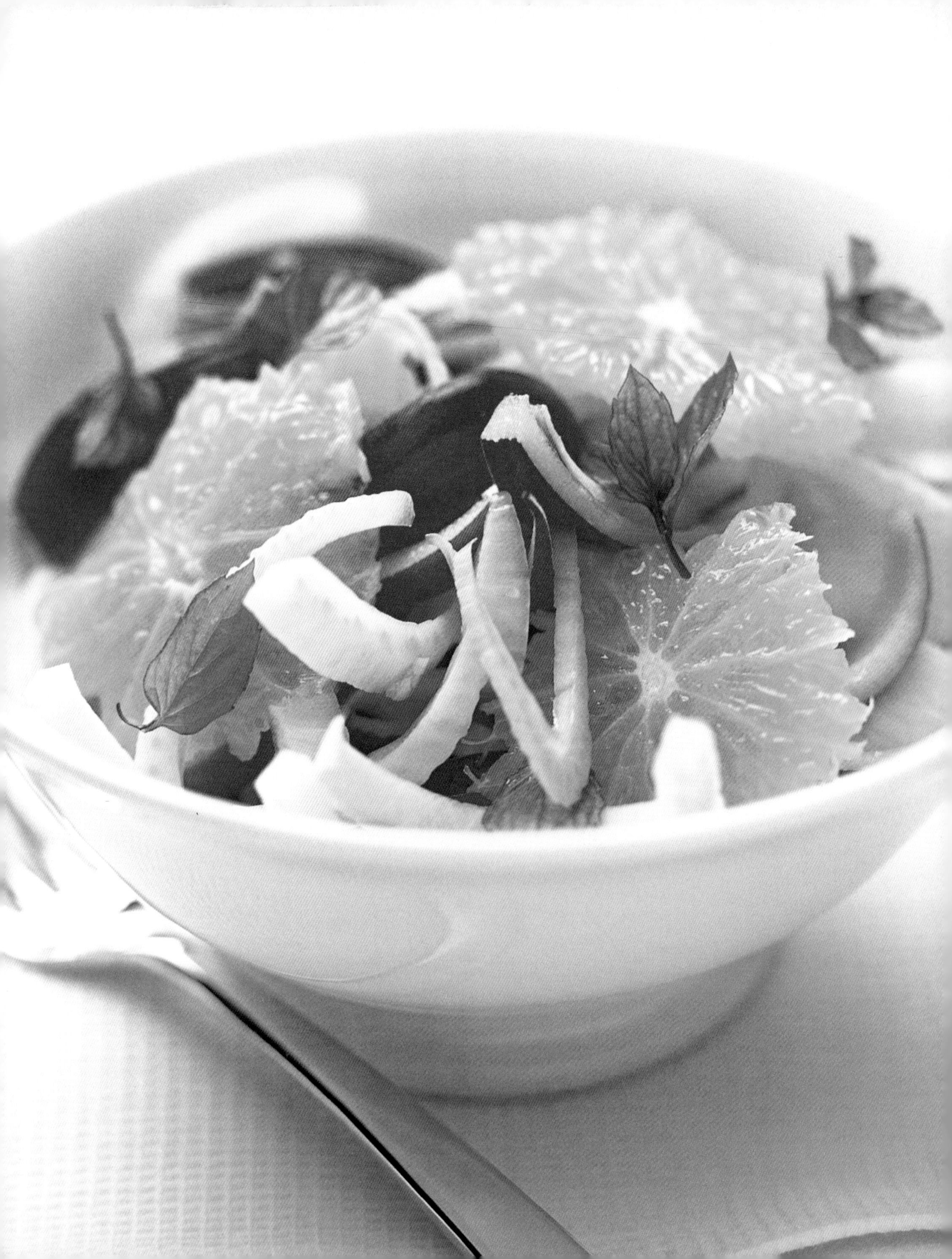

the complete **superfoods** cookbook

michael van straten

MITCHELL BEAZLEY

the complete superfoods cookbook

Michael van Straten

First published in Great Britain in 2007 by Mitchell Beazley, an imprint of Octopus Publishing Group Limited, 2–4 Heron Quays, London E14 4JP.

A CIP catalogue record for this book is available from the British Library.

ISBN 10: 1 84533 087 0

ISBN 13: 978 1 84533 087 3

Commissioning Editor: Rebecca Spry

Executive Art Editor and Designer: Nicky Collings

Copy Editor: Jamie Ambrose

Senior Editor: Hannah McEwen

Proofreader: sandseditorial.co.uk

Photography: Peter Cassidy, Nicki Dowey, Francesca Yorke

Stylist: Katherine Ibbs, Louise Mackaness

Production: Angela Couchman

Index: John Noble

Printed and bound by Toppan Printing Company in China

Typeset in Myriad

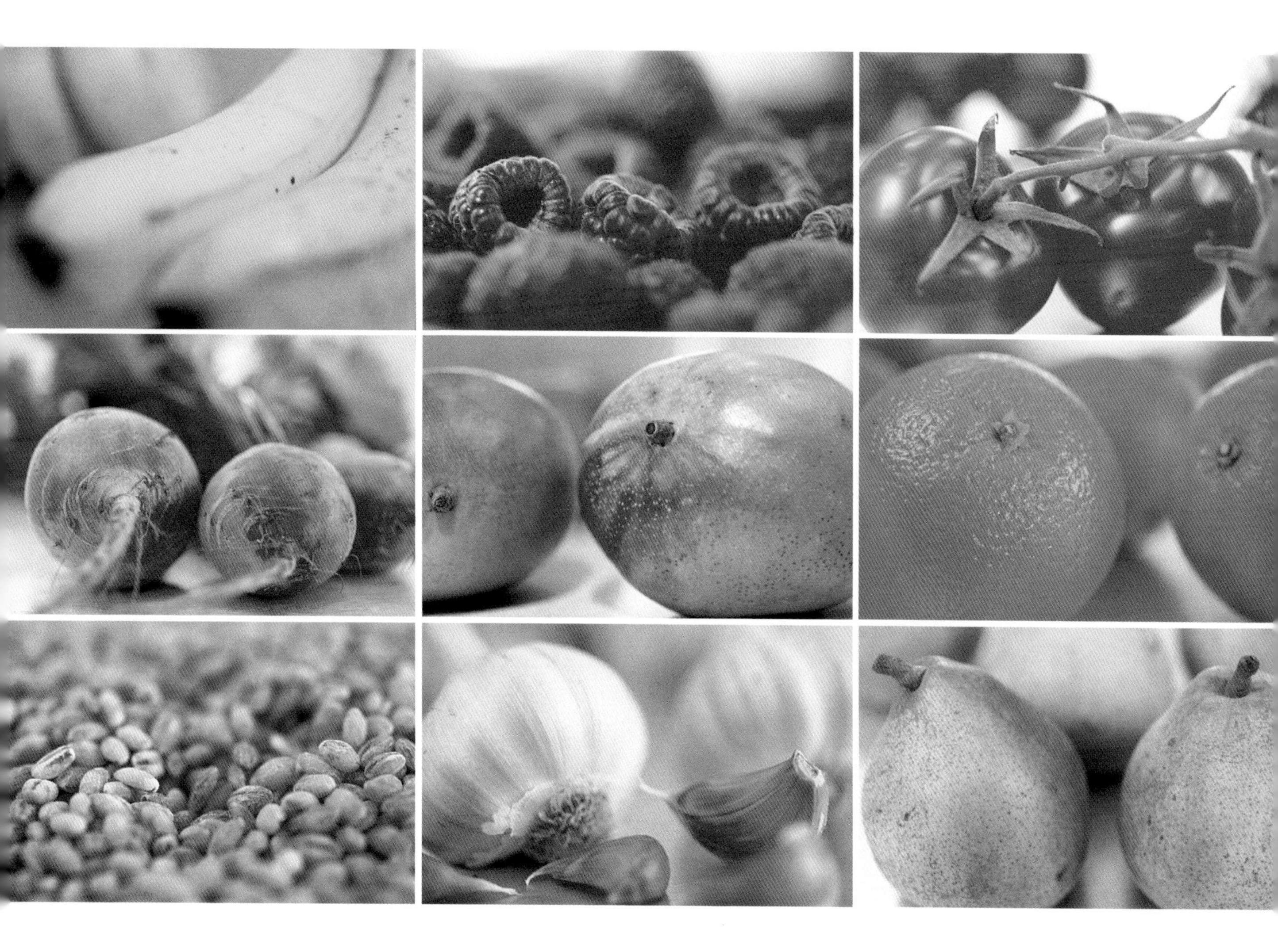

contents

"Superfoods" is the new buzz-word, but what does it mean? Can fruits and vegetables slow down ageing, lower blood pressure or even prevent some forms of cancer? As a complementary health practitioner; broadcaster, author and journalist concerned with natural health, food and healing; and an organic gardener since meeting Rachel Carson, author of *Silent Spring,* way back in the 1960s; I have become totally convinced that there are superfoods with the power to enhance and extend life.

With my colleague Barbara Griggs, I coined the term "superfoods" back in 1990 and personally, I don't grow much in my organic garden that I can't eat, because fresh produce has the most nutrients and the best flavour. If it's organic, you get even more nutrients and avoid environmental- and health-damaging chemicals.

A superfood must have substantial levels of one or more essential vitamins and minerals and/or be a rich source of the unique "phytochemicals" – powerful natural substances that protect the body's cells from damage. Surprisingly, the two don't always go together.

Celery, for example, is pretty useless nutritionally: ninety-five per cent water, only seven energy-giving calories in 100g and you burn more chewing it. But it has been valued as a medicinal vegetable since ancient Rome. The phytochemicals it contains provide flavour and calming properties. As a natural diuretic, it gets rid of surplus fluid, so it is perfect for women with monthly bouts of puffy hands, feet or breasts.

Superfoods affect whole populations and are the reasons why southern European men have a fifty per cent lower risk of prostate cancer than the British – Spaniards, for example, eat more than twice as much fruit and vegetables as the average Brit. Their superfood diet also means fewer strokes, and less heart disease, bowel cancer and other ills.

As a practising naturopath for more than forty years I base most of my advice for patients on the links between food and health. However, I'm not a member of the "food police" and certainly don't believe that one bar of chocolate, a cup of coffee, a jam doughnut or a dollop of cream on your strawberries will put your health at risk for the next twenty years.

I worry desperately about the many people I see – mostly women – who have become so obsessed with food that they angst about every forkful that goes in their mouths. Of course, it's great to eat organic food if you can, and it's important to consume less animal fat, salt and sugar, and more fruit, vegetables and wholegrain cereals, but the quest for healthy eating should never become a holy grail. The world has suddenly become inhabited by hordes of people convinced, only on the basis of extremely bogus and questionable tests, that they're allergic to dairy products, wheat, coffee, tea and a hundred other staple foods.

These poor obsessives come to your house for dinner with a brown paper bag containing a handful of sprouted mung beans, three grated carrots and a sprinkle of sesame seeds. They've suddenly become macrobiotic believers, vegans, fruitarians or, God preserve us, breatharians, who believe they can survive on fresh air.

For optimum energy, resistance to disease, protection of the heart, slower ageing and an extension of the vital faculties – such as reproduction, hearing, sight, memory, reasoning and, above all, the ability to revel in the joy of living – we all need superfoods.

If you think superfoods are all the exotic expensive things that ordinary people can't afford, you couldn't be more wrong. Here are ten everyday foods and the reasons why they're super. You'll find them all spread around the recipes in the rest of the book.

apples: Pectin and vitamin C reduce cholesterol; pectin protects against pollution by eliminating heavy metals; malic and tartaric acids relieve indigestion and break down fats; traditional with cheese, duck and goose; two a day help arthritis, rheumatism and gout; grated apple stops diarrhoea.

advocado pears: Potassium relieves fatigue, depression and poor digestion; vitamins A, B, C and E make it an anti-cancer food; healthy monounsaturated oil; stimulates production of collagen; eat for circulation, skin and fertility. Ignore all rumours that this nutritional powerhouse is fattening.

bananas: Perfect fast food with potassium, zinc, iron, folic acid, calcium, vitamin B_6 and fibre. Good for digestion and menstrual difficulties; essential for athletes; perfect food for old and young. With apples, rice and dry toast, it makes up the BRAT diet, the ideal treatment for sickness and diarrhoea.

cabbage: Iron, chlorophyll, vitamin C, sulphur compounds and healing mucilaginous substances. Powerfully anti-cancer; vital for anaemia, stomach inflammation and ulcers; protective against stress, infection and heart disease. Best eaten slightly steamed.

carrots: Super-rich in betacarotene – one supplies enough for a day; anti-cancer, especially of the bowel; puréed for infant diarrhoea; juiced for liver problems; also contains vitamins C and E which ease circulatory disease, chest infections, and skin and eye problems. Eat carrots two or three times a week lightly cooked.

garlic: The king of healing plants. Modern science proves it reduces cholesterol, lowers blood pressure, stops blood from clotting and improves the circulation. It's antibacterial, antifungal, antiviral, anti-cancer, and good to relieve chest infections and stomach bugs too. Eat at least a clove each day.

oats: Protein, polyunsaturated fats, B vitamins, calcium, potassium, magnesium, silicon and vitamin E. They're easily digested and soothing to the digestive tract. Oats help depression and reduce cholesterol – a daily bowl can lower levels by twenty per cent. They also help regulate sugar metabolism, so they're good for diabetics. They are the best and cheapest of all breakfast cereals.

oily fish: The only source of all the essential fatty acids. These are vital during pregnancy and breast- feeding for the proper development of the brain in babies and infants. In children and adults, oily fish maintain brain function and can help in the treatment of dyslexia and attention deficit hyperactivity disorder (ADHD). They're also the most important source of vitamin D, essential for strong bones and many hormone functions. Great for the relief of arthritis.

onions: Protect the circulatory system and are a powerful antibiotic. They're good for chest, stomach and urinary infections, and their diuretic activity helps with arthritis, rheumatism and gout. A recent study in Newcastle gave a traditional fry-up breakfast to volunteers, but half of them got fried onions too; the onion eaters' blood was much less likely to clot than the others – research in America shows that half a raw onion a day raises the amount of good fats in the blood by thirty per cent.

potatoes: Even when boiled or baked, this wonderful vegetable is a source of fibre, B vitamins, minerals and enough vitamin C to keep scurvy at bay. They are best baked in their skins since lots of nutrients, especially potassium and fibre, are in the skin. At less than a calorie per gram, cheap and very filling, potatoes are good news for slimmers, and all the bad things you read about them are unfair and wrong, unless you only want to eat chips.

ten facts about superfoods

1. Two apples a day can reduce cholesterol by ten per cent.

2. 400g of fruits, vegetables and salads daily halve your risk of heart and circulatory disease.

3. Eating one portion of any of the cabbage family daily significantly reduces the risk of lung, colon and breast cancer.

4. Two portions a week of spinach, sorrel or beetroot tops reduces the risk of adult macular degenration (AMD) by fifty per cent.

5. The equivalent of six ripe tomatoes daily – whole fruit, purée, sauce, soup, ketchup, sun-dried or juice – halves the risk of prostate cancer in men and helps prevent blood clots and high blood pressure.

6. One clove of garlic daily reduces cholesterol and makes the blood less sticky, preventing blood clots.

7. Southern Europeans get twice as much of their energy (ten per cent) than we do in the UK (four-and-a-half per cent) from the protective fruit and veg superfoods.

8. The Mediterranean diet, with its high level of superfoods, means less disease and longer life expectancy – for example, Greeks have the lowest amount of bowel cancer in the whole of Europe.

9. Vitamin pills are not a substitute for superfoods. All the studies using pills to replicate the benefits of the Mediterranean diet for heart disease have failed.

10. Superfoods explain 'the French Paradox' – cheese, pâté, sausage, wine and cigarettes but massive intakes of superfoods means sixty per cent less risk of premature death from heart disease than the UK.

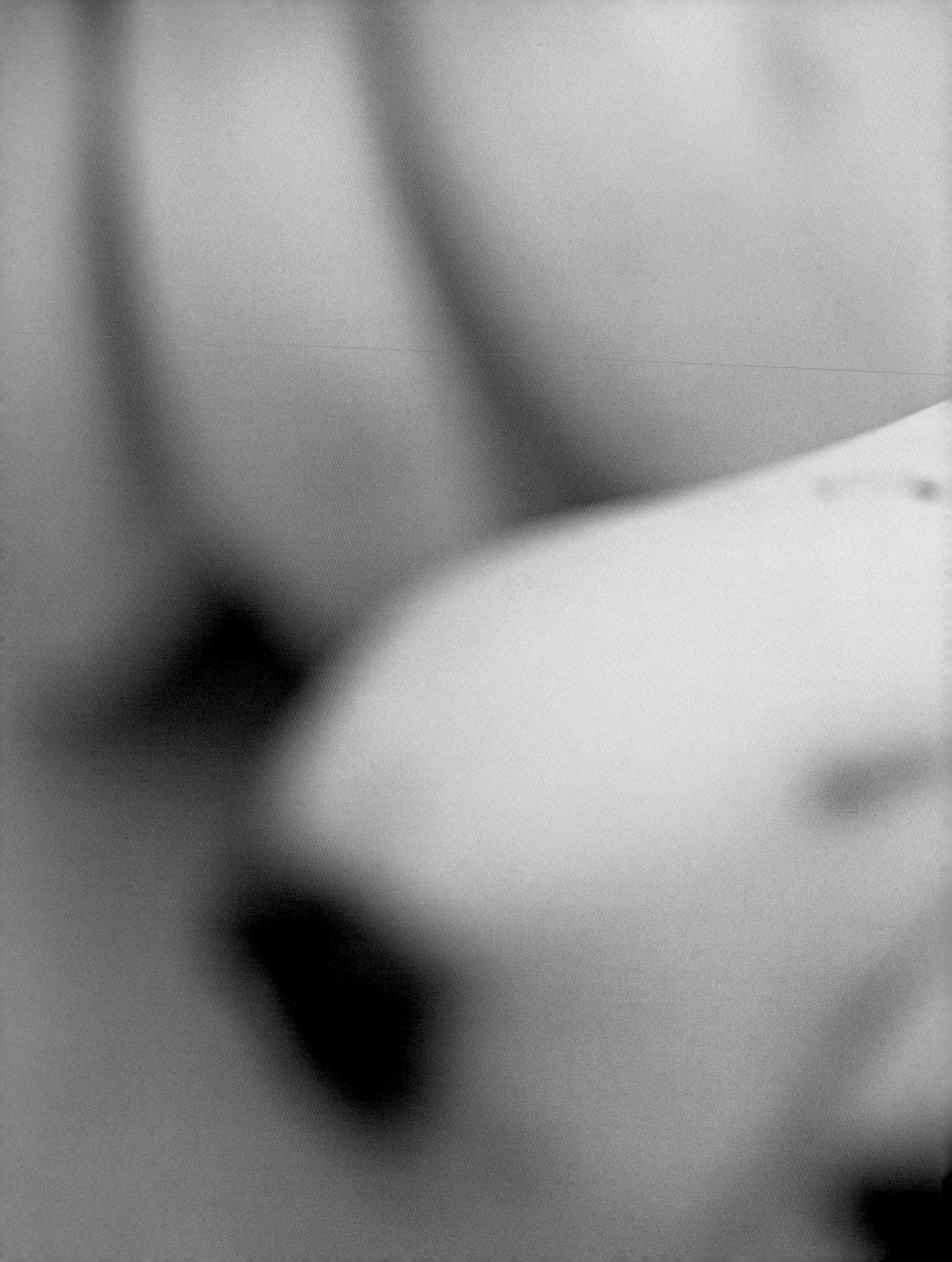

energy

Everybody feels lethargic at times. Too many late nights, a gruelling day at the office, family problems, travel frazzle or just the simple need for a break… all of these can wear us down. Yet victims of chronic fatigue often have no idea why they feel listless, never have any surplus energy, even wake up tired. If that sounds familiar, then here are some of the answers.

Exhaustion may have a psychological or physical cause but is often a combination of the two. Among common psychological causes are stress, anxiety, depression, dissatisfaction, relationship problems, anger, frustration or just plain boredom. Physically, specific illnesses can cause chronic fatigue. Anaemia is a common and often unrecognized cause, particularly among menstruating women. The problem is common, too, in careless vegetarians who stop eating meat and don't substitute it with other good sources of iron. Thyroid, hormone problems and heart disease are yet more common causes of a constant lack of energy, as is poor posture, which is often the result of badly designed seating. So, too, is chronic pain, such as backache, arthritis, rheumatism, tension, headaches and migraines. Viral infections and their lingering after effects, surgery and all major illnesses inevitably result in fatigue. Post-viral fatigue syndrome, otherwise known as ME, is now recognized as a genuine physical problem.

Allergy, or sensitivity, to foods and environmental pollutants is another major cause of fatigue. According to Dr Stephen Davies, chairman of the British Society of Nutritional Medicine, "waking tired" is one of the classic symptoms of food or chemical sensitivity. If you suspect this could apply to you, see a consultant in allergy medicine, as well as trying out the recipes in this chapter.

In addition, people who suffer from tiredness often lack the energy for active exercise, without which the body's absorption of iron and other vital minerals is poor. They become trapped in a vicious circle of dwindling energy, which leads to less exercise, resulting in even less energy.

Millions of people the world over wake up every morning wondering how on earth they'll get through the day ahead. Once a thorough check with your doctor has established that there is no serious underlying illness to cause your lack of energy, the cure is often to be found in your own hands, and self-help can be remarkably successful. All the energy you need comes from what you eat and drink. But choosing the right food is crucial to maintaining your health and vitality. Any form of fatigue is exacerbated by a poor diet. When you're tired and lethargic generally, shopping, cooking and planning meals become daunting chores. Snack meals of bread and cheese, sandwiches, tea and biscuits, which replace healthy eating, will further deplete nutritional reserves and start another downward spiral.

In this chapter you will find simple but energizing recipes that use the best of the high-octane "super-foods". Beans and barley in soups; potatoes, rice, eggs and blood-nourishing beetroot; fish, beef and lamb for strength-building protein; herbs, spices and special juices... each recipe is designed to provide the winning combination of instant and long-term energy release to lift you out of the trough of fatigue and keep you going at peak performance levels. All those who feel they haven't got the energy to cope with life will benefit from the recipes in the following pages.

energy checklist

• Try to refuse all refined carbohydrates. White sugar, white flour and processed foods made with them – cakes, biscuits, packet puddings etc – are a heavy tax on your digestion, using up energy you can ill afford to spare. These are high glycaemic index (GI) foods, which may give you an instant lift but will leave you with a terrible blood-sugar deficit soon afterwards. They also trigger the release of enormous quantities of insulin, and excessive consumption is the first step on the road to Type 2 diabetes.

• Fats in excess are a similar drain on the body's resources. Hidden fats are found in processed foods and in most fast foods.

• Alcohol has the most pernicious effect of destroying the B vitamins that are particularly needed for stamina and for the health of your nervous system in general.

• Caffeine, found in tea, coffee, colas and chocolate, inhibits the uptake of iron – a crucial mineral – when consumed at the same time as sources of this nutrient. If you drink tea or coffee, don't do so at meals featuring good sources of iron such as eggs, wholewheat cereals and meat.

• Red meat itself, though supplying valuable iron, is hard work for your digestive system. You're better off getting your iron from other sources for the time being.

• High-energy drinks, marketed as giving energy to the listless, are rich in glucose. They may give you a deceptive lift, but they contain nothing of real value to help combat fatigue at the root of the problem.

vegetable and bean soup

In the middle of winter, you not only need the warming properties of this typical peasant soup, but you'll also benefit from the **antibacterial** effects of the garlic and onion. A bowlful of this delicious combination will keep you going when you have to shovel the snow away from your door.

- 4 tbsp extra-virgin olive oil
- 1 large onion, finely chopped
- 2 garlic cloves, peeled, finely chopped
- 2 large courgettes, trimmed and grated
- 4 new potatoes, scrubbed and grated
- 1 large carrot, peeled and trimmed if not organic, grated
- 1.5 litres or 55 fl oz vegetable stock (page 252)
- 2 x 240g cans (drained weight) flageolet beans

In a large saucepan, heat the oil. Add the onions and garlic and sweat gently for about five minutes.

Add the grated vegetables and continue heating for five more minutes, stirring continuously and adding a little more oil if necessary.

Pour in the stock and simmer for ten minutes, then whizz in a food processor or blender until smooth. Return to the pan.

Rinse the beans thoroughly. Add to the pan and bring back to a simmer. Heat gently for five more minutes and serve.

Serves 4

Ideal for a nutritional **energy boost**, as beans and potatoes supply masses of **slow-release energy**. Carrots are rich in immune-boosting **vitamin A**.

thick barley and vegetable soup

Barley is a staple food in the Middle East; in ancient Rome it was used in soups to feed gladiators. Sadly, it's mostly ignored in Western cooking. This recipe uses whole pot barley, a real **winter tonic,** available in most supermarkets and health-food stores. In contrast, refined pearl barley provides only calories.

- 2 tbsp extra-virgin olive oil
- 1 large onion, finely chopped
- 1 large carrot, peeled and trimmed if not organic, finely cubed
- 1 large leek, trimmed, washed and very finely diced
- 1 litre or 35 fl oz vegetable stock (page 252)
- 3 bay leaves
- 5 tbsp pot barley
- 1 large handful of chopped fresh parsley

In a large saucepan, heat the olive oil. Add the carrots, leek and onion, and heat gently for five minutes.

Add the vegetable stock and bay leaves.

Bring to the boil and add the barley.

Simmer for about one hour.

Remove the bay leaves and serve with the parsley sprinkled on top.

Serves 4

This soup provides a great supply of vital nutrients. Pot barley is rich in **fibre, calcium, potassium** and **B vitamins**.

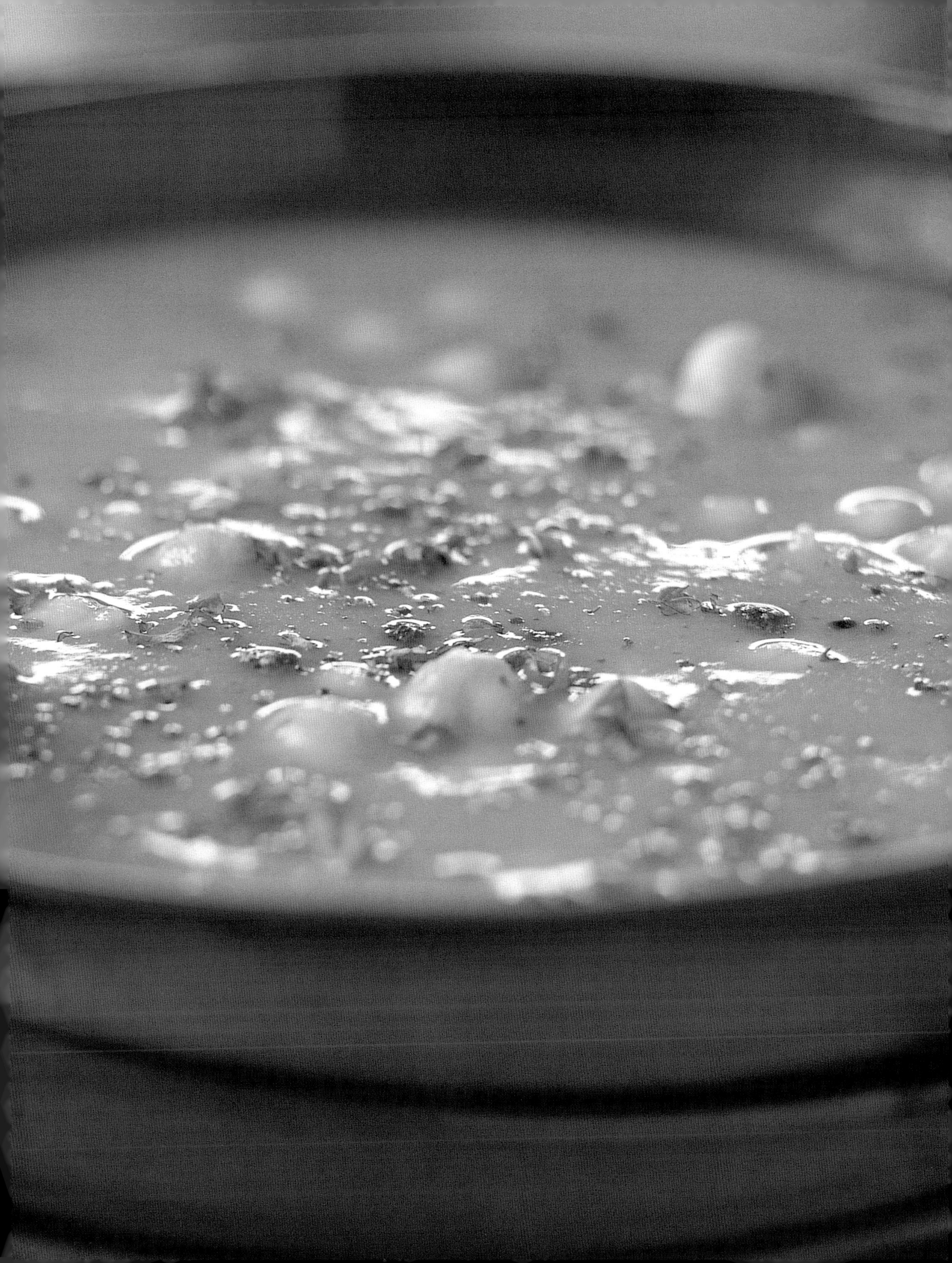

leek and potato soup

Potatoes are at their healthiest and most nutritious when eaten with their skins – something you can do safely only by using **organic** produce. As well as providing **high levels of energy**, leeks make this soup a useful treatment for gout, arthritis, rheumatism, chest infections and sore throats.

- 60g or 2oz butter
- 1 garlic clove, chopped
- 2 leeks, chopped
- 375g or 13oz small new potatoes, unpeeled and unquartered
- 1 large onion, sliced
- 900ml or 32 fl oz vegetable stock (page 252)
- 2 tbsp fresh parsley, finely chopped
- freshly ground black pepper, to taste
- 150ml or 5 fl oz double cream

Melt the butter in a large saucepan, then sweat the garlic in it for two minutes.

Add the leeks, potatoes and onions and cook on a medium heat for ten minutes.

Add the stock and simmer for twenty minutes, or until the vegetables are tender.

Liquidize in a blender or food processor, then finish by adding the parsley, pepper and cream.

Serves 4

This recipe contains lots of **potassium**, half the daily requirement of **vitamin C**, and useful amounts of iron, **zinc**, selenium, iodine, folic acid, betacarotene and **fibre**.

celtic broth

If ever there were a liquid mixture of health and energy, this is it. Oats provide **slow-release energy** as well as a good dose of soluble fibre, which reduces cholesterol levels. Broccoli is packed with heart- and circulatory-protective nutrients in addition to cancer-fighting agents.

- 1 tbsp extra-virgin olive oil
- 5 spring onions, chopped
- 450g or 1lb broccoli florets
- 60g or 2oz porridge oats
- 1 litre or 35 fl oz half-and-half vegetable stock (page 252) and semi-skimmed milk
- freshly ground black pepper, to taste
- ground nutmeg, to taste
- 1 tbsp each fromage frais and chopped chives

Pour the oil in a large saucepan and cook the spring onions until soft. Add the broccoli and stir for two minutes, then add the oats and stir for two minutes more.

Slowly add the stock and milk and stir. Cover and simmer gently for twelve minutes.

Add the pepper and nutmeg to taste and serve with a swirl of fromage frais and a sprinkling of chopped chives.

Serves 4

Organic oats are rich in essential **B vitamins**. This is a good source of protein that is low in fat and contains plenty of fibre, calcium, **potassium**, trace minerals and vitamins A, B and C.

chicken yum-yum

What could be more of a pick-me-up than a mug full of this crystal-clear, **energizing**, **warming**, and immune-boosting chicken broth? In different cultures around the world, chicken broth functions like Jupiter: the bringer of jollity.

- 1 chicken quarter (not a breast)
- 1 leek, washed and quartered
- 1 fennel bulb, quartered
- 1 large handful of mixed summer herbs
- 1 carrot, sliced lengthways
- 1 onion, halved, with skin left on
- 850ml or 30 fl oz water

Trim any fat off the chicken, and place in a large saucepan. Add the vegetables and water.

Simmer, covered, for forty minutes. Strain off the chicken and vegetables and serve the yum-yum immediately.

Note: this can be kept in the refrigerator for up to three days. If you do this, skim off any residue of cold fat and heat on a stove or in a microwave before serving.

Serves 3

Root vegetables are an abundant source of **minerals**, **carotenoids**, and other phytochemicals, together with the immune-boosting and **antiviral** components from the chicken.

welsh rarebit

A good Welsh rarebit is a traditional and tasty teatime treat. Some of the best cheese-makers in England, Ireland, Scotland and Wales send their **organic farmhouse produce** to Randolph Hodgson at his famous Neal's Yard Dairy, Covent Garden, London, so get some if you can.

- 4 slices bread, sourdough or wholemeal
- butter, for spreading
- 4 tsp sharp fruit chutney
- 85g or 3oz organic farmhouse cheese (lancashire or cheshire)

Lightly toast the bread on both sides and spread thinly with the butter.

Spread each slice with a heaped teaspoon of chutney; slice the cheese finely, then crumble it on the top of each slice. Pile it high and make sure it comes right to the edges.

Place under a hot grill until the cheese is nicely melted. Serve with a simple green salad for a wonderful quick and healthy supper.

Serves 4

As well as a mixture of quick and slow-release energy, this provides loads of **protein** and plenty of calcium, not to mention some iron, lots of selenium, folic acid and ten per cent of the recommended daily requirement of **vitamin E**.

aubergine and courgette layer

A non-meat dish with the **power punch** of a mule. The unique flavour and texture of the aubergine, the giant, misshapen tomatoes and the ever-present smell of marjoram make this the perfect winter pick-me-up. It's delicious hot or cold – even your most carnivorous friends won't notice the absence of meat.

2 medium aubergines
a pinch or two of salt, to taste
150ml or 5 fl oz extra-virgin olive oil
2 red onions, chopped
3 garlic cloves, finely chopped
6 large courgettes
450g or 1lb buffalo mozzarella
4 beef tomatoes, slicing variety
3 medium bay leaves, finely crushed
3 tbsp marjoram, finely chopped
1 tbsp dandelion leaves, finely chopped
6 tbsp raclette, grated

Peel and slice the aubergines, sprinkle both sides with a little salt and put on an oiled baking sheet in a preheated oven at 200°C (400°F/gas mark 6) for ten minutes. Sweat the onions and garlic in olive oil for ten minutes. Cut the courgettes, mozzarella and tomatoes into medium-sized slices.

Pour the onion mixture into an ovenproof dish. Layer with the aubergines, then the tomatoes, courgettes and mozzarella, finishing with a mozzarella layer on the top.

Mix the crushed bay leaves, chopped marjoram, dandelion and raclette and sprinkle over the top of the mozzarella. Cover with aluminium foil, return to the oven and bake at 200°C (400°F/gas mark 6) for fifty minutes. Remove the foil and bake for a further ten minutes, or until slightly crisp.

Serves 4

Provides calcium from the cheese; protein, fibre and vitamins galore from the vegetables; extra **iron** and carotenoids from the dandelion; heart-boosting lycopene from the tomatoes.

cheese and bread pudding

This savoury bread pudding takes a few minutes to prepare and half an hour to cook and it is another **high-energy** lunch or light evening meal. You can vary the flavour by trying any variety of hard organic farmhouse cheese.

60g or 2oz butter
4 slices wholemeal bread (no crusts)
3 shallots, finely chopped
175g or 6oz mature cheddar or gruyère cheese, grated
4 medium free-range eggs
600ml or 20 fl oz milk
freshly ground black pepper, to taste
¼ tsp paprika
2 tomatoes, thinly sliced

Butter the bread and cut it into small squares. Place a layer in a buttered pie dish. Make another layer with the shallots, then add the cheese and top with more of the bread.

Beat the eggs, milk and pepper and pour into the dish; sprinkle with the paprika. Cover with the tomatoes and bake in an oven preheated to 200°C (400°F/gas mark 6), until brown on top (approximately thirty minutes).

Serves 4

Provides almost half the daily requirement of protein, well over half the requirement of **calcium** and vitamin A, and plenty of **folic acid**. Lots of iodine, selenium and **vitamin C** make this a sustaining, energizing and bone-building meal.

free-range spanish omelette

The deep, rich, yellow eggs and the vivid red peppers make this dish a visual delight. It may take longer to make than a conventional omelette, but the result is an **energizing**, sustaining dish.

4 tbsp extra-virgin olive oil
1 large potato, peeled and diced
1 medium onion, finely sliced
½ red pepper, deseeded and cut in thin strips
1 courgette, unpeeled and thinly sliced
freshly ground black pepper, to taste
4 free-range eggs, well beaten

In a large, thick-bottomed frying pan, heat the oil and the potatoes and fry briskly for five minutes, stirring constantly. Turn down the heat, add the onions and cook for five minutes. Add the peppers and cook for four minutes, then add the courgettes and cook for another three minutes until the vegetables are soft (but the onions are not brown).

Add the pepper to the eggs and pour into the pan; turn the heat down and stir thoroughly. Leave to cook very slowly. As it sets, the edge will curl away from the pan. Shake the pan occasionally to keep the omelette moving; as soon as the underside starts to brown, remove from the heat. Put under a grill for two to three minutes to finish cooking. Hold a large plate over the pan and turn upside down; the omelette should drop out.

Serves 4

The sustaining, slow-release energy in this recipe is good for the entire body. It supplies a fifth of the recommended daily requirement of **protein**, lots of potassium, a quarter of daily iodine and a good supply of **folic acid**, vitamin C and betacarotene.

organic pasta with raw courgette

Wholemeal pasta contains fibre and B vitamins, so choose your favourite – as long as it's organic. Combined with the fresh, clean flavours of the courgette, the parmesan helps make this a delicious and healthy easy-to-cook meal.

1 tsp extra-virgin olive oil
a couple of pinches of salt
450g or 1lb spaghettini
200g or 7oz courgettes, washed, unpeeled and finely grated
10g or ¼oz butter
2 tbsp finely grated fresh parmesan
freshly ground black pepper, to taste

Add the olive oil and salt to a large saucepan full of water and bring to the boil. Add the pasta and stir for a few seconds to prevent sticking.

Fill a serving dish with boiling water to warm it.

When the pasta is cooked, drain. Empty the water from the serving dish; put in the pasta, add the courgette, butter, parmesan and pepper, and mix thoroughly.

Serves 4

A good source of **protein, fibre, folic acid** and energy, together with useful amounts of vitamins A and C.

complete eastern risotto

Here's a complete meal in under half an hour, and one that offers all the **heart** and **circulatory** benefits of onions and garlic into the bargain. Bulgur wheat gives this dish a very different texture and flavour to rice. Serve it in the traditional Middle Eastern way, with yogurt, onions and a green salad.

60g or 2oz unsalted butter
1 large onion, finely chopped
2 garlic cloves, chopped
250g or 9oz bulgur wheat
450ml or 16 fl oz chicken or vegetable stock (pages 252–3)
1 pinch of sea salt

for the garnish
1 large onion, sliced into rings
1 tbsp peanut or rapeseed oil
about 125ml or 4 fl oz natural, live yogurt

Over a low heat, melt the butter in a large, heavy-bottomed saucepan. Add the chopped onion and garlic and cook gently until they start changing colour.

Add the bulgur wheat and stir until coated with butter.

Add enough stock to cover the mixture, then add a pinch of salt, bring to the boil, cover and simmer gently for ten minutes, or until the liquid is absorbed (add more stock if it seems to be drying out too quickly).

While the bulgur is cooking, fry the onion rings until they begin to crisp. Serve the bulgur decorated with onion rings and yogurt.

Serves 4

A good **carbohydrate** dish packed with plenty of protein, fibre, iodine and vitamin A, as well as useful amounts of iron, vitamin B_1, niacin and folic acid.

smart sage fish cakes

These delightfully light fish cakes are quick, easy to make and **nutritious**. The tuna is enhanced by the combination of sage and marjoram, making these a smart choice for everyone, particularly when served with a fresh, green salad. They make a good carbohydrate/protein boost for athletes.

150ml or 5 fl oz extra-virgin olive oil
1 medium onion, very finely chopped
1 x 250g can tuna
250g or 8oz potatoes, boiled and roughly mashed
1 tsp fresh marjoram, finely chopped (½ tsp dried)
1 tsp fresh sage, finely chopped (½ tsp dried)
2 eggs, beaten

Sauté the onion gently in olive oil. Allow to cool and mix thoroughly with the tuna. Add the potatoes and herbs and mix well. Add half the beaten egg and mix again.

Form the mixture into eight flat cakes.

Dip each cake in the remaining egg. Shallow-fry gently in olive oil for seven minutes each side.

Serves 4

This high-power dish offers brain-boosting **protein** from the fish and slow-release energy from the potatoes. It's also rich in **essential fatty acids**, zinc and selenium, and very low in saturated fats. Sage acts as a hormone booster. Marjoram stimulates the metabolism.

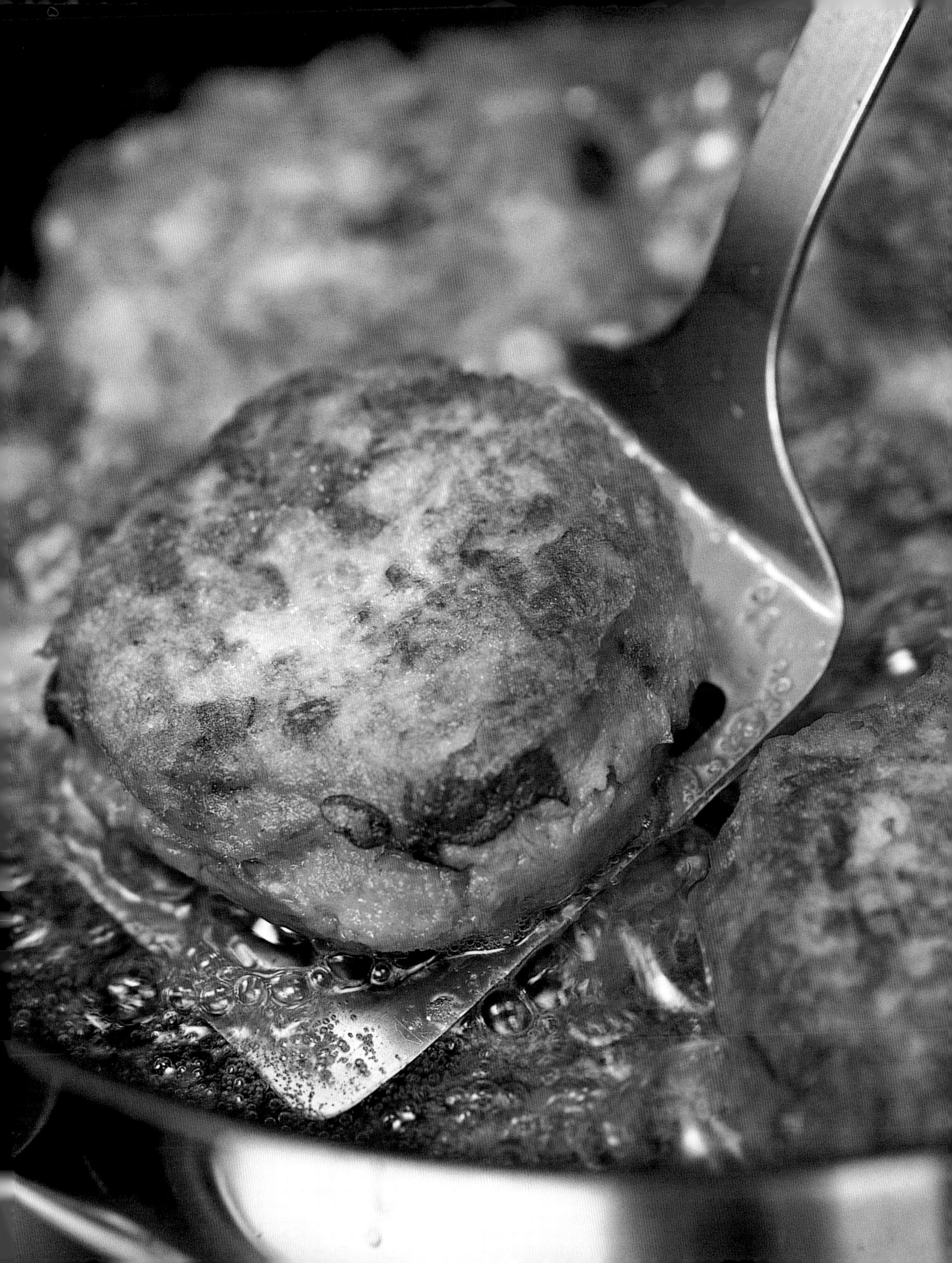

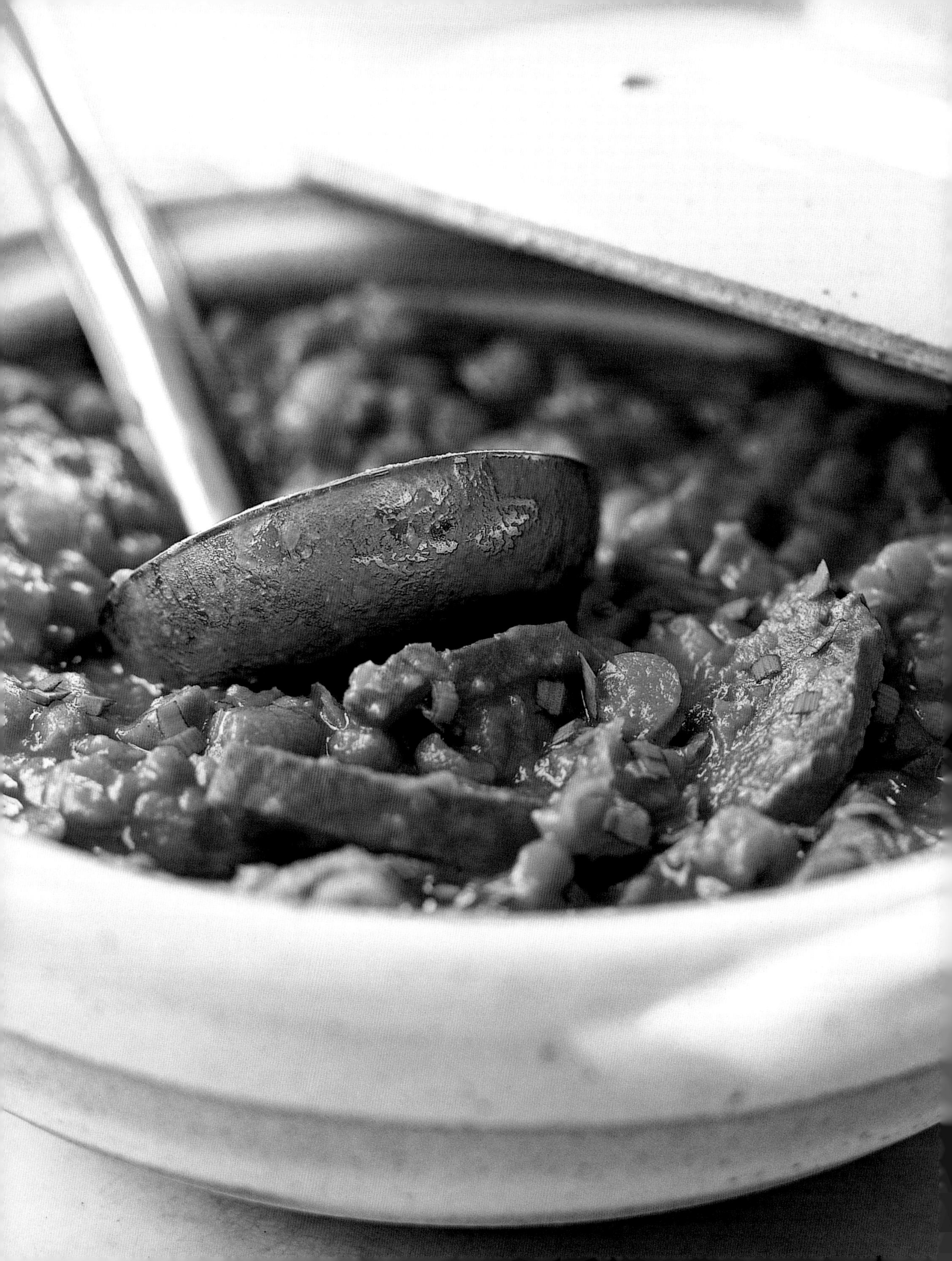

southernwood eggs

The aromatic flavour of southernwood combines perfectly with creamy mayonnaise and salty anchovies in this delicious recipe. In addition, crunchy beans make a great foil for the soft, delicate eggs. As well as being a **power herb**, southernwood has been used since medieval times as an insect repellent.

4 organic eggs
1 x 100g can or jar anchovies
150ml whole milk
8 tbsp home-made mayonnaise (or best commercial quality)
4 tbsp southernwood leaves, finely chopped
1 x 200g or can kidney beans, rinsed thoroughly

Boil the eggs for ten minutes. Rinse immediately in lots of cold water and leave to rest for five minutes. Remove the shells and cut in half lengthwise.

Soak the anchovies in milk for ten minutes. Drain.

Mix the mayonnaise with the southernwood leaves.

Arrange the egg halves on plates, surrounded with kidney beans.

Place the anchovies on the eggs in a criss-cross pattern and top with the herb mayonnaise.

Serves 4

Rich in **protein**, essential fatty acids, fibre, **calcium** and **iron**. Southernwood contains the volatile oil abrotanin, which improves digestion and the absorption of nutrients, thus aiding in energy production. Southernwood should not be eaten during pregnancy.

dutch pea soup with smoked sausage

Another of the great peasant recipes of Central Europe. Split peas give this soup its unique character and its thick, porridge-like consistency. A bowlful with a chunk of bread and a crisp winter salad is all you need for a **nourishing** and **energizing** lunch or supper.

300g or 10½oz split green peas
40g or 1½oz unsalted butter
200g or 7oz smoked back bacon, finely chopped
1 medium onion, coarsely chopped
1.5 litres or 55 fl oz vegetable stock (page 252)
500g or 1lb 2oz smoked sausage, rind removed, cut into chunks

Soak the peas in plenty of water overnight.

In a large saucepan, melt the butter and sauté the bacon gently for two minutes. Add the onion and continue heating for four more minutes.

Stir in the soaked peas, add the stock and simmer, covered, until the peas are soft – between one and two hours.

Mix in the sausage and simmer for another ten to fifteen minutes.

Serves 4

A soup tailor-made for warmth and energy. Split peas are rich in **fibre** and **minerals**, while sausage supplies vital **protein**.

spanish bean and chorizo soup

Good neighbours make a huge difference to your life. My wife Sally and I are blessed with the best. Denzil lived for some years in Spain and passed this recipe on to his wife, Vee, who often arrives on our doorstep with a steaming pan of this taste of Spanish sun to **chase away winter blues**.

2 tbsp extra-virgin olive oil

1 medium onion, finely chopped and diced

2 garlic cloves, peeled, finely chopped

1 tbsp plain flour

1.2 litres or 40 fl oz chicken stock (page 253)

1 x 450g can butter beans, rinsed

100g or 3½oz broad beans

250g or 9oz thin chorizo sausage, finely cubed

Heat the olive oil in a large saucepan. Sweat the onion and garlic gently in the oil until softened – about ten minutes. Stir in the flour and continue stirring for about five minutes.

Pour in the stock very slowly, stirring until the flour takes up the liquid completely. Add the butter beans and broad beans.

Simmer until the beans are almost tender – about ten minutes.

Add the chorizo and heat through.

Serves 4

This soup will help fight off winter depression. Butter-beans and broad beans contain fibre, **protein, minerals** and natural plant hormones that help elevate mood.

robust rosemary lamb

Super charged power radiates from this lovely lamb dish. What's more, even though it takes a few hours to cook, the preparation couldn't be simpler. The classic flavour of rosemary is sure to please and it enhances the rest of the power nutrients contained in the vegetables and meat.

6 tbsp extra-virgin olive oil

1 large onion, chopped

2 garlic cloves, chopped

4 lean lamb chops or 8 cutlets

2 large carrots, peeled and diced

4 baby turnips, peeled and sliced

1 fennel bulb, cut into chunks

4 medium bay leaves

1 large sprig rosemary

900ml or 30 fl oz vegetable stock (page 252)

500g or 1lb spinach or Swiss chard, washed and torn into shreds

Heat the oil and gently sweat the onion and garlic. Remove from the pan.

Wash the lamb, dry thoroughly, season with salt and pepper and gently sauté it in the oil, sealing it all over. Place into a large casserole dish along with the onion and garlic. Add the vegetables, bay leaves, rosemary and stock to the casserole.

Bring gently to the boil, adding more water if necessary, then put into an oven preheated to 200°C (400°F/gas mark 6) for two hours, checking the stock level occasionally.

Half an hour before the dish is ready, add the spinach or Swiss chard, making sure the leaves are covered with the stock.

Serves 4

Bursting with minerals, **betacarotene**, fibre, protein and other important carotenoids, this dish also features **circulation-boosting** phytochemicals from the garlic and onions.

chickpea and spicy beef sausage soup

The perfect soup if you're suffering from the winter blues, because it helps improve everything from **circulation** to mood. The combination of chickpeas and spicy sausage protects your bones during the dark days of winter, **improves blood flow** and promotes balanced blood-sugar levels.

3 tbsp extra-virgin olive oil

1 large onion, finely chopped

1 large garlic bulb, peeled and finely chopped

300g or 10½oz spicy beef sausage, cut into chunks

1.2 litres or 40 fl oz vegetable stock (page 252)

2 x 240g cans (drained weight) chickpeas

In a large saucepan, heat the oil. Add the onion and garlic and sweat them until softened. Add the sausage. Pour in the stock and chickpeas and simmer until tender – about fifteen minutes.

Remove four tablespoons of the chickpeas and liquidize the rest of the mixture in a food processor or blender.

Return to the heat until boiling.

Serve with the whole chickpeas floating on top.

Serves 4

A soup that provides all-round nutrition. Chickpeas are **rich in calcium**, while the beef in the sausages provides protein, **iron** and B vitamins, all of which nourish the nervous system.

mediterranean steak

A **power-packed** dish to please the fussiest carnivore. Steak isn't a principal part of the Mediterranean diet, but when they do it, it's a **veritable feast**. Here, the flavours of the meat blend seamlessly with the garlic, sage and marjoram in the rice, made more interesting by the pungent, minty pennyroyal.

4 beef fillet steaks

300ml or 10 fl oz red wine

2 medium bay leaves

1 medium onion, chopped

2 garlic cloves, chopped

8 tbsp extra-virgin olive oil

250g or 8-9oz arborio rice

500ml or 18 fl oz vegetable stock

1 tbsp each sage, parsley and marjoram

1 small pinch pennyroyal

Marinate the steaks in the wine with the bay leaves, and half the onion, garlic and olive oil for one hour.

Sweat the remainder of the onion and garlic in the rest of the olive oil. Add the rice and stir until coated.

Mix the herbs into the stock. Add the stock gradually to the rice and simmer until each addition is absorbed. Add the wine marinade, minus the bay leaves.

Grill or fry the steaks for five to six minutes each side, depending on taste.

Serves 4

Rich in iron, B vitamins – especially B_{12} – and plenty of good energy calories from the rice. Volatile oils are provided by the pennyroyal, which also contains bitter phytochemicals that **stimulate** gastric juices and improve the digestion of meat.

lively chicory liver

The melt-in-the-mouth consistency of organic calves' liver is the perfect foil for the crisp, fried sage leaves; and the iron it provides (enhanced by the wild chicory) makes this a **power dish extraordinaire**. Note to expectant mothers: avoid this dish due to its high vitamin A content.

- 6 tbsp sunflower oil
- 16 medium sage leaves
- 75g or 2oz unsalted butter
- 4 thin slices calves' liver
- 4 tsp fresh wild chicory leaves
- 2 limes, cut in half

Heat the sunflower oil and fry the sage leaves for around one minute, or until they're crisp. Drain the leaves on kitchen roll and keep warm.

Melt the butter in a frying pan. Sprinkle the liver with chicory leaves and cook for two minutes on each side, until cooked to your liking.

Serve scattered with the sage leaves, with the lime halves on the side.

Serves 4

A feast of **power-boosting iron** comes from the liver, together with protein, **vitamin** B_{12} and a massive dose of vitamin A. There's also a day's dose of **vitamin C** from the lime juice, all **brilliantly digested** thanks to the phytochemicals in wild chicory.

mother's yorkshire pudding with apples

Here's a dessert that tastes good and does you good – a sweet you can eat without guilt. As well as loads of energy, this delicious recipe supplies **heart-protective** pectin, which helps reduce cholesterol. It also offers **digestive benefits** from the volatile oils present in cloves and cinnamon.

- 450g or 1lb dessert apples
- 30g or 1oz seedless raisins
- 1 tbsp lemon juice
- 30g or 1oz soft brown sugar
- 2 whole cloves
- 1 tsp ground cinnamon

for the batter

- 170g or 6oz wholemeal flour
- 60g or 2oz white flour
- 90g or 3oz soft brown sugar
- 2 medium free-range eggs
- 600ml or 20 fl oz milk

Layer the peeled, cored and sliced apples on the bottom of a lightly greased ovenproof dish.

Add the raisins, lemon juice, sugar and whole cloves and sprinkle with the cinnamon.

Mix together all the batter ingredients, beating thoroughly, and pour over the top.

Place in a preheated oven at 170°C (330°F/gas mark 3) and cook for one hour.

Serves 4

Organic apples tend to have a much higher vitamin content than non-organic ones. Provides plenty of protein, **fibre**, calcium, potassium and vitamin B_{12}, together with useful amounts of iron, zinc, iodine and **vitamin E**.

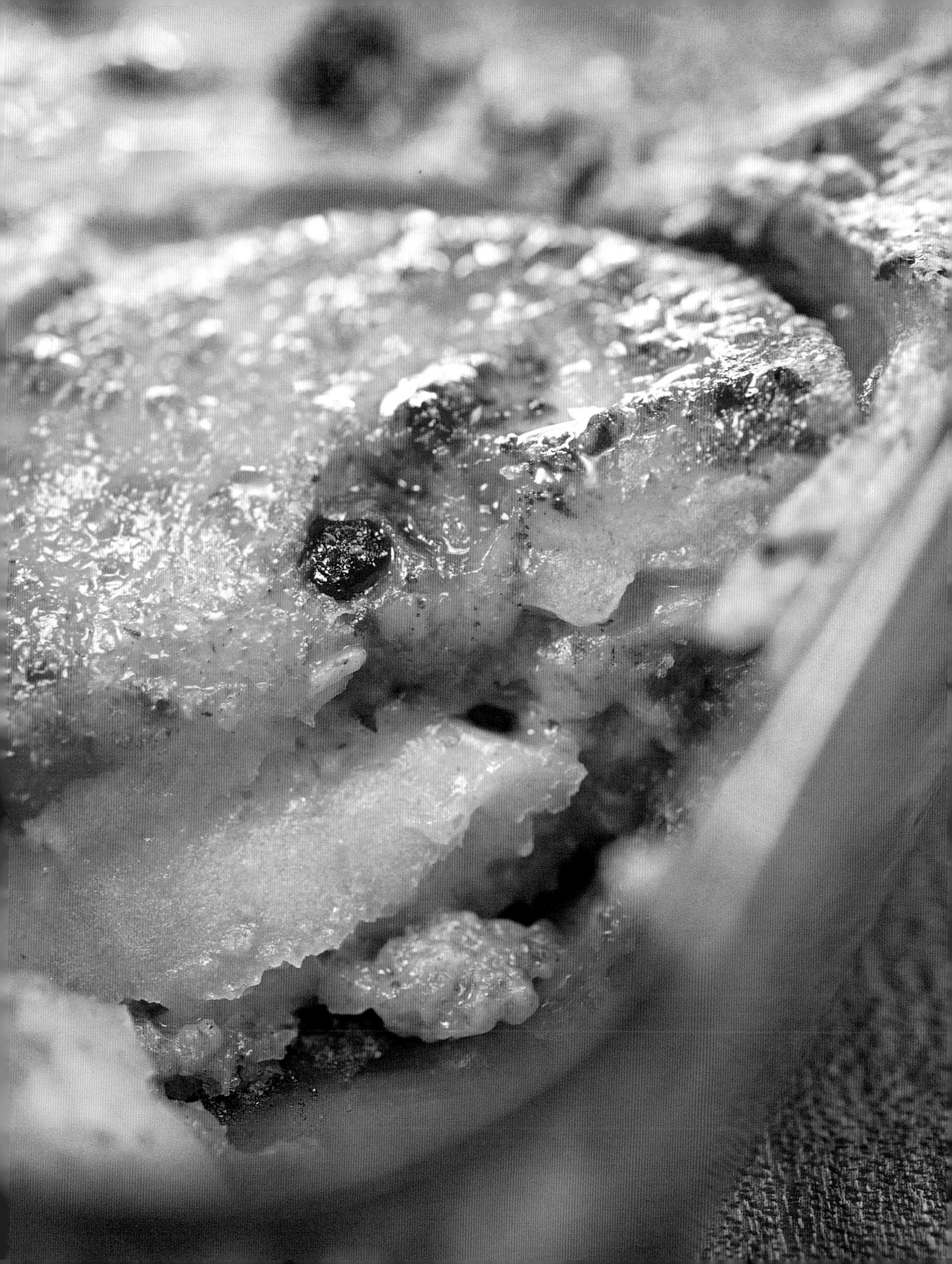

lychee, buttermilk and honey

Fresh lychees are a taste sensation. They have the most delicate flavour and are also a useful source of **nutrients**. Using buttermilk rather than yogurt or ordinary milk provides a different texture, as well as an unusual taste, to this energy-giving recipe.

10 lychees, peeled and stoned
125ml or 4 fl oz buttermilk
3 level tbsp runny honey
2 redcurrant sprigs (for garnish)

Put the lychee flesh into a blender and whizz.

Add the buttermilk and honey and whizz again.

Serve with the redcurrant sprigs draped over the edge of the glasses.

Serves 1–2

Lychees are a good source of **vitamin C**; they also contain some **calcium**, potassium, and phosphorus: important for energy conversion. The protein and **extra calcium** from the buttermilk means you avoid "insulin rush", getting instead a sustained increase in vitality.

spiced smoothie

One of the most common causes of chronic fatigue is zinc deficiency. The zinc supplied by pumpkin seeds is often the first step on the road to feeling more **vital** and **healthy**. Regular consumption of live yogurt is also a tremendous boost to the immune system, thanks to the beneficial bacteria it contains.

300ml or 10 fl oz natural, live yogurt
1 tbsp tahini
½ tsp allspice
a little milk (optional), for thinning
ice cubes
1 tsp pumpkin seeds

Put the yogurt, tahini and allspice in a blender or food processor and whizz until combined.

Thin with the milk until you achieve the consistency you require.

Serve over ice cubes with the pumpkin seeds scattered on top.

Serves 1–2

Live yogurt is not only an excellent source of calcium, but it is the best source of the **probiotic bacteria** responsible for producing the essential B vitamins that nourish the nervous system and help **banish anxiety**, stress and fatigue. Add the slow-release calories, even more calcium from the tahini, **zinc** from the pumpkin seeds and the mood-enhancing benefits of allspice, and you've got a great recipe for improved vitality.

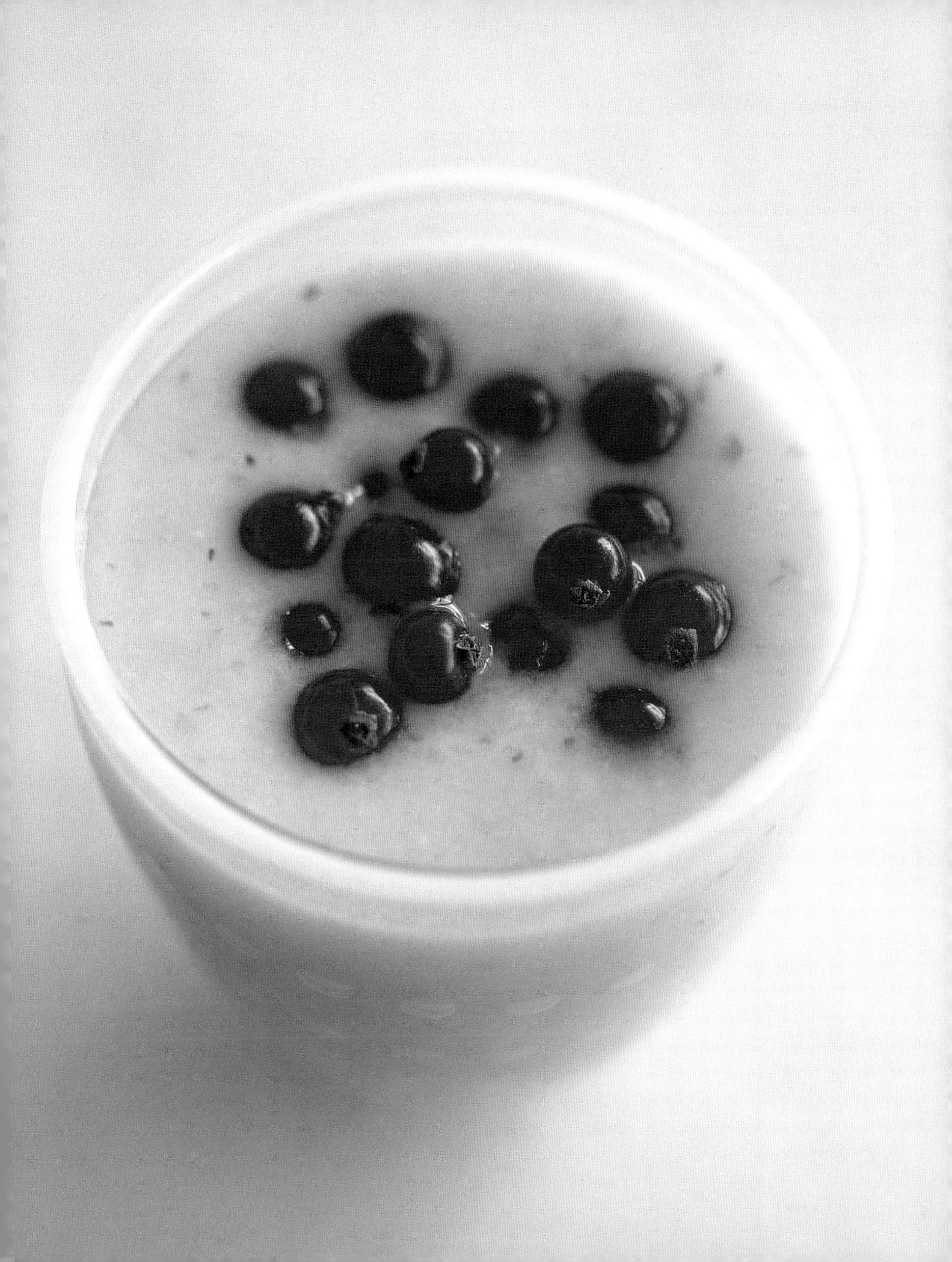

guava delight

The ideal combination of instant and **slow-release energy** with the added kick of the Brazilian rainforest herb known as guarana. All the tropical fruits are rich in natural sugars for an instant lift, while the banana provides lots of complex carbohydrates for a more gradual release of usable energy.

1 guava, peeled
1 mango, peeled and stone removed
1 banana, peeled
5g or 1 tsp guarana powder

Put the guava and mango through a juicer.

Whizz the banana with the juice in a blender or food processor.

Add the guarana and whizz again.

Chill before serving.

Serves 1–2

Guavas and mangoes are rich in **betacarotene**, vitamin C, natural sugars and protective antioxidants. Banana contains large amounts of **potassium** – important for preventing cramp. So if you need extra vitality for sport and exercise, this is the drink for you.

a punch of power

A super vitality juice with plenty of essential nutrients and some potent natural phytochemicals from the coriander and spinach. It makes an excellent drink for the active as it provides **instant energy** from the natural sugars in the carrots and kiwi fruit. It's also a good source of potassium.

4 carrots, peeled and trimmed if not organic
1 kiwi fruit, washed and unpeeled
1 small handful fresh coriander, with stems
1 handful baby spinach leaves

Put all the ingredients into a juicer, reserving a few coriander leaves.

Mix well and serve with coriander leaves on top.

Serves 1–2

This vitality drink provides a double dose of betacarotene and potassium from the carrots and kiwi fruit, along with **extra magnesium** and plenty of vitamin C. The spinach adds extra carotenoids and a powerful boost of cancer-fighting plant chemicals. The coriander contains **heart- and circulatory-protective coumarins**.

high flyer

If you've a busy day ahead and little chance of a good meal, set yourself up with this blood-building, vitamin-laden **energy-booster**. A massive health-protector and life-extender, the High Flyer will keep your mental faculties in top gear. As a bonus, it slows skin ageing and prevents sun damage.

6 spinach leaves

3 carrots, peeled and trimmed if not organic

1 apple, unpeeled and uncored

1 medium beetroot, unpeeled, with leaves

Wash all the ingredients and peel, top and tail the carrots (unless they're organic).

Put all the ingredients into a juicer. Mix well and serve.

Serves 1–2

Super-rich in **carotenes** and **potassium,** this is also bursting in vitamin C and contains **B vitamins**. Beetroot increases the oxygen-carrying power of blood; it also **increases brain power,** aiding concentration and memory.

the red-eye special

Had one too many nights on the tiles? Then this is the **detoxifying** juice for you. The natural oils in parsley and mint will soothe the stomach and calm jangley nerves. With clear eyes, no headache and no puffiness or gritty skin, you'll get through the day in better shape than you ever imagined possible.

6 mint leaves, with sprigs

6 spinach leaves

1 medium-sized, yellow-fleshed, melon, peeled and deseeded

1 handful parsley, with stalks

Wash all the ingredients (except the melon) and put through a juicer.

Mix well and serve.

Serves 1–2

Super-rich in potassium and **vitamin A**, this is also a detoxifying juice, thanks to the parsley. Both parsley and mint have a healing effect on the entire digestive system and are calming to the central nervous system. Melon juice also overflows with **healing betacarotenes** and is exceptionally curative and cooling.

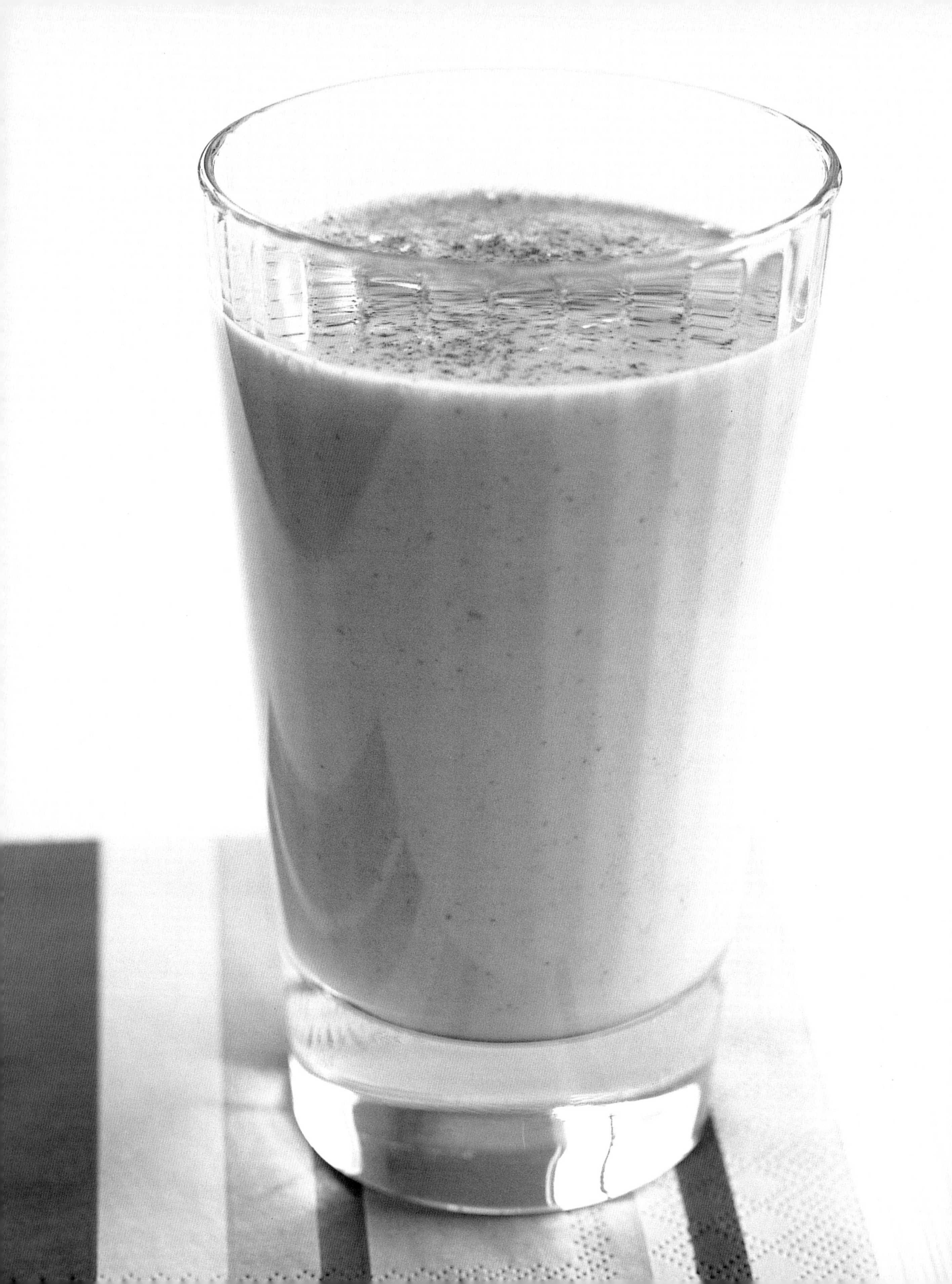

wake-up call

Here's a combination of quick- and slow-release energy, essential nutrients, protein and fibre that is a great early-morning starter or a before-sport **booster** for your **vitality**. Peanut butter provides slow-release energies which prevent a fall in blood sugar.

- 2 dessert apples, washed, cored and quartered
- 1 pear, washed, cored and quartered
- 2 bananas, peeled
- 1 heaped tbsp smooth peanut butter
- 150ml or 5 fl oz crème fraîche
- 1 tsp cinnamon

Put the apples and pear through a juicer.

Put the juice, peanut butter, crème fraîche and bananas into a liquidizer or blender and whizz.

Serve with the cinnamon sprinkled on top.

Serves 1–2

The peanut butter provides slow-release energy and helps **reduce cholesterol** and insulin levels. Add the banana for more slow-release energy and lots of potassium to prevent cramp, and you've got the basis for a great vitality drink. The rest of the fruit provides **vitamin C** and **soluble fibre**, while the crème fraîche gives you **calcium** and B vitamins.

peak performer

Few people realize the nutritional value that may be found in a ripe pear of any variety. If you're a bit sluggish, then the soluble fibre found in the pears and apples – together with the rich supply of natural sugars in grapes and pineapple – are just the thing to aid digestion and provide **instant energy**.

- 12 black or white grapes
- 4 pears, unpeeled, uncored and quartered
- 2 apples, unpeeled, uncored and quartered
- 2 pineapple slices, peeled

Put all the ingredients through a juicer, mix well and serve.

Serves 1–2

Rich in potassium, pectin (soluble fibre) and **natural healing enzymes**, this juice contains vitamin C, **calcium** and traces of B vitamins. In addition, the tannins, **powerful flavones**, and other aromatic compounds harboured in grapes combine to make it energizing and **cancer-fighting** – all this in a superjuice that tastes as great as it smells!

primary pepper punch

Ripe red and yellow peppers are sweet and succulent. What's more, they combine beautifully with the other vegetables to make this a cocktail with a difference. You'll obtain ultimate **antioxidant** power from the massive dose of betacarotenes and other carotenoids that colour these vibrant vegetables.

- 2 carrots, peeled and trimmed if not organic
- 1 small beetroot, unpeeled, with leaves
- 1 celery stick, with leaves if possible
- ½ yellow pepper, deseeded
- ½ red pepper, deseeded

Put all the ingredients through a juicer, mix well and serve.

Serves 1–2

Super-rich in betacarotene, vitamins A and C, folic acid, and potassium. The **iron-rich** beetroot tops help prevent anaemia, so this is a primary **power juice** for women. It also declares war on the damaging free radicals present in our environment, making it ideal for city dwellers.

pumping iron

A power-pumping **iron tonic** in a glass. While its nutritional content is very low, cucumber is nonetheless regarded as an important **healing vegetable** in natural medicine. Here, its cool, refreshing flavour contrasts superbly with the astringency of beetroot, spinach and watercress.

- 2 apples, unpeeled, uncored and quartered
- 1 small beetroot, unpeeled and quartered, with leaves
- 1 medium cucumber, cut into chunks
- 1 handful spinach leaves
- 1 handful watercress

Put all the ingredients through a juicer, mix well and serve.

Serves 1–2

Super-rich in iron, vitamin C and folic acid, this juice is also rich in betacarotene and other **carotenoids**, which protect against cancers. The vitamin C aids the absorption of iron by the body. All this, plus its instant supply of **natural sugars** makes Pumping Iron the perfect juice for serious exercisers, body-builders, vegetarians and women planning pregnancy.

boxer's beverage

Overflowing with instantly available essential nutrients, Boxer's Beverage provides **power, energy** and **stamina.** The minerals, vitamins and easily utilized calories make it the perfect partner for a high-carbohydrate snack shortly before physical exercise. It's also a great reviver after exertion.

4 carrots, peeled and trimmed if not organic

1 kiwi fruit, washed and unpeeled

1 small handful fresh coriander, with stems

1 handful baby spinach leaves

Put all the ingredients through a juicer, reserving a few coriander leaves.

Mix well and serve with extra coriander leaves on top.

Serves 1–2

This vitality drinks provides a double dose of betacarotene and potassium from the carrots and kiwi fruit, along with **extra magnesium** and plenty of vitamin C. Spinach adds extra carotenoids and a powerful boost of **cancer-fighting** plant chemicals. The coriander contains heart- and circulatory-protective coumarins.

horse power

As well as the **instant energy** from carrots' and apples' natural sugars, horseradish adds a new dimension. You'll get very little juice from three ounces of horseradish, but what you do get is instant **circulation stimulation.** With the blood coursing through your veins, you'll be ready for anything.

4 carrots, peeled and trimmed if not organic

2 apples, unpeeled, uncored

85g or 3oz fresh horseradish

Put all the ingredients through a juicer, mix well and serve.

Serves 1–2

Super-rich in vitamins A, C and E, potassium and **vitamin B_6**, this juice contains some calcium and traces of other **B vitamins.** With just under three hundred calories a glass, it's a good quick-energy source. In addition, horseradish contains sinigrin, a powerful natural antibiotic that also **protects against infections.**

ginger it up

This spicy variation on the traditional Indian lassi will give an instant lift to anybody's flagging vitality. The stimulating effects of ginger, the beneficial bacteria in the yogurt, and the **digestive benefits** of mint all work together to give your **vitality** a welcome lift just when you need one.

4cm or 1½in piece fresh ginger, peeled
250ml or 9 fl oz natural, live yogurt
about 10 mint leaves (and 4 small sprigs for garnish)
chilled sparkling mineral water, to taste

Grate the ginger.

Put the yogurt, ginger and mint leaves in a blender and whizz until smooth.

Mix with the mineral water to your desired consistency.

Pour into glasses and serve with the mint sprigs floating on top.

Serves 1–2

It's the **circulatory-enhancing** effect of zingiberene and **gingerols** that makes ginger such a powerful stimulant. Its hotness is offset by the cool yogurt, which supplies valuable calcium, some protein, B vitamins and **probiotic bacteria**, which are so essential for immunity and good digestion. Add digestive mint, and you have a cooling, revitalizing smoothie.

melon and mango tango

Just smelling this wonderful juice first thing in the morning awakens the brain, opens the eyes and quickens the blood. Quick and easy to make, this cool, refreshing drink will **kick-start** your metabolism and help shrug off that early-morning sluggishness. One glass, and you'll be running at full power.

1 mango, peeled and stone removed
½ yellow-fleshed melon (cantaloupe, musk, ogen), peeled and deseeded

Put all the ingredients through a juicer, mix well and serve.

Serves 1

Super-rich in vitamins, this juice provides more than your daily needs of both **vitamins A and C**. Melon helps gets rid of morning puffiness. As a bonus, it also contains adenosine, a substance that makes blood less sticky, thus reducing the risk of blood clots and heart attack. The mango is a super-rich source of **instant energy** and nutrients. The combined vitamin A content of melon and mango juice is a boost to the immune system and helps protect the body from cancer.

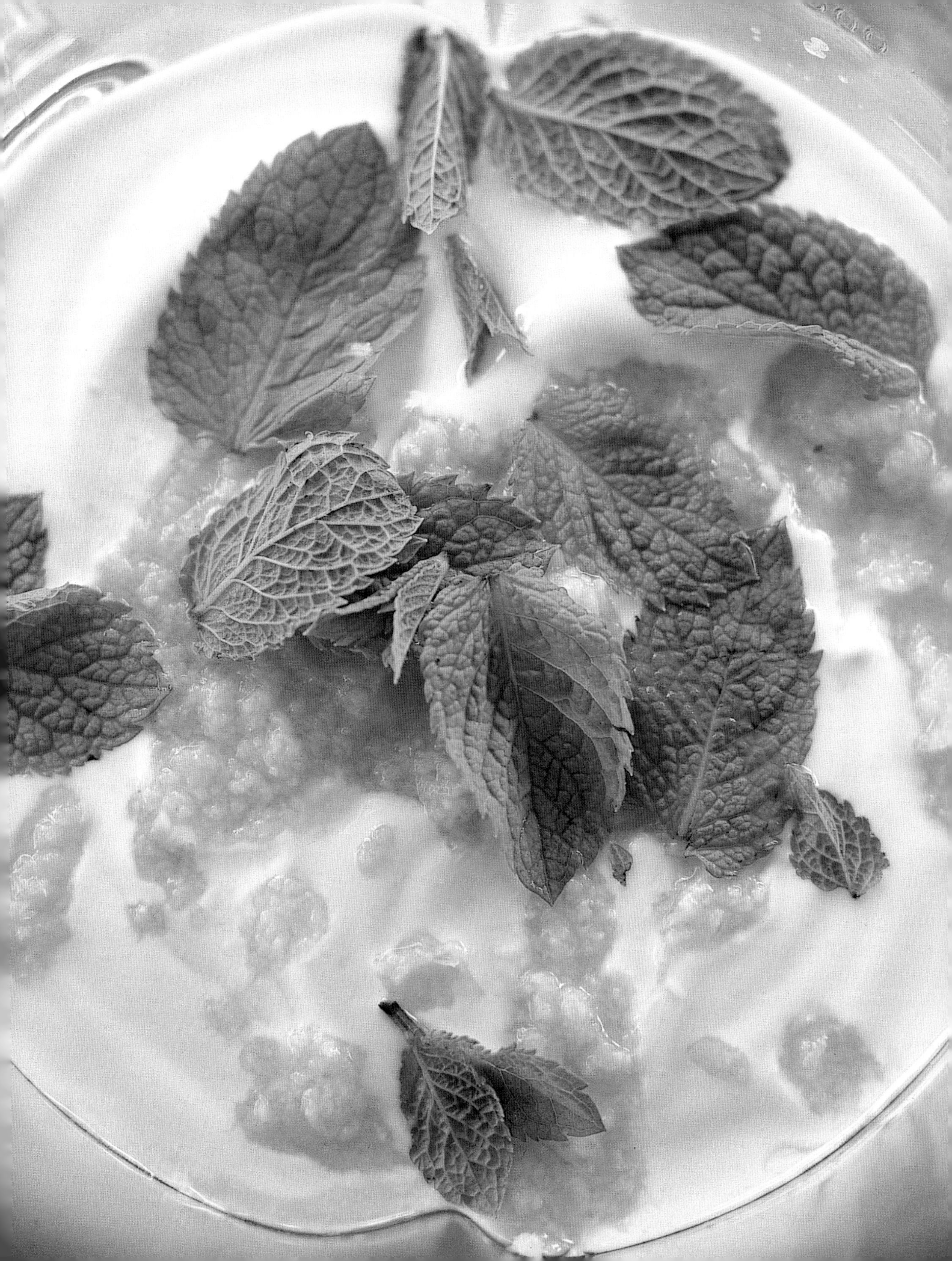

spinach spectacular

The perfect **midday power booster**. Taken with a light lunch, it will see you through a mentally or physically arduous afternoon and still leave you with reserves for an evening on the town. As a bonus, both spinach and watercress contain powerful substances that protect against cancer.

1 apple, unpeeled, uncored and quartered

1 celery stick, with leaves, chopped into chunks

85g or 3oz fresh young spinach leaves

1 handful watercress

Put all the ingredients through a juicer, mix well, and serve.

Serves 1–2

This juice is super-rich in **vitamins A** and **C**, folic acid and **riboflavin** (B_2). While rich in iron, spinach is hard to make the most of due to the oxalic acid in its leaves, which stops absorption. Placed in this superjuice, however, the other vitamins and nutrients it contains would have given Popeye **superpowers** even he never dreamed of!

green apple power punch

A **zappy cleanser** to start your day, the Green Apple Power Punch is ideal for stimulating the digestive system and replacing lost minerals following physical activity. Take this on an empty stomach, and don't eat or drink anything else for half an hour to let its natural fruit sugars do their work.

6 sorrel leaves

2 large granny smith apples, unpeeled, uncored and quartered

1 lime, peeled (unless key lime)

1 mint sprig, with stems

1 handful parsley, with stalks

Put all the ingredients through a juicer, mix well and serve.

Serves 1–2

Try this one for some real health power in a glass. It's super-rich in **vitamins A, C, E** and **B_6** and folic acid, as well as being rich in magnesium and potassium. It also contains some calcium and iron. Soluble fibre in apples and natural oils in mint are good for the entire digestive system; sorrel has been used by Native Americans for centuries as an **anti-cancer food**, while the lime's natural pigment, known as limonine, protects against cancer, too.

mediterranean muscle

Throughout the southern Mediterranean, the combination of tomatoes and basil is inseparable, not only for taste but also for the wonderful combination of aromas. This juice is **rich in minerals** to renew tired muscles, and contains essential oils from the basil that act specifically on tired minds.

4 large, ripe plum tomatoes

1 carrot, peeled and trimmed unless organic

1 celery stick, with leaves, cut into large chunks

1 handful basil

the juice of ½ lemon

Put everything apart from the lemon juice through a juicer. Mix well, squeeze in the lemon juice and serve.

Serves 1–2

A juice that is super-rich in vitamins A, C, E, **folic acid** and potassium, and rich in iron and **magnesium**. Low in calories, it's perfect for weight-watchers. It also gets a five-star rating for **peak power** of mind and body, and is delicious, calming and mildly diuretic. It also contains lycopene, a powerful **natural antioxidant** which protects against heart disease.

hot and smooth prune

The prune is the butt of too many jokes. Yes, it does contain natural chemicals that have a mild laxative effect, but prunes are far more than this. Combined here with live yogurt, the juice makes a surprisingly delicious and enjoyable **revitalizing** drink.

450ml or 16 fl oz prune juice

30ml or 1 fl oz thick-set natural, live yogurt

In a medium saucepan, warm the prune juice gently.

Pour into two mugs.

Serve with the yogurt floating on top.

Serves 2

Weight for weight, prunes are by far the richest food source of **protective antioxidants** and provide a **massive boost** to natural resistance and vitality. Don't wait until you feel you need to use this kitchen remedy; enjoy it when you're at risk of being attacked by any bugs around.

peanut butter surprise

To many people, peanut butter means piling on the pounds. Nothing could be further from the truth – especially if you choose organic, low-salt brands. The **vitality** boost from this drink comes from the combination of instant and **slow-release energy**.

4 level tbsp smooth peanut butter
300ml or 10 fl oz natural, live yogurt
150ml or 5 fl oz milk
runny honey, to serve (optional)

Blend the peanut butter together with about half the yogurt.

Pour into a saucepan with the rest of the yogurt and the milk.

Warm, stirring continuously, until well combined, but don't boil it or you'll kill the good bacteria.

Serve in mugs or heatproof glasses. Drizzle over with runny honey, if desired.

Serves 2

As well as **natural carbohydrates,** yogurt contains millions of beneficial live bacteria, which have a profound effect on the immune system, boosting resistance and enhancing the conversion of food into energy. Peanuts provide health-giving lignans, vitality-boosting monounsaturated fatty acids and a bonus of minerals and fibre.

desert island juice

Drinks made from milk have long been associated with growth, health and **vitality**. Milk is an excellent source of calcium, protein, B vitamins and energy from its natural lactose (milk sugar). Mixed here with health-boosting dates, it's a great vitality drink.

8 dates, stoned and ready to eat
200ml or 7 fl oz milk
200ml or 7 fl oz coconut milk, or the equivalent in coconut cream diluted with hot water to the consistency of milk – about 4 heaped tsp

Cut the dates into eight pieces each. Put into a small bowl and just cover with freshly boiled water. Leave for ten minutes.

Purée the dates, with the water, in a small blender until completely smooth.

Heat the milk and coconut milk (or cream mixture). Add the puréed dates.

Froth with a whisk or cappuccino wand and serve.

Serves 2

For anyone who can't tolerate dairy milk, this recipe is just as good a vitality booster if made with soya milk. Dates are a key to the benefits of this drink and have been part of man's staple diet since 3,000BC. Some varieties are an extremely rich source of **iron**, particularly Gondela from Sudan and Khidri from Riyadh, in Saudi Arabia. All dates are vitality food as their ease of digestion and instant energy are acceptable even to the weakest invalids.

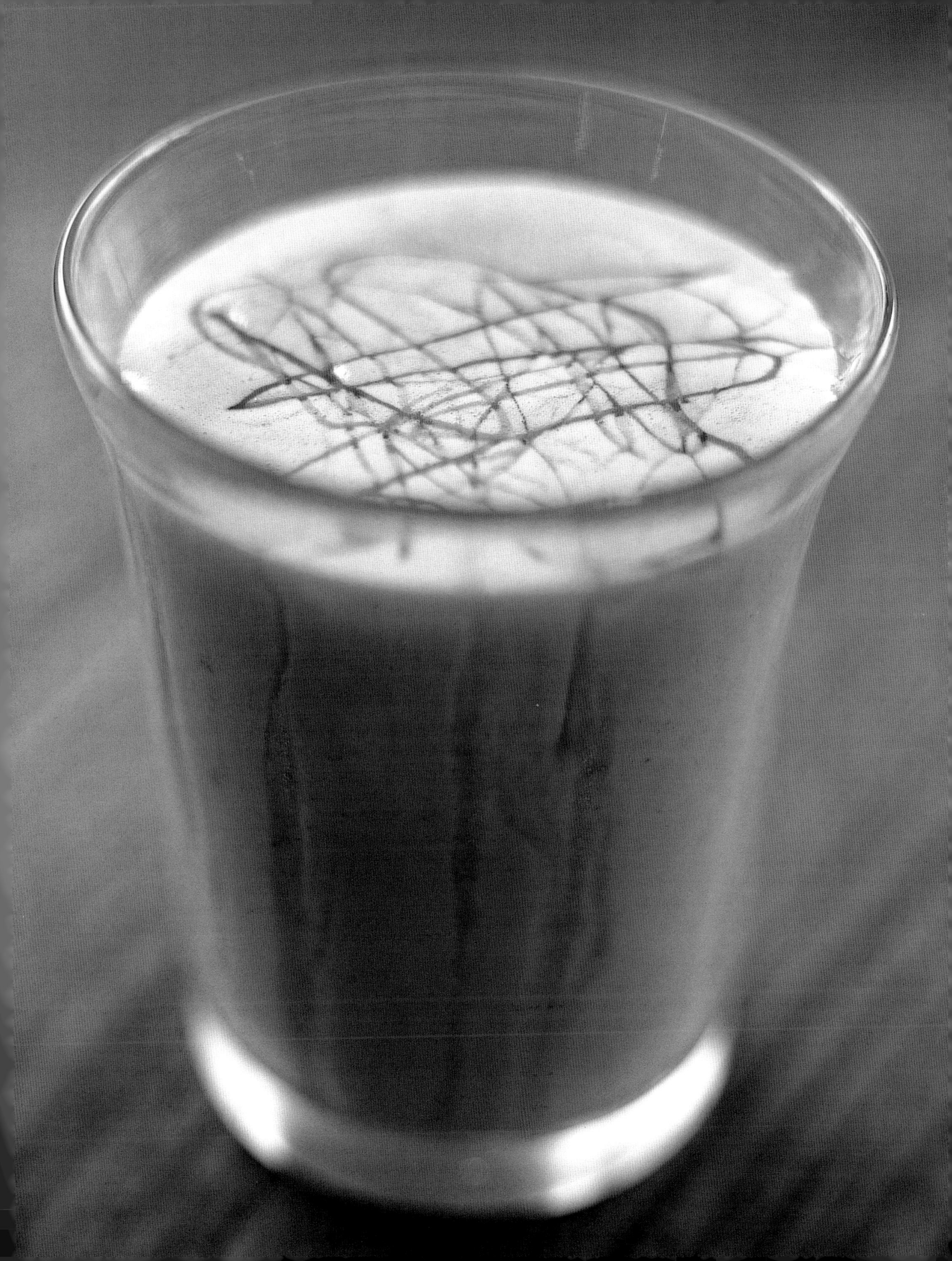

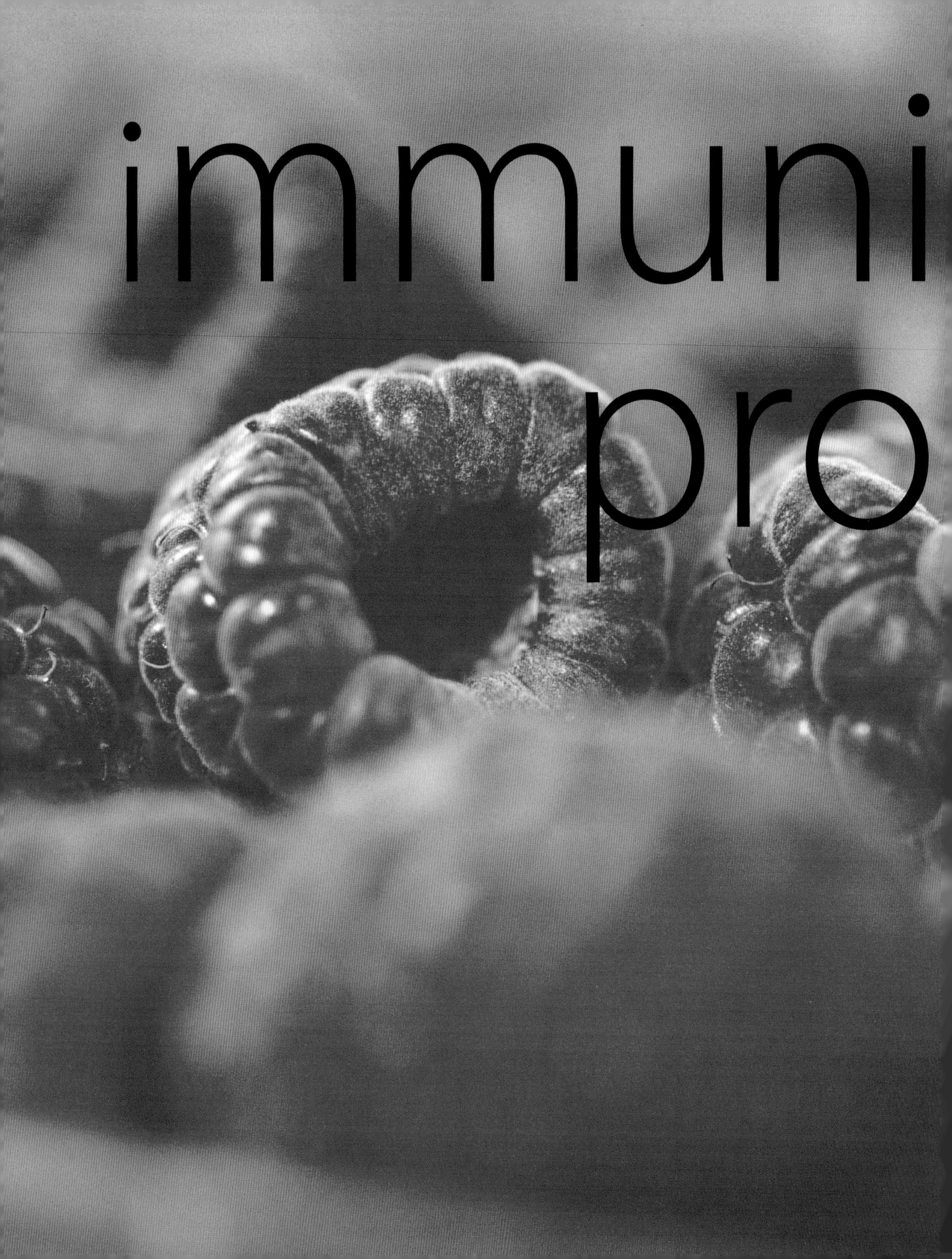
immuni
pro

ty &
tection

Have you ever wondered why there's always someone you know who never catches the flu, never goes down with mystery viruses and travels all over the world without Delhi belly or Montezuma's revenge? These are people who have a highly effective immune system. How do they get it? Well, it's partly nurture and partly nature. Inheriting the right genes from your parents gets you off to a good start, as does exposure to bacteria at an early age – this kick-starts the immune system and actually strengthens it in the long run. Yet, even with a strong genetic background, eating a healthy diet rich in all the vitamins and minerals that help build strong immunity is vital.

The body has its own natural defence mechanisms they protect it from infections and against the internal damage created by free radicals. This immune system depends on an adequate consumption of essential vitamins and minerals, a sufficient amount of natural protective plant chemicals and an adequate supply of antioxidants to mop up damaging free radicals.

Yet, in order to function at its optimum level, the immune system also needs to be protected against antinutrients. High intakes of fats, sugars, alcohol, caffeine; exposure to heavy metals such as cadmium, lead and mercury; smoking and general atmospheric pollution... all these can compromise natural immunity and make disease more likely.

Unfortunately, the human body faces another obstacle to health in the form of food production. Due to modern intensive methods of farming and horticulture, including monocropping, intensive rearing, synthetic fertilizers, insecticides and pesticides, much food may be nutrient-deficient and contaminated with residues. Even a sensible diet of these foods may not supply the optimal nutrient needs of the immune system, so it is important to include regular amounts of high-nutrient foods in your diet. By altering food intake to increase the amount of beneficial nutrients, and choosing organic food whenever you can, it is possible to improve the effectiveness of natural resistance.

An adequate consumption of good protein is essential, so opt for fish, poultry, lean meat, low-fat dairy products, cereals and legumes. A selection of vitamin A- and betacarotene-rich foods should be eaten every day; a deficiency impairs immune responses, but only a small increase in consumption improves them. Carrots, spinach, sweet potatoes, melon and a small portion of liver a week is sufficient.

Deficiencies of the vitamin B complex are known to interfere with natural immune responses. White fish, oily fish, poultry, spinach, peas, kidney beans, chickpeas, brown rice and bananas should all be on the daily menu. Citrus fruits and all fresh produce are needed to supply vitamin C, large amounts of which appear to increase levels of immunoglobulin, whereas deficiency causes a delayed reaction of the immune system.

Another reason for including large amounts of oily fish in the diet is their high content of vitamin D, which is also essential for the immune system. They are also rich suppliers of the important vitamin E, together with olive oil, nuts, avocados and wholegrain cereals.

One of the commonest and least recognized nutrient deficiencies that affects the immune system is zinc. Shellfish, pumpkin seeds, lean beef and, best of all, oysters all contain this mineral.

Essential fatty acids present in fish oils and cold-pressed safflower and linseed oils are other vital components in the integrity of the body's defences.

Surprising but vital immune boosters are the natural probiotic bacteria that live in your gut – two kilograms if you're healthy. These come from fermented foods like live or bio-yogurts, the Japanese milk drink Yakult or natural supplements. These good bugs not only improve your digestion, but have a powerful strengthening effect on your natural defences. You need the good bugs to kill off the bad ones. Don't forget that whenever you are prescribed a course of antibiotics, you must eat live yogurt every day or take one of these probiotic supplements – antibiotics kill the good bugs as well as the bad.

Immunity checklist

- Eat more oily fish for omega-3 fatty acids; poultry and lean meat for protein; spinach, sweet potatoes and carrots for betacarotene; chickpeas and wholegrain cereals for B vitamins and folic acid; olive oil, safflower oil, nuts, seeds and avocados for vitamin E; citrus fruits, cherries and berries for vitamin C and bioflavonoids; and low-fat dairy products for calcium and vitamin D.
- Eat less animal fat, sugar, alcohol, caffeine, highly processed carbohydrates and all processed, prepacked, ready-made foods.

green-and-white delight

There's more than visual appeal to this simple but powerful **immunity boosting** salad. Watercress belongs to the same valuable plant family as cabbages, broccoli and Brussels sprouts. It contains some iodine, lots of potassium and the strong mustard oil known as benzyl, which is an effective antibiotic.

1 large bunch watercress, large stalks removed

2 white onions, finely sliced

2 tbsp extra-virgin olive oil

1 tbsp walnut oil

Thoroughly wash the watercress – even if it's "ready-washed".

Dry the watercress and put it in a bowl, laying the onion slices on top.

Drizzle with both oils – and enjoy!

Serves 4

Natural chemicals found in watercress make it specifically protective against lung cancer. Add the antibacterial, circulatory and **cholesterol-lowering** properties of onions and you have a salad that should be eaten regularly, especially by smokers. A simple yet powerful dose of natural protection.

viva españa bread salad

A sunny salad with an **antibacterial** punch. Nothing could be quicker, easier or more delicious than this typical Spanish salad. Followed by fresh fruit and a piece of cheese, it's an instant summer meal bursting with Mediterranean sunshine, but use really ripe tomatoes and stale, coarse wholemeal or country bread.

3 tbsp extra-virgin olive oil

2 garlic cloves, chopped

4 thick slices of bread, cubed (crusts removed)

6 ripe plum tomatoes

1 red onion, sliced

1 tbsp lemon juice

a pinch of coarse sea salt

freshly ground black pepper

1 handful torn fresh basil leaves

Heat the oil in a frying pan and add the garlic and bread cubes. Stir until the bread becomes crispy. Remove with a slotted spoon and drain on kitchen paper.

Wash and roughly chop the tomatoes. Put the bread cubes into a bowl.

Add the tomatoes, onion, lemon juice, coarse sea salt, plenty of freshly ground black pepper and the basil.

Toss well and serve.

Serves 4

Ripe tomatoes are rich in lycopene, which protects against prostate and breast cancer as well as heart disease. Bread provides **B vitamins**; onions and garlic help lower cholesterol and boost natural immunity, as they contain both antibacterial and **antifungal agents**. Basil is one of the most calming and mood-enhancing of all herbs.

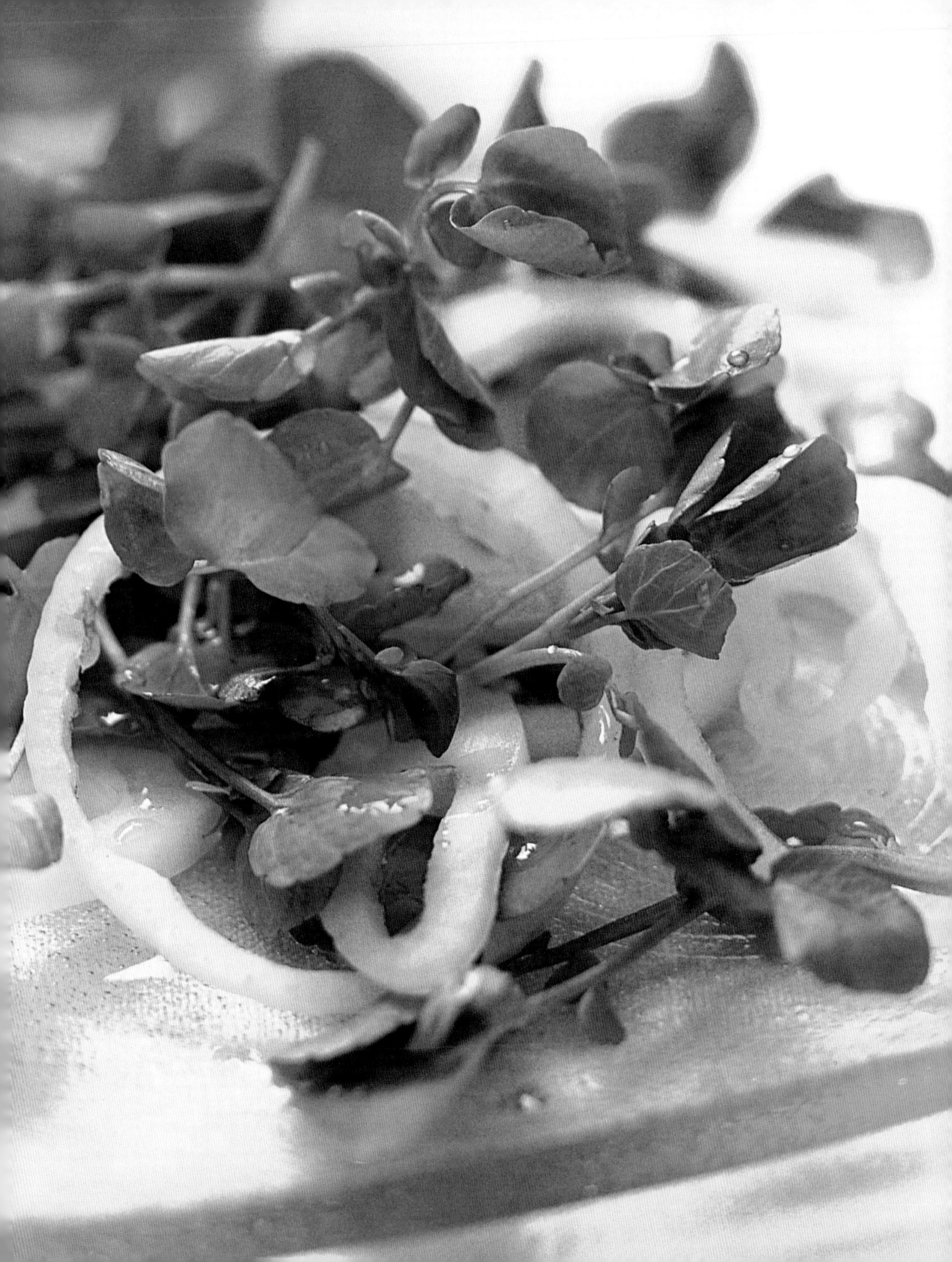

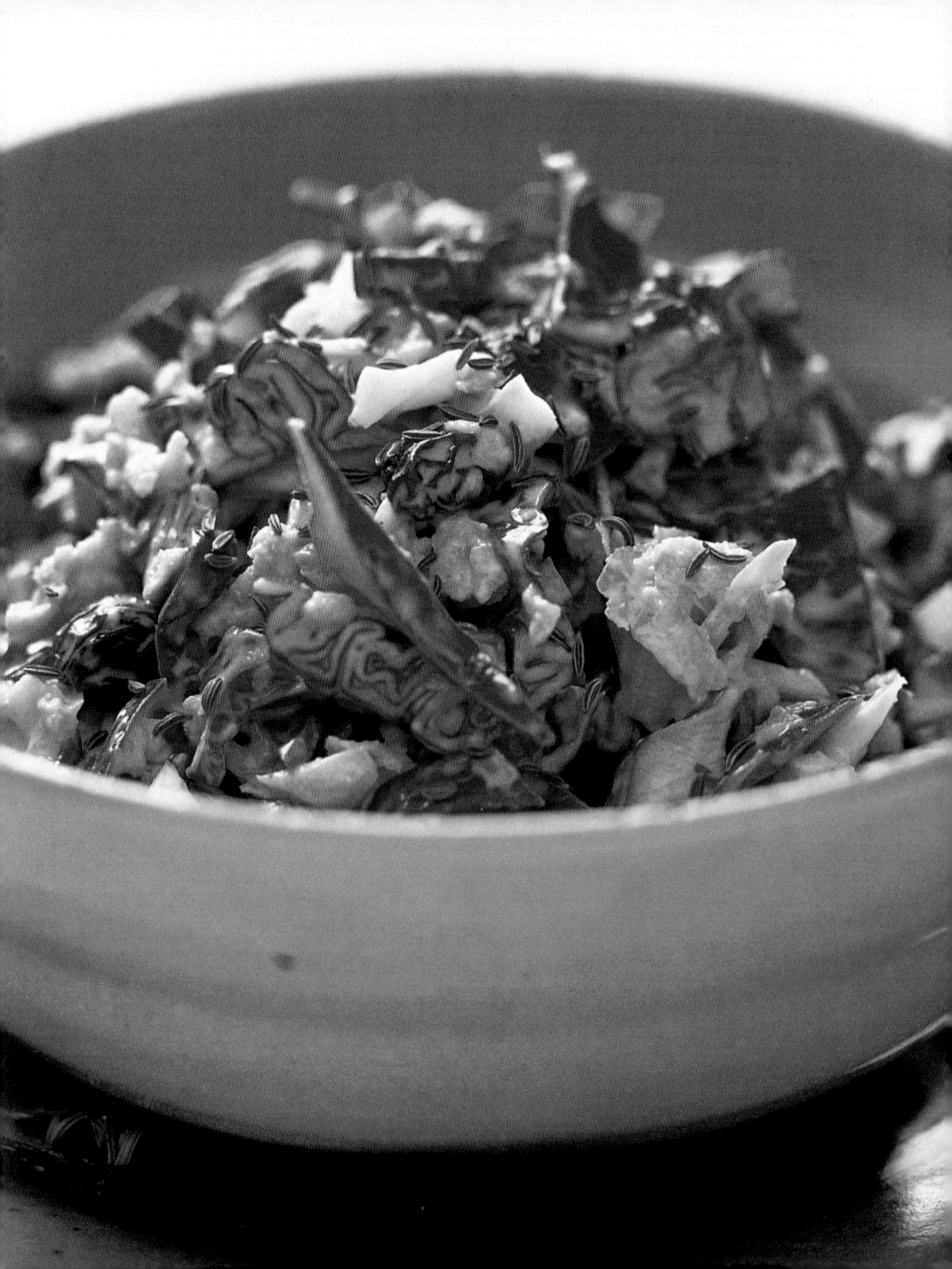

back to the roots

Rich in vitamin A and natural sulphur for **maximum immunity**. Sadly, root vegetables are ignored in many homes today – more's the pity. They are cheap, easy to use, and a powerhouse of immune-enhancing nutrients. All in all, a great immune-boosting salad with an interesting texture and flavour.

- 2 large, old carrots, peeled and grated
- ½ medium celeriac, peeled and grated
- 2 small turnips, thinly sliced
- 6 radishes, trimmed and thinly sliced
- 4 spring onions, trimmed and thinly sliced
- 1 handful fresh parsley, chopped
- 3 tbsp standard salad dressing

Put the carrots into one bowl and the celeriac into another bowl. Mix some of the dressing with the carrot and celeriac. Press each into two timbale pots (or small jelly moulds) and chill for half an hour.

Turn out onto a large plate and decorate with the turnip slices, radishes and spring onions. Sprinkle with the parsley and drizzle with the remaining dressing.

Serves 4

Old carrots are super-rich in **betacarotene**, which the body converts into vitamin A, a vital part of the **natural defence mechanism**. Turnips contain the sulphurous compound raphanol, which is antibacterial; as a bonus, turnips are good for gout, too. Celeriac is a major source of the phytochemical apigenin, which is protective against many types of cancer.

caraway coleslaw

A traditional healing salad with a yogurt twist, this combines all of the **healing powers** of cabbage with the digestive benefits of caraway seeds.

- ½ small red cabbage
- ½ small white cabbage
- 1 large dessert apple
- 1 handful seedless raisins
- 1 x 150g carton natural, live yogurt
- juice and zest of 1 unwaxed lemon
- 1 tsp caraway seeds
- freshly ground black pepper

Wash and finely shred both cabbages. Wash and coarsely grate the unpeeled apple.

Mix the cabbage with the apple and add the raisins.

Combine the yogurt, lemon juice and zest. Mix into the cabbage mixture and stir thoroughly.

Sprinkle the caraway seeds on top and season to taste with black pepper.

Serves 4

All cabbages are rich sources of **vitamin C** and sulphur – a protective and antibacterial combination – and red cabbage contains large amounts of **betacarotene**. Live yogurt means a massive injection of beneficial bacteria, which play a vital role in natural immunity.

hot or cold italian bake

A versatile dish to **ward off** a variety of **ills**. This combination of tomatoes, courgettes, oregano and emmenthal cheese is equally delicious as a hot supper dish, or served warm or cold as a salad to accompany a jacket potato, cold chicken or cold roast beef or lamb.

2 tbsp extra-virgin olive oil
1 medium onion, finely chopped
2 garlic cloves, finely chopped
4 medium fresh tomatoes, thinly sliced
4 courgettes, thinly sliced
1 x 400g can chopped tomatoes
2 tsp fresh oregano leaves
freshly ground black pepper
85g or 3oz grated emmenthal cheese

Gently heat the oil, then add the onion and garlic and sweat until soft but not brown. Add the chopped canned tomatoes and stir until warmed through.

Tip the contents of the pan into an ovenproof dish and add a layer of courgettes, a layer of tomatoes, a sprinkle of oregano and black pepper; repeat until you've used all the tomatoes and courgettes.

Cover with grated cheese and bake in an oven preheated to 180°C (350°F/gas mark 4) for thirty minutes.

Serves 4

Immensely rich in **lycopene,** one of the natural chemicals that protect against heart disease and prostate cancer. Oregano is full of **antibacterial volatile oils** that help ward off coughs, colds and other infections. Cheese contains valuable protein and masses of calcium.

creamy watercress soup

In addition to having a wonderful peppery flavour, watercress is one of the most important **immune-protectors** you can eat. If you smoke, eat this soup twice a week, as it may well reduce your chances of lung cancer. There's an additional benefit from the protective probiotic bacteria in live yogurt.

100g or 3½oz unsalted butter
4 large spring onions, trimmed and finely sliced
350g or 12oz watercress
1 litre or 35 fl oz vegetable stock (page 252)
1 bouquet garni: 3 sprigs each parsley, thyme, and rosemary, tied together, or a good commercial bouquet garni bag
200ml or 7 fl oz natural, live yogurt

In a large pan, melt the butter, then gently sweat the onions for three minutes.

Pull the leaves off any thick watercress stalks; discard the thicker stalks. Add the watercress to the pan and stir briskly for one minute. Add the stock and bouquet garni. Simmer for ten minutes, then remove the bouquet garni. Liquidize until smooth and return to the pan.

Add the yogurt and stir thoroughly. Serve hot with herb croutons. Alternatively, serve cold as a delicious summer soup.

Serves 4

Watercress contains antibacterial mustard oils, lots of **betacarotene** and a phytochemical that protects the cells of lung tissue against the carcinogenic effects of smoking.

white onion soup

Onions have a long tradition in folk medicine, particularly for helping the body overcome the effects of chest infections. In this recipe, this **healing property** is combined with the protective essential oils from bay leaves, thyme and rosemary to make a delicious and health-giving, flavour-packed soup.

55g or 2oz unsalted butter

500g or 1lb 2oz white Spanish onions, very finely sliced

3 level tbsp flour

1 litre or 35 fl oz full-cream milk

4 bay leaves

10 peppercorns, slightly crushed

1 bouquet garni: 3 sprigs each parsley, thyme, and rosemary, tied together, or a good commercial bouquet garni bag

1 medium bunch flat-leaf parsley, washed and finely chopped

Melt the butter over a very low heat. Add the onions. Cover and stir until thoroughly coated, then allow to sweat gently for ten minutes.

Sift in the flour and continue cooking for a further five minutes, stirring continuously. Pour in the milk and add the bay leaves, peppercorns and bouquet garni.

Simmer very gently for about ten minutes, until the onions are quite soft.

Remove the bay leaves and bouquet garni, and strain out the peppercorns.

Serve garnished generously with chopped parsley.

Serves 4

For fighting chest infections. Onions offer **antiviral** and **antibacterial protection**. Parsley, a natural diuretic, aids the natural cleansing process.

bread and garlic soup

There are many variations of this soup throughout Spain; to judge from the number I've tried, every family has its favourite recipe. This is mine. If garlic's potency puts you off, take heart: cooking it this way seems to prevent the residual garlic breath, so be brave and give it a try if you want a bowlful of **super** immunity.

5 tbsp olive oil

1 medium head garlic, split into cloves, peeled and finely chopped

4 thick slices wholemeal bread (crusts removed), made into breadcrumbs

1.5 litres or 55 fl oz vegetable stock (page 252)

½ handful fresh oregano or 2 generous pinches dried oregano

4 medium organic eggs

Heat the oil gently in a large pan. Add the chopped garlic and sweat slowly, covered, for three minutes. Tip in the breadcrumbs, vegetable stock and oregano. Keep covered and simmer for two minutes, adding more stock if the mixture gets too thick.

Beat the eggs. Add them to the pan and simmer very gently for two more minutes.

Serves 4

A soup to help fight bacteria. Garlic contains powerful **antibacterial substances**. Oregano adds antiseptic thymol. Eggs provide health-giving B vitamins.

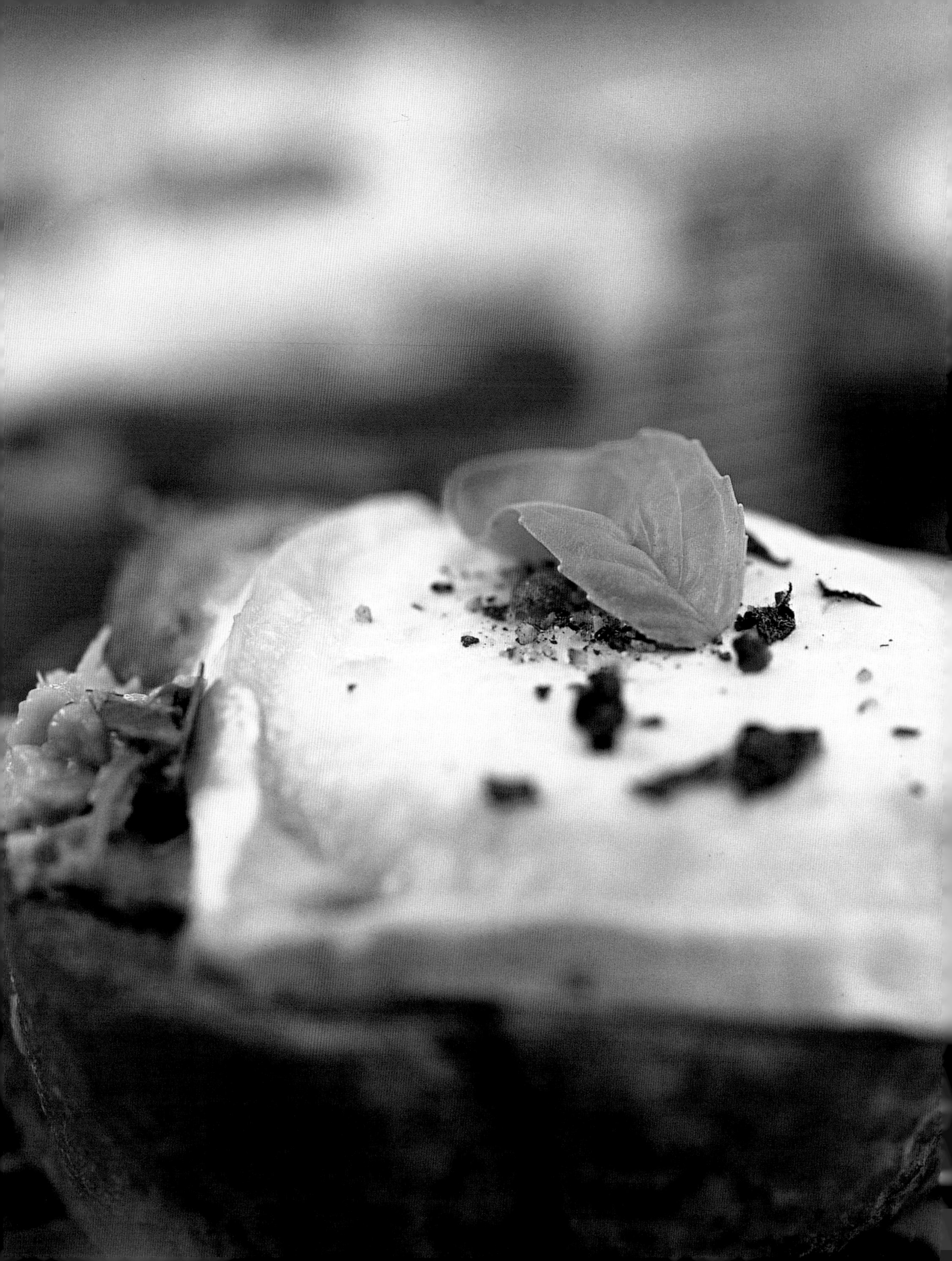

savory fava salad

This instant, inexpensive meal is as full of health benefits as it is of good hearty flavour. All beans are bursting with **nutrients**, but the combination of broad (fava) beans and kidney beans contains more than most. Canned beans are more delicious than other preserved vegetables; just be sure to rinse them thoroughly.

approximately 500g or 1lb fresh broad beans (shelled and cooked) or canned

1 x 400g can kidney beans

4 spring onions, finely chopped

3 tomatoes, coarsely chopped

1 cucumber, peeled and diced

6 tbsp extra virgin olive oil

2 tbsp balsamic vinegar

1 tbsp (combined) chopped savory and thyme

Rinse the canned beans in running water.

Combine all ingredients up to and including the cucumber in a large bowl and mix well.

Combine the herbs, oil and vinegar and mix into the salad. Cover and leave for thirty minutes to allow the flavours to blend together.

Serve with crusty wholemeal bread.

Serves 4

Packed with **protective isoflavones**, natural phyto-oestrogens that protect against breast cancer, osteoporosis and the uncomfortable symptoms of menopause. Savory's carvacrol reduces flatulent effects while thyme's antibacterial essential oils add extra protection.

mediterranean rarebit

This colourful, tasty Mediterranean treat is a **protective feast** for all the senses. The green and red of basil and tomato set against the creamy white cheese make it inviting to the eye, while the pungent, unmistakable odour of oregano and the delicate scent of basil create an explosion of flavours.

1 wholemeal baguette, cut into 2.5cm (1in) slices

2 garlic cloves, halved

1 small avocado

1 small bunch parsley

3–4 tomatoes, sliced thinly enough to cover each slice of bread

goat's cheese, sliced, as for tomatoes

basil, as many leaves as slices of bread

about 2 tsp oregano, dried

Toast the bread slices gently on both sides. Rub one side with the cut section of a clove of garlic.

Mash the avocado with the parsley and spread thinly on the bread. Top with tomato slices, then the goat's cheese. Sprinkle with oregano.

Grill for about five minutes, or until the cheese starts to run. Add the basil leaves to each slice and grill for an extra minute.

Serves 4

Low in saturated fat, yet rich in healthy **monounsaturated fats** and **vitamin E**, this dish provides heart, lung and skin protection, good fibre, plenty of calcium and B vitamins. Oregano is a powerful antibacterial, and the linalool in basil relieves acne.

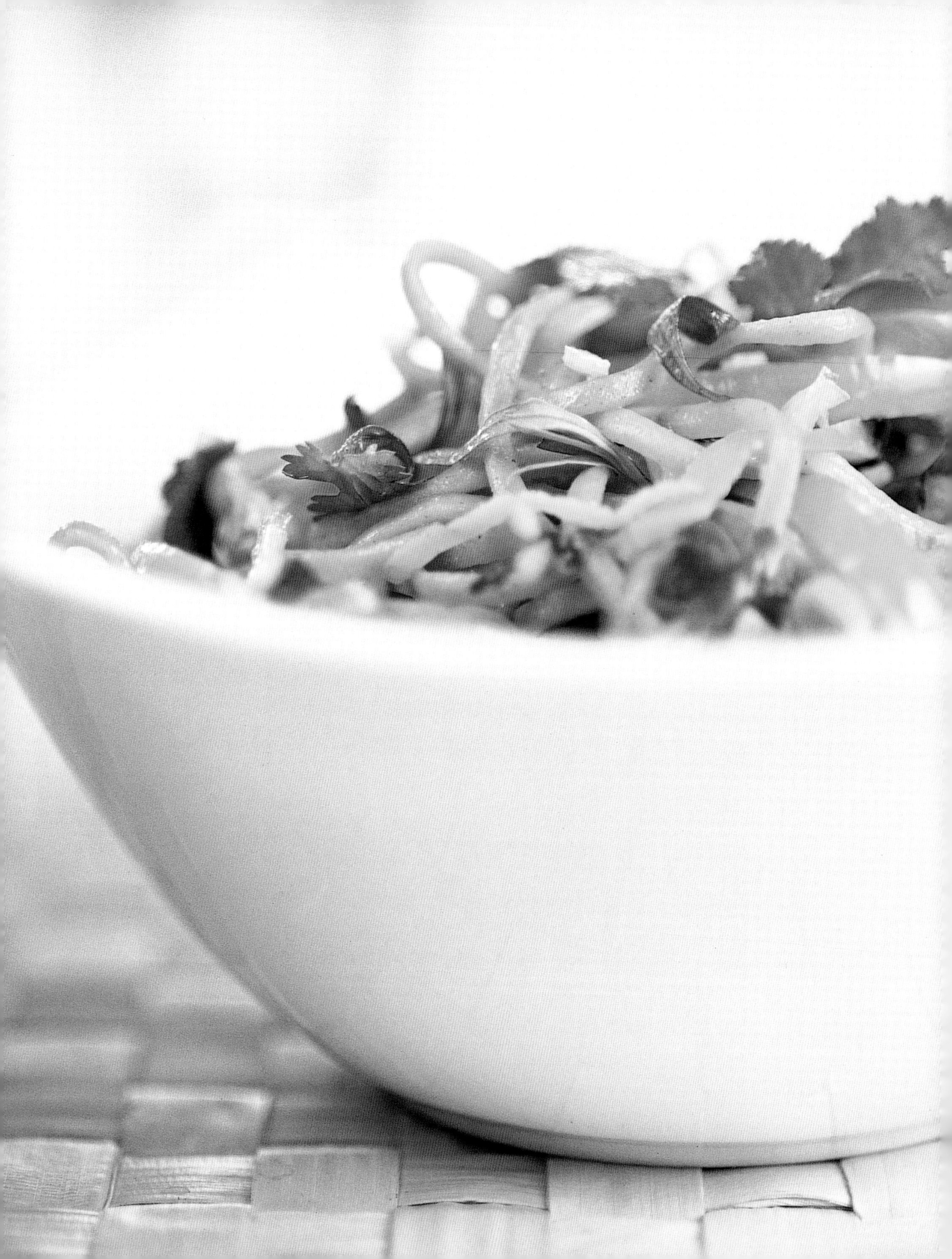

welsh minestrone with rice and leeks

It's no wonder that the leek is the national emblem of Wales, a nation renowned for its singing. When **coughs, colds, flu** and **sore throats** abound, nothing could be better than this wonderfully thick cornucopia of germ-fighting nutrients. What's more, it tastes terrific.

3 tbsp extra-virgin olive oil
3 welsh onions, chopped
2 leeks, trimmed and finely sliced
300g or 10½oz mixed root vegetables, washed, peeled, and diced finely
1.2 litres or 40 fl oz vegetable stock (page 252)
100g or 3½oz long-grain rice
100g or 3½oz peas, fresh or frozen
100g or 3½oz green beans, cut into 2cm or ¾in slices

Heat the olive oil and gently sweat the onions and leeks for five minutes.

Add the diced vegetables. Stir until thoroughly coated with oil.

Pour in the stock and rice and simmer for fifteen minutes.

Add the peas and beans and continue simmering until tender.

Serves 4

For protection against colds and flu. Root vegetables offer a **mineral boost**. Beans and peas provide natural plant hormones. Leeks add protective phytochemicals.

summer noodles

Everyone knows how good it is to wake up in summer with the sun streaming through the windows. This recipe imparts that **warm feeling**, whatever the weather. Sunny, orange marigold petals combined with the fresh green of tarragon and coriander give an added lease of life to the noodles.

250g or 8oz egg noodles
2 tbsp rapeseed oil
2 garlic cloves, chopped
1 large yellow pepper, deseeded and sliced very thinly
zest and juice of ½ lemon
1 tbsp coriander, chopped
1 tbsp tarragon, chopped
1 tbsp marigold petals
1 tbsp garlic oil

Cook the noodles according to the instructions on the packet.

Heat the rapeseed oil in a large wok or frying pan. Add the garlic and yellow pepper and stir-fry for one minute.

Add the noodles and stir-fry for three minutes.

Stir in the lemon juice, zest and herbs and continue stir-frying for one minute.

Add the garlic oil and mix in thoroughly – and serve.

Serves 4

Egg noodles provide carbohydrates and some **protein**. Combined with the antioxidants, carotenoids and **vitamin C** from the garlic and peppers, they become this delicious dish, an instant protector of the heart and immune system.

protective egg shell

The smooth yogurt, the soft, delicate eggs, the crush of the capers and the bite of the horseradish make this an intriguing starter as well as a good boost to the **immune system.** The nasturtium flowers and anchovies aren't just for decoration, either; they contribute to this dish's therapeutic benefits.

8 eggs, hard-boiled, shelled and halved lengthways

1 tsp fresh horseradish, grated (or preserved); or 2 tsp ready-made sauce

12 capers

1 large carton natural, live low-fat yogurt

1 small can anchovies, drained, soaked in milk for 10 minutes and patted dry

1 handful nasturtium flowers

Place the eggs, cut-side down, on a large oval serving dish.

Mix the horseradish and capers with the yogurt, and pour over the eggs.

Decorate with the anchovies.

Scatter with the nasturtium flowers. Serve, and enjoy!

Serves 4

Eggs supply protein, yogurt offers **probiotic bacteria** and anchovies give essential fatty acids, lots of calcium, iodine and **vitamin D**. Sinigrin, from horseradish, protects mucous membranes, and nasturtium flowers supply powerful antibacterial properties. Capers stimulate the appetite, improve absorption of nutrients and are gently laxative.

pasta melissa

Lemon balm (its Latin name is *Melissa*) is a remarkable herb, traditionally used as a heart-relaxer and wound-healer. Its volatile oils, flavonoids and tannins also help **fight depression**, stress and indigestion. Looking at the ingredients, you might think this recipe can't possibly work, but it does – deliciously.

2 x 50g cans anchovy fillets

2 garlic cloves, chopped

juice of 1 lemon

4 tbsp extra-virgin olive oil

400g or 14oz spaghetti

3 tbsp lemon balm, chopped

3 medium tomatoes, coarsely chopped

2 tbsp parsley, chopped

Put the anchovy fillets, with some oil still clinging to them, in a mortar and crush with a pestle until they break down. Add the garlic and keep crushing.

Remove to a medium-sized bowl, add the lemon juice and mix well. Slowly drizzle in the olive oil and mix well.

Cook the pasta according to the packet instructions. Drain well. Stir in the anchovy and oil mixture. Add the lemon balm and mix again. Serve sprinkled with tomato pieces and parsley.

Serves 4

Rich in heart-protective **omega-3** fatty acids from the anchovies, monounsaturated fat from olive oil and garlic, and with the bonus of vitamin C from lemon juice, tomatoes and parsley. Lemon balm has strong **antiviral properties** and is protective against the cold-sore virus.

caperbility fish

I've never understood why John Dory is probably near the bottom of the list of popular fish. Since being introduced by my neighbourhood fishmonger to this extremely ugly but perfectly textured and wonderfully flavoured fish, I have become quite the fan. Enjoy this **protective** dish.

4 john dory fillets
4 generous knobs butter
4 dill sprigs
1½ glasses dry white wine
1 tbsp capers, rinsed
freshly ground black pepper, to taste

Wash the fish and place on a large sheet of foil in an ovenproof dish. Put a knob of butter and a sprig of dill on each fillet. Pour the wine on top.

Scatter the capers over the fish. Season generously with black pepper.

Pull aluminium foil over the fish and secure firmly at the top and sides.

Bake in a preheated oven at 180°C (350°F/gas mark 4) for twenty minutes.

Serves 4

Another meal rich in protein and full of **B vitamins** and the **minerals** you'd expect from deep-water sea fish. The particular protective value of capers comes from capric acid, which increases the flow of gastric juices, stimulating appetite and making digestion more efficient.

baked fish with organic tomato, onion and garlic

This recipe comes from my favourite fishmonger, David Blagdon, in Marylebone. Deep-water fish remains one of the **healthiest** foods in the world – as long as you don't overcook it. This dish is a healthy choice due to its low fat content and, thanks to the tomatoes, onions and garlic, it helps prevent heart disease.

4 tomatoes, finely chopped
2 garlic cloves, finely chopped
1 large onion, finely chopped
4 x 175g or 6oz fresh fish fillets: halibut, hake, cod etc
freshly ground black pepper, to taste
2 dessertspoons extra-virgin olive oil

Tear off four pieces of aluminium foil large enough to make a loose parcel around each fillet.

Mix together the tomato, garlic and onion and spread a layer in the centre of each piece of foil. Put the fish on the mixture and sprinkle what's left on top of each fillet. Season with pepper and a drizzle of the oil.

Wrap each fillet into a loose parcel and bake in an ovenproof dish in an oven preheated to 200°C (400°F/gas mark 6) for twenty minutes.

Serves 4

Provides lots of protein, phosphorus, **potassium**, folic acid and useful amounts of **minerals**, B vitamins and vitamin C. Tomatoes supply heart-protective lycopene, while onions and garlic are **naturally antibiotic**.

earl's fish

The **distinctive flavour** of bergamot is commonly associated with Earl Grey tea. It combines brilliantly with fish, particularly the blander varieties. In combination with the exotic spiciness of myrtle leaves, this recipe is equally suitable for hake, cod and white tuna – perfect to set before a king, let alone an earl.

2 tbsp extra-virgin olive oil
60g or 2oz unsalted butter
4 swordfish steaks
1 tbsp chopped bergamot leaves
1 glass rosé wine
8 whole myrtle leaves
freshly ground black pepper, to taste

In a large frying pan, heat the oil and butter. Fry the fish with the bergamot leaves for around twelve minutes, turning once, until just crisp on each side.

Remove the steaks with a slotted fish slice, leaving the juices in the pan.

Turn up the heat. Add the wine, then the myrtle leaves and boil briskly for one minute.

Pour the sauce over the fish, season with the pepper and serve.

Serves 4

This low-fat, **high-protein** fish is an excellent source of minerals, especially iodine. Bergamot contains **heart-protective** and cancer-fighting essential oils, especially limonene and linalyl, which aid digestion and relaxation. Myrtle leaves protect the urinary system from infection.

salmon maundy

Chervil, tarragon and chives are three of the strongest **protective herbs** around, and this simple dish contains them all. It also has real visual appeal, which makes for a great starter or, in more substantial quantities, a perfect light lunch or supper.

3 tbsp extra virgin olive oil
1 tbsp balsamic vinegar
3 tbsp chives, finely snipped
1 tbsp tarragon, coarsely chopped
2 tbsp chervil, coarsely chopped
250g or 8oz cold poached salmon fillet
250g or 8oz cooked basmati rice, cold
2 large tomatoes, roughly chopped
1 red pepper, thinly sliced
freshly ground black pepper, to taste

Mix the oil, balsamic vinegar and most of the herbs together and stir the mixture into the rice.

Flake the salmon, discarding any skin, and stir into the rice along with the chopped tomato and red pepper.

Add a generous grind of black pepper and stir again.

Sprinkle with the remaining herbs and serve.

Serves 4

Contains **essential fatty acids**, protein, and minerals (especially iodine) with lots of B vitamins from the salmon. Tomatoes and red peppers supply betacarotene and vitamin C. Chervil, tarragon and chives provide antibacterial and antiviral volatile oils. Chervil also helps to lower blood pressure, and it contains useful amounts of iron.

venetian kebabs

Served on a bed of herb-flavoured rice, this is a simple but showy **protective** dish. Use organic chicken livers to avoid antibiotics, and the best-quality prunes, preferably pruneaux d'Agen. If you can't get shallots, substitute pieces of red onion.

- 250g or 8oz chicken livers
- 25g or 1oz butter
- 12 sage leaves, washed
- 6 small and firm prunes, soaked, dried, pitted and halved
- 12 shallots, peeled
- 12 cherry tomatoes
- 12 small brown-cap mushrooms

Wash and dry the chicken livers. Fry in butter for no more than two minutes.

Remove the livers with a slotted spoon, but reserve the butter.

Cut each liver into three pieces and thread on to four long skewers with the remaining ingredients: a sage leaf, a liver, a prune, a shallot, a tomato, a mushroom, a sage leaf and so on.

Brush each kebab with some of the reserved butter and cook under a very hot grill, turning frequently until done, approximately five minutes.

Serves 4

The liver supplies iron, **B vitamins** and protein, while the prunes offer fibre and a massive helping of protective antioxidants. Add the **antiviral** and **bacterial benefits** of onions, and the anti-inflammatory and antiseptic qualities of the sage, for a protective powerhouse.

chicken and noodle soup

You'll obtain plenty of health benefits from the traditional immune-strengthening properties of chicken soup. In addition to the **health-promoting** benefits of chard and chilli, the egg noodles provide a little iron and easily absorbed energy – always important in the body's fight against infection.

- 3 tbsp extra-virgin olive oil
- 1 large onion, finely chopped
- 1 medium red chilli, deseeded and very finely chopped
- 1.2 litres or 40 fl oz chicken stock (page 253)
- 150g or 5½oz chard, stalks torn from the leaves
- 250g or 9oz egg noodles

Heat the olive oil and sweat the onion and chilli gently for five minutes.

Add the stock, bring to the boil, turn down the heat and simmer for ten minutes. Strain into a clean saucepan.

Slice the chard stalks very finely, add to the pan and simmer for ten minutes.

Tear the chard leaves roughly and add to the pan with the noodles.

Simmer until tender – usually not more than three minutes.

Serves 4

A soup that aids the fight against infection. Chard is an amazing source of **betacarotenes**, and chillies contain capsaicin, which stimulates the circulation.

chinese pak choi and chicken

Pak choi is a member of the cabbage family that is now widely available and easy to prepare. Combined with spring onions, garlic and chicken stock, it creates a **power-packed** supersoup.

- 6 large spring onions
- 4 tbsp rapeseed (canola) oil
- 2 garlic cloves, peeled and crushed
- 1.2 litres or 40 fl oz chicken stock (page 253)
- 2 chicken breasts, skinned and shredded finely along the grain of the flesh
- 4 heads pak choi, thick stems removed and reserved, leaves finely chopped
- 150g or 5½oz Chinese noodles or vermicelli (optional)
- 1 tsp tamari or light soy sauce

Chop the white parts of four of the spring onions very finely; cut the others lengthwise almost to the root and reserve.

Heat the oil very gently. Add the chopped onion and garlic and sweat for just two minutes. Pour in the stock. Bring slowly to a simmer and remove the garlic. Continuing to simmer, add the chicken and reserved pak choi stems, and cook for ten minutes, until the chicken is almost tender. Remove the pak choi stems.

Add the pak choi leaves, noodles or vermicelli, and tamari or soy sauce and simmer for five minutes. Serve with the reserved spring onions floating on top.

Serves 4

A recipe that will strengthen the immune system. Pak choi contains protective **thiocyanates**, as well as large amounts of **betacarotene** for good cell health.

duck soup with prunes

Duck, like chicken, is a delicious source of a whole host of vitamins and minerals. The prunes make this soup an extremely high source of **protective antioxidants.**

- 2 large carrots, peeled and trimmed if not organic, and coarsely chopped.
- 1 cooked duck carcass, some flesh still attached, all skin and fat removed
- 2 bay leaves
- 1 bouquet garni
- 1 large onion, finely chopped
- 2 stalks of celery, coarsely chopped
- 10 whole peppercorns
- up to 1.5 litres or 55 fl oz vegetable stock (page 252)
- 200g or 7oz prunes, stoned

Put all the ingredients except the prunes into a large saucepan. Bring to the boil and simmer for an hour. Strain into a bowl.

Set aside the duck. Discard the bouquet garni and push some of the vegetables through a sieve into the stock, depending on how thick you like the soup. Add vegetable stock at this stage to give the quantity and texture you prefer. When the duck is cool enough to handle, scrape off the remaining meat and add to the stock.

Chop or snip the prunes into peanut-sized pieces. Add to the pan and simmer gently for twenty minutes.

Serves 4

Duck is rich in **body-building protein**, protective enzymes and **B vitamins**. Bay leaves provide cineole and laurenolide, essential oils that fight respiratory infections.

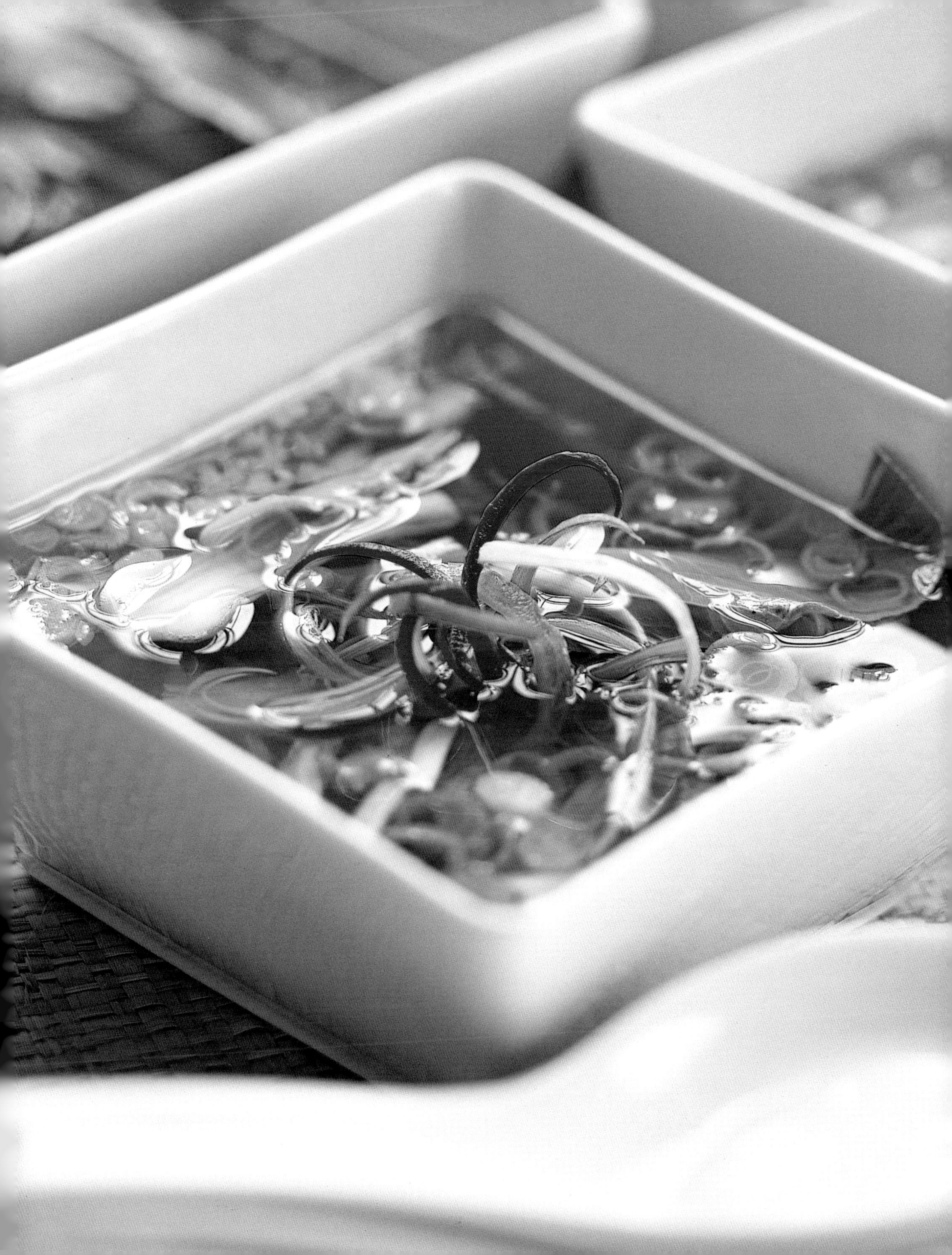

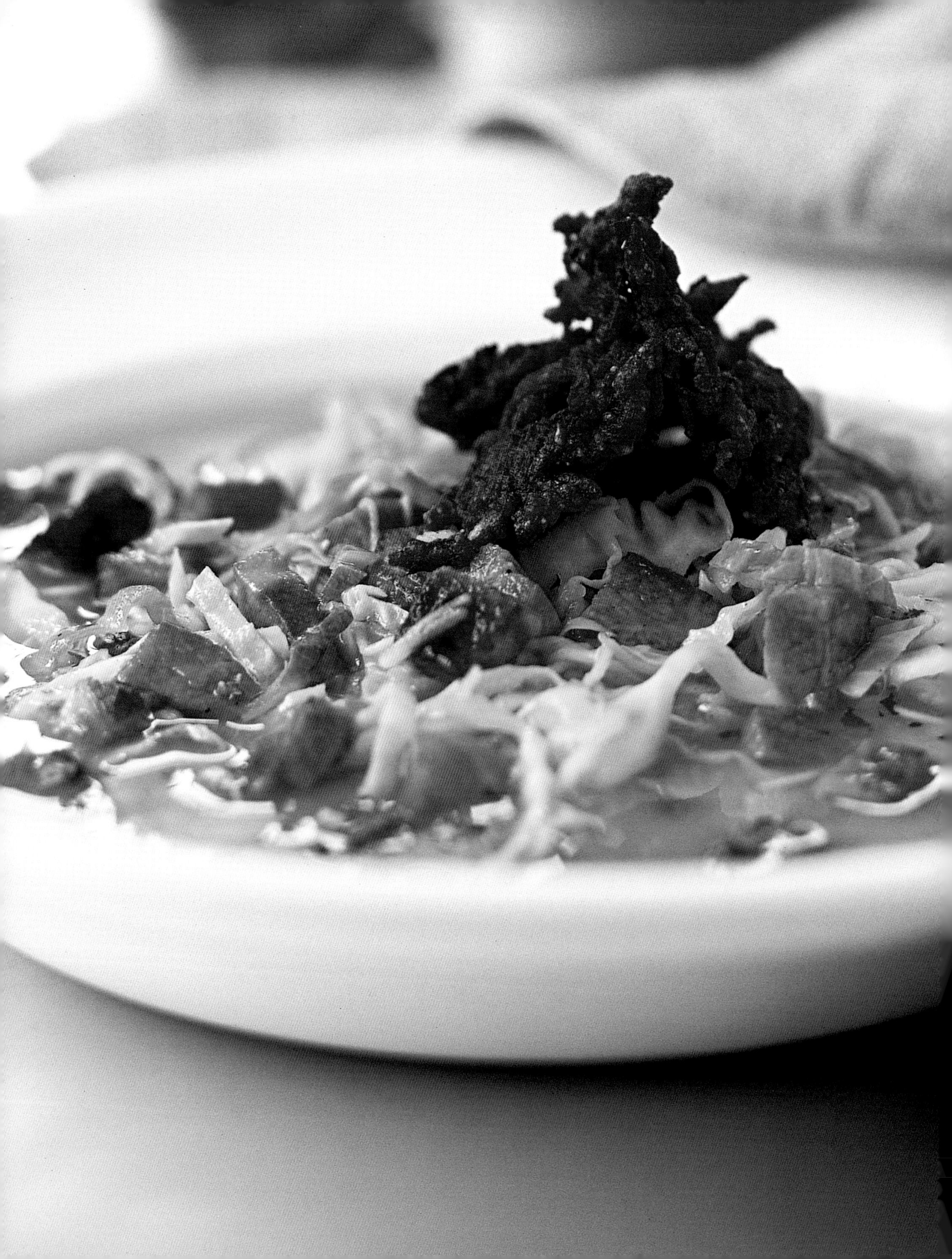

posh hyssop hotpot

Adding mint to lamb comes from the days when most sheep were eaten as mutton. The **digestive benefits** of mint are as important as its flavour. The unique taste of this recipe also depends on the sage, parsley, lemon juice and spices – which naturally give it even greater nutritional value.

1kg or 2–3lb scrag end of lamb

2 tbsp rapeseed or peanut oil

1 large onion, thinly sliced

400ml or 14 fl oz vegetable stock (page 252)

1 bunch parsley, mint and hyssop, tied together

juice of 1 lemon

1 tsp fresh ginger root, grated

1 generous pinch each nutmeg and ground cloves

Cut the lamb into serving-size pieces. Heat the oil in a large ovenproof casserole and fry the meat, sealing it all over.

Add the onions and fry gently for two minutes.

Add the remaining ingredients.

Transfer to a preheated oven and cook at 180°C (350°F/gas mark 4) for two hours.

Serves 4

True peppermint (*Mentha piperita*) is rich in **essential oils**. It also contains cancer-fighting limonene and is a valuable source of carotenes. As well as protecting the digestive system, it is a **powerful antiviral**. The unusual addition of hyssop – rich in many volatile oils – makes this recipe good protection against coughs, colds and the flu.

cabbage soup with gammon

Of all the vegetables, cabbage and its relatives must be regarded as among the most important for their **medicinal value**. This soup also provides a good dose of protein from the gammon and immune-enhancing carotenoids from the vegetable stock.

300g or 10½oz gammon (or more for a very robust soup), fat removed

4 tbsp extra-virgin olive oil

2 red onions, finely chopped

1.5 litres or 55fl oz vegetable stock

300g or 10½oz potatoes, peeled and cubed

500g or 1lb 2oz organic savoy cabbage, finely shredded

200g or 7oz noodles or spaghettini

Cube the gammon, dry-fry until cooked through, and reserve.

Heat the oil. Sweat the onions in the oil. Add the stock and the potatoes and simmer until the potatoes are just tender. Whizz in a food processor or blender until smooth.

Return to the pan and bring back to a simmer. Add the cabbage and cook for five minutes.

Stir in the noodles or spaghettini and the gammon and continue cooking for about three to four minutes until the pasta or noodles are *al dente*.

Serves 4

A dish designed for prevention and protection. Cabbage is rich in **antibacterial sulphur** and **cancer-fighting thiocynates**. Potatoes provide vitamin C.

pastami salad

No, the title isn't a mistake; it's a description of this delicious pasta and salami salad. In spite of using these wonderful meats in vast quantities, our Continental neighbours suffer far **less heart disease** than we do. That's due to eating huge amounts of heart-protective foods, including the herbs used here.

- 250g or 8oz pasta, any small variety
- 1 cucumber, cut into julienne strips
- 125g or 4oz salami, skinned and diced
- 250g or 8oz tomatoes
- 3 tbsp extra virgin olive oil
- 1 tbsp balsamic vinegar
- 1 tbsp fresh parsley, chopped
- 1 tbsp fresh marjoram, chopped
- 2 welsh onions stems, finely snipped

Drop the tomatoes into boiling water for two minutes, remove with a slotted spoon, allow to cool, and peel, deseed and chop.

Cook the pasta according to the directions on the packet; drain and cool. Mix the pasta together with the cucumber, salami and tomatoes.

Combine the oil, vinegar and parsley, pour over the mixture and chill well, turning at least once.

Just before serving, stir in the lettuce and sprinkle with the marjoram and Welsh onions.

Serves 4

Welsh onions are rich in natural chemicals that help lower blood pressure. Marjoram contains **flavonoids**, which function as antiviral antioxidants. Tomatoes are rich in heart-protective lycopene, while iceberg lettuce supplies folic acid, another heart-protector.

double-six stew

A genuine one-pot meal, as everything cooks together in a fragrant, mouthwatering blend. Lovage's unusual taste combines well with the bay leaf and marjoram to make this dish delicious and **protective**.

- 500g or 1lb lean stewing steak, cubed
- 4 tbsp plain flour, seasoned to taste
- 3 tbsp extra-virgin olive oil
- 2 garlic cloves, chopped
- 500g or 1lb combined weight onion, celery, carrots, broad beans, swede, and parsnip, chopped and peeled as necessary
- 300ml or 10 fl oz Guinness
- 1 bouquet garni: a bay leaf and a sprig each of marjoram, parsley and thyme
- 1 tbsp lovage leaves, chopped

Toss the cubed meat in the seasoned flour, and brown in the olive oil and garlic in a large casserole dish.

Add the vegetables and stir briskly for two minutes.

Add the Guinness, the bouquet garni and water, if necessary, to cover.

Bring to the boil. Cover and simmer for two-and-a-half to three hours, adding more water if necessary.

Stir in the lovage leaves just before serving, and enjoy with some good, chunky wholemeal bread.

Serves 4

Enormous **immune-boosting properties** come from the six herbs and six vegetables. **Antioxidants**, cancer-protective phytochemicals, heart-protective and antibacterial herbs combine to provide super protection. In addition, lovage is antimicrobial.

beef gaulloise

Modest amounts of best-quality organic lean beef make a valuable contribution to the diet. The typical Gallic flavour of this casserole is redolent of holidays in France; just inhaling its aroma is sure to **lift the spirits**.

- 2 garlic cloves, chopped
- 30ml or 1 fl oz extra-virgin olive oil
- 750g or 1½lb lean chuck steak, cubed
- 1 x 400g can chopped tomatoes
- 75g or 3oz pitted black olives
- 1 small red pepper, deseeded and thinly sliced
- 1 sprig fresh thyme (or 1 tsp dried)
- 1 or 2 glasses red wine, to taste

In an ovenproof casserole, sauté the garlic gently in the olive oil.

Add the meat and fry until brown all over.

Add the remaining ingredients, including the sauce from the tomatoes and enough red wine to cover.

Cover the casserole and transfer to a preheated oven.

Cook for about two hours at 150°C (300°F/gas mark 2).

Serves 4

The combination of the allicin from garlic and the powerful antiseptic thymol from thyme offsets the fat in the beef. Super-rich in **protein**, betacarotene and lycopene, which offers extra heart protection, this dish is also an excellent source of easily absorbed iron.

blueberry booster

This is mega-health insurance on a plate. In addition to the **antioxidant protection** this provides, there's also beneficial bacteria in live yogurt, which play a vital role in the body's defences against infection. Winter or summer, this is a fruit salad that will help you avoid coughs, colds and flu.

- 6 fresh mint leaves
- 2 x 300g cartons natural, live yogurt
- 1 tbsp runny honey
- zest of ½ unwaxed lemon
- 1 ripe pineapple, peeled, cored and sliced
- 150g or 5½oz blueberries, washed
- 4 kiwi fruits, peeled and slices

Chop the mint and stir it into the yogurt, along with the honey and lemon zest.

Arrange the pineapple slices on a large platter and fill the centre of each with blueberries.

Surround with the kiwi fruit slices and pour the yogurt dressing on top.

Serves 4

Blueberries provide **antioxidant protection**, pineapple adds the healing enzyme bromelain, while kiwi fruit offers betacarotene and vitamin E, along with a vast amount of **vitamin C**.

cicely surprise

A delicious variation on baked apples. The natural combination of mint and apple is enhanced by the **intriguing hint** of aniseed that is imparted by sweet cicely. Together with the added sweetness and succulence of the honey and butter, these herbs create a beguiling mixture of fragrance and flavour.

- 4 medium dessert apples, cored but with the bottom intact
- 8 mint leaves
- 1 tsp sweet cicely leaves, finely chopped
- 4 tsp runny honey
- 4 very small knobs butter

Place each apple on a large square of foil and fill with mint leaves, a pinch of cicely, a teaspoon of honey and a knob of butter.

Wrap each apple securely in its foil. Bake in a preheated oven at 180°C (350°F/gas mark 4) for twenty to thirty minutes, or until soft. This recipe also works brilliantly on a barbecue.

Serves 4

Two apples a day supply sufficient **fibre** and natural plant chemicals to reduce cholesterol and blood pressure. Add the digestive and **antiseptic volatile oils** in mint and the antibacterial properties of cicely for an all-round protective sweet.

moorish rice pudding

A better-than-average rice pudding that not only tastes good, but **does you good**. For a bit of extra dash, sprinkle a few pure, deep-blue borage flowers on top. Its health benefits are listed below, but it does contain a toxic alkaloid and should not be eaten on a regular basis.

- 500ml or 16 fl oz whole milk
- 1 tsp shredded borage leaves
- 2 pinches crushed coriander seeds
- 60g or 2oz pudding rice
- 75g or 2½oz dried apricots, chopped
- 1 tbsp brown sugar

Put the milk, borage leaves and coriander into a saucepan. Bring slowly to the boil, then turn off the heat and leave until cool.

Strain the milk and pour it into an ovenproof dish, then add the remaining ingredients.

Transfer to an oven preheated to 150°C (300°F/gas mark 2) – and leave for two hours, stirring occasionally during the first forty-five minutes.

Serve hot or cold.

Serves 4

Calcium and **vitamin D** from whole milk make this dish a good bone-protector. Borage is a useful sickroom herb as it reduces fevers and is soothing to the whole respiratory tract. It is also mildly diuretic and helps reduce fluid retention.

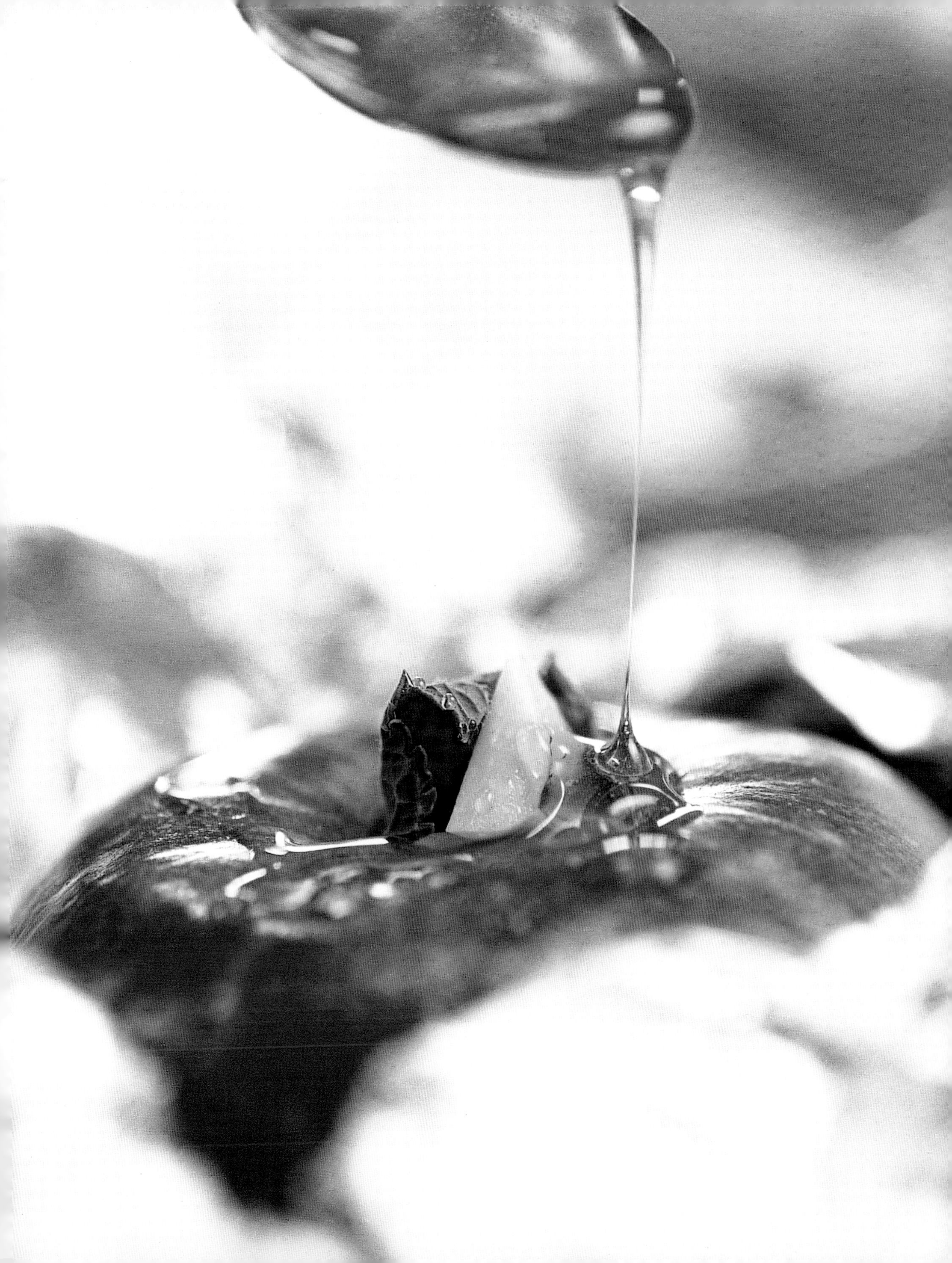

flowery rhubarb delight

Hot or cold, this makes a **delightful combination**. The delicate taste of elderflower contrasts with the more astringent flavour of rhubarb, its acidity tempered beautifully by the creamy yogurt. Gather elderflowers for free from any hedgerow, but don't plant a tree in your garden unless you want a forest!

750g or 1lb 10oz rhubarb, washed and cut into 2cm/1in pieces

2 tbsp brown sugar (or to taste)

1 handful fresh elderflowers, well washed

1 x 600ml or 20 fl oz carton natural, live yogurt

4 mint leaves, chopped, plus 4 whole leaves, to garnish

1 tsp cinnamon

zest of ½ lemon

Put the rhubarb and sugar in a large saucepan with just enough water to cover. Place the elderflowers in a piece of muslin, tie into a bag and add to the rhubarb.

Cover and bring slowly to the boil. Simmer for ten to fifteen minutes, or until cooked, stirring occasionally. Remove the bag of elderflowers.

Whisk together the yogurt, chopped mint, cinnamon and lemon zest. Serve the rhubarb covered with yogurt and decorated with the remaining mint leaves.

Serves 4

Traditionally used to treat and prevent respiratory infections, elderflowers are also helpful for catarrh, hayfever and children's ear infections. In combination with mint, they are also useful for the **relief of flu** and its symptoms.

cucumber soother

To help prevent, as well as cure, sore throats, tonsillitis, laryngitis and sinusitis. The healing properties of carrots combine with cucumber to soothe mucous membranes, and the diuretic action of celery **reduces swelling** of the **tonsils**, **adenoids** and **throat**. Sage adds a powerfully antiseptic kick.

3 carrots, peeled and trimmed unless organic, chopped into rough chunks

2 celery sticks, with leaves

1 small pineapple, peeled and roughly chopped

6 fresh sage leaves

15cm or 6in cucumber

Put all the ingredients through a juicer, mix well and serve.

Serves 1–2

Super-rich in betacarotene, **potassium** and natural enzymes, this juice also contains **vitamin C** and **folic acid**. The natural enzyme bromelain in pineapple is especially healing to the lining of the mouth and throat; it is also a great aid to digestion. Sage is a valuable antiseptic thanks to its high content of the essential oil known as **thujone**.

pro-bonus 1

The earlier women start to build healthy bones, the less likely they are to develop **osteoporosis** in later life. Pro-Bonus 1 and 2 are good sources of easily absorbed calcium and magnesium, both of which are essential for bone development. They're a great **bone tonic** for women throughout life.

3 apples, unpeeled, uncored and quartered

2 celery sticks, with leaves, if possible

1 medium beetroot, with leaves

½ small round cabbage, cut into wedges

Put all the ingredients through a juicer, mix well and serve.

Serves 1–2

Super-rich in **calcium**, **magnesium** and **vitamin C**, rich in folic acid and potassium, this juice also contains iron and phosphorus. The extra nutrients from the beetroot tops, the cancer-fighting nutrients in the cabbage and the calming influences of celery make this a powerful tonic.

pro-bonus 2

Not so rich in calcium as Pro-Bonus 1, but it provides a treasure trove of other micronutrients vital for healthy bones. Ideal at any age, but it is especially good for women approaching, going through or after the **menopause**, as it ensures the best utilization of other calcium sources in the diet.

4 carrots, peeled and trimmed unless organic, chopped into rough chunks

3 large chard leaves, with stalks

2 apples, unpeeled, uncored and quartered

2 small broccoli heads, purple sprouting, with leaves and stalks

1 small red pepper, deseeded and quartered

1 handful watercress, with stalks

Put all the ingredients through a juicer, mix well, and serve.

Serves 1–2

Super-rich in **vitamins A**, C, E, and B_6, folic acid, potassium and **magnesium**, this juice also contains vitamin K, calcium, boron, some other **B vitamins** and iron. Calcium alone isn't the answer to strong, healthy bones; trace minerals and vitamins are essential to the absorption process – and this superjuice has an abundance of them all.

mangobano smoothie

Make this a family favourite for breakfast, and you'll send them all off to school, college or work with a shot of natural resistance. This is valuable during the autumn and winter months, when we're all exposed to other people's **flu-** and **cold-causing organisms**.

1 large mango, peeled and stone removed

2 bananas, peeled and sliced

400ml or 14 fl oz natural, live yogurt

Put all the ingredients into a blender and whizz until smooth.

Serves 2

You'll get lots of resistance-building **betacarotene**, flavonoids, potassium, **antioxidants** and vitamin C from the mango; plenty of potassium, fast- and slow-release energy and **vitamin B_6** from the bananas; and more resistance-building bacteria from the yogurt.

green tea with apples

If you're not a regular drinker of green tea, you'll find its flavour a lot weaker than your usual tea blend. The subtle taste goes well with the sweetness of the apple juice and the tartness of lemons. Green tea has been used medicinally in the Far East as an **immunity-building** drink for thousands of years.

2 green-tea tea bags

1 small dessert apple, preferably cox's orange pippin

½ lemon

75ml or 3 fl oz apple juice

Put the tea bags into two large heatproof glasses. Half-fill with boiling water and leave to brew for ten minutes. Remove the tea bags. Leave to cool completely.

Core the apple and cut into thin slices. Squeeze the juice from the lemon.

Add the lemon and apple juices to the tea.

Serve with the apple slices on top.

Serves 2

Green tea contains immune-boosting antioxidants. Apples supply cholesterol-lowering **pectin**, a special type of soluble fibre; they also contain **malic acid** for digestion and **potassium** to keep blood pressure down. Add the **vitamin C** in the juices and you have a great health-giving beverage.

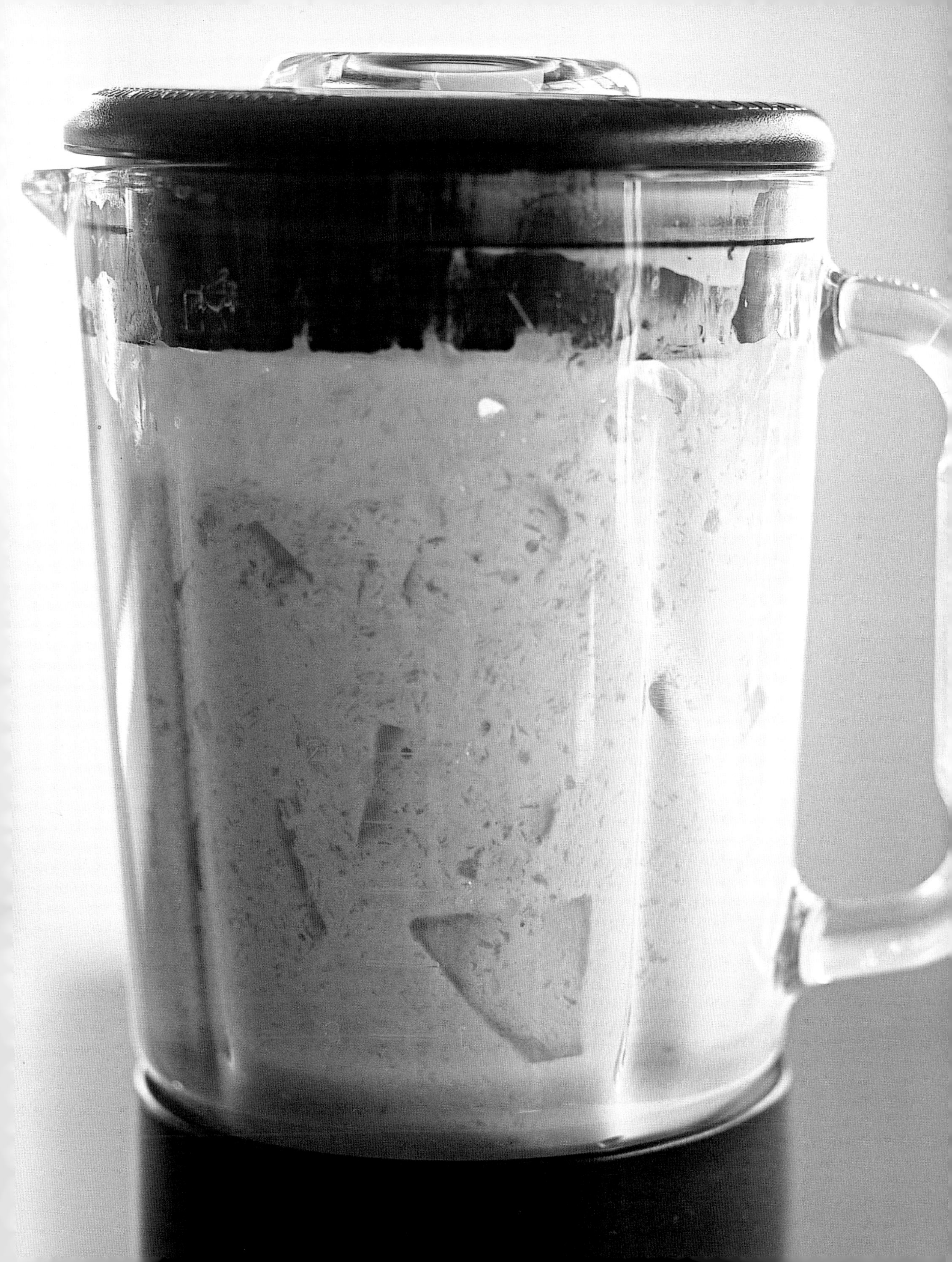

cranberry cup

Apart from tasting great, this mixture of cranberry juice and star anise is doubly **protective** because it's hot. Served cold, the essential oils from the star anise would not be extracted, so you'd get neither the benefit nor much flavour.

4 whole star anise
300ml or 10 fl oz cranberry juice

In a medium saucepan, add the star anise to the cranberry juice.

Bring slowly to just under boiling point.

Leave the star anise floating on top to serve.

Serves 2

Surely there can't be a woman in the Western world who doesn't know that the juice of the amazing cranberry is both a treatment for and a protector against urinary infections. Star anise is rich in **essential oils** that improve digestion and protect against coughs and colds.

tango smoothie

This tastes and smells wonderful. The **unique taste** of lime contrasts well with the sweeter, heavier flavours of the other fruits, and when yogurt is added it takes on a wonderful creamy consistency. For a thicker smoothie, try using traditional Greek yogurt or adding some mascarpone or crème fraîche.

2 large peaches, stones removed
2 large mangoes, peeled and stones removed
1 lime
450ml or 16 fl oz natural, live yogurt

Put the peaches and mango through a juicer.

Cut two or three slices from the lime, then squeeze the juice from the rest.

Mix the lime, peach and mango juices with the yogurt.

Serve with the reserved lime slices on top.

Serves 2

The peaches and mangoes provide a large injection of **betacarotene** and other **carotenoids**, which protect the skin and mucous membranes and help boost immunity, while an extra **vitamin C** boost comes from the lime. The yogurt provides resistance-boosting friendly bacteria that live in the intestine, where they both help destroy unwanted bugs and have a direct effect on the general immune system.

veggie wake-up call

Pawpaws and vegetable juice may sound a bit strange, but there's nothing odd about the finished drink. Your **immune system benefits** from some of the healthiest of fruits, the nutrients in the mixed vegetable juice, the spiciness of ginger and the creamy smoothness of a good, live, natural yogurt.

2 pawpaws, peeled and deseeded
150ml or 5 fl oz vegetable juice
150ml or 5 fl oz apple juice
1 tsp ground ginger
50ml or 2 fl oz natural, live yogurt

Put all the ingredients into a blender or food processor and whizz until smooth.

Serves 2

As well as the **carotenoids** you'd expect from pawpaws, there's a special benefit from the digestive enzyme **papain**, which they also contain. The ground ginger is a surprising immune-booster, as its gingerols will help "ginger up" your entire system.

spuds 'r' us

The sweet potato really is one of the most **immunity-building** and **cancer-preventative** foods around. Mixing sweet potatoes with kiwi fruit and orange juice makes a delicious combination that is a powerful protector against short-term infections and long-term disease.

1 large sweet potato, washed
3 kiwi fruits, peeled
300ml or 10 fl oz freshly squeezed orange juice

Put the potato and kiwi fruits through a juicer.

Add the orange juice and mix well.

Serves 2

Huge amounts of **vitamin C** from the kiwi fruit and orange juice are coupled with betacarotene and a range of **essential carotenoids**, as well as the cancer-fighting **phytochemicals**, in the sweet potato. The orange juice also provides bioflavonoids, which play an important role in protecting blood vessels. This mixture is an all-round protector that increases your natural resistance to bugs and degenerative diseases.

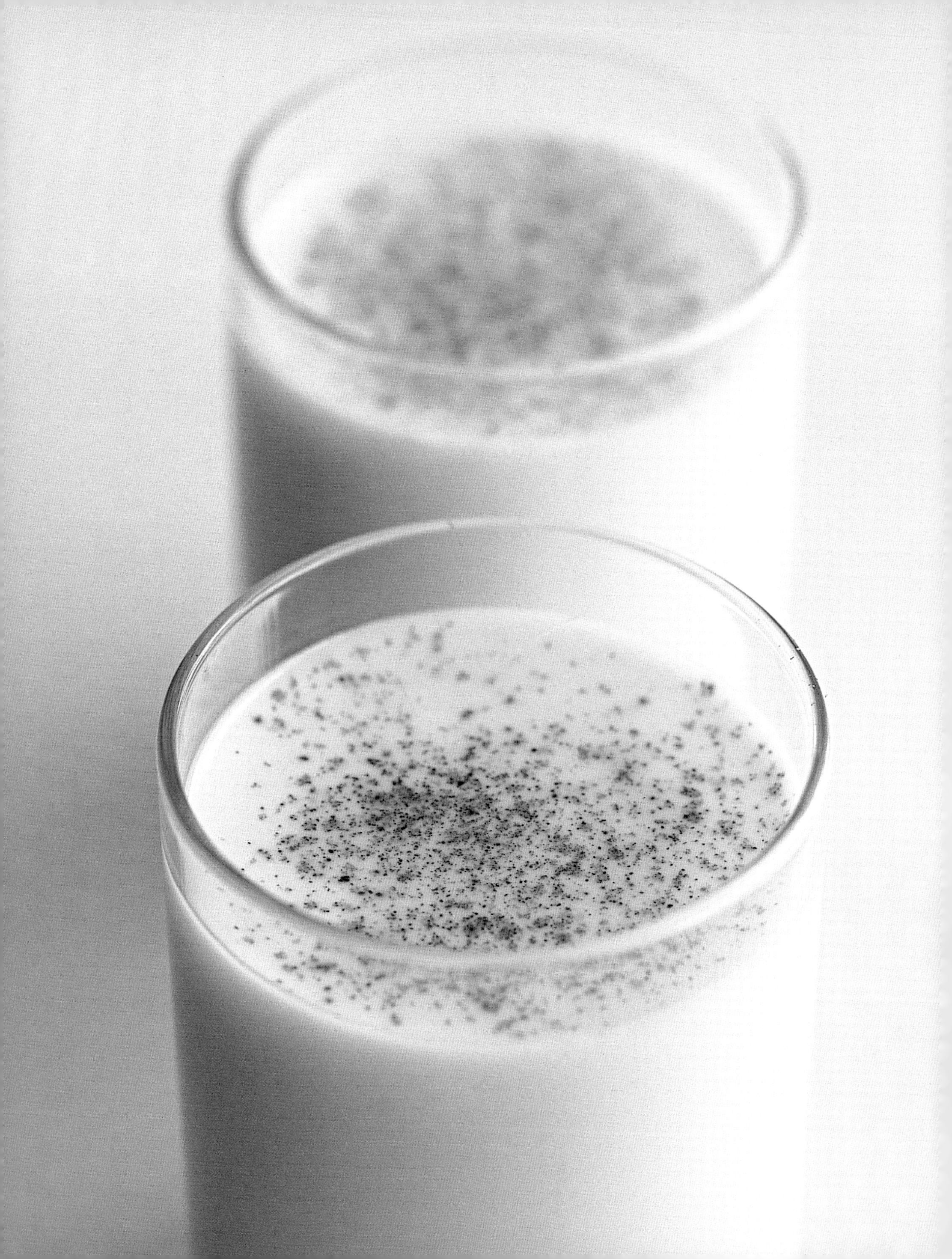

spiced coconut

Coconut milk is easily available even in your local supermarket, so there's no excuse for not trying this exotic, spicy way to **protect** yourself from all sorts of **infections**. This takes just seconds to prepare, but do take the time to savour the taste and soak up the benefits.

- 300ml or 10 fl oz coconut milk
- 150ml or 5 fl oz full-fat milk
- 1 tbsp runny honey
- 2 tsp ground cloves, plus a little to serve

Put the coconut milk, ordinary milk, honey and cloves in a blender and whizz well.

Serve with an extra pinch of ground cloves on each glass.

Serves 2–3

Coconut and whole milk provide **calcium, magnesium,** potassium, protein and modest amounts of vitamins B and D. Cloves add aromatic **essential oils** that are both healing and antibacterial. Honey contains traces of natural antibiotics produced by bees – which is why honey never goes mouldy.

mulled pawpaw

A large punch-bowlful served to your friends before dinner will give them all a glow of well-being – without alcohol. Like many tropical fruits, the pawpaw is rich in protective enzymes and vitamins, and when combined with these tropical spices, it provides a huge **boost** to the **immune system**.

- 10 cloves
- 1 cinnamon stick, broken into 3 pieces
- 150g or 5½ oz demerara sugar
- 1 litre or 35 fl oz pawpaw juice
- 1 litre or 35 fl oz apple juice
- 1 tsp allspice
- 3 pinches of nutmeg
- 1 small pawpaw, peeled, deseeded and cut into small slices

Tie the cloves and cinnamon in a muslin bag.

Put the sugar and juices into a large saucepan. Add the muslin bag, allspice and nutmeg.

Bring slowly to the boil and simmer for ten minutes. Fish out the muslin bag.

Serve in a punch-bowl or other large, heatproof bowl with the pawpaw slices floating on top.

Serves 10

An average pawpaw provides twice the daily requirement of **vitamin C** and a quarter of the **vitamin A**; both are essential for the proper functioning of the immune system and natural defences. Additional nutrients come from the pawpaw and apple juices, immune-boosting properties from cinnamon and allspice, and a feel-good factor from nutmeg.

black beauty

The American Concord grape is one of the most powerful antioxidant and protective foods, so this drink is a major weapon in the fight against free radicals that accelerate ageing and damage cells. Cinnamon, cloves and allspice are **antibacterial** and **antiviral**, and help to protect against winter infections.

750ml or 26 fl oz American Concord purple grape juice
1 cinnamon stick
a generous grating of nutmeg
1 pinch allspice
10 whole cloves
1 unwaxed lime
1 unwaxed orange
15ml or ½ fl oz molasses
2 sprigs curry plant

Put the grape juice into a stainless-steel, glass or enamel (not aluminium) pan, then add the cinnamon, nutmeg and allspice. Press the cloves into the lime and add to the juice.

Remove as much of the peel from the orange as possible, leaving the pith behind. Cut the peel into very thin strips and add to the pan, along with the juice of the orange.

Heat slowly, stirring in the molasses when the liquid starts to simmer. Keep simmering gently for ten minutes. Put a sprig of curry plant into two large, heatproof glasses, then strain this invigorating, alcohol-free punch into each.

Serves 2

Bursting with **protective antioxidants**, and the orange peel is high in **bioflavonoids**. You'll also get a big boost of **vitamin C** from the lime and orange juice, as well as important levels of carotenoids. Molasses adds useful doses of essential trace minerals.

hot bloody mary

It's not often that processing increases the protective value of fresh produce, but this is true of tomatoes. This juice is hugely **protective** against **prostate** and **breast cancer** and it also helps prevent age-related macular degeneration (AMD), the most common cause of blindness in the elderly.

300ml or 10 fl oz tomato juice
2 dashes tabasco sauce
2 small measures vodka (about 15ml or 1 tbsp)
2 cinnamon sticks

Warm the tomato juice and pour it into two decorative, heatproof glasses.

Add the Tabasco sauce and vodka.

Serve immediately, with the cinnamon sticks for stirring.

Serves 2

Fully ripe tomatoes are the richest source of the **carotenoid lycopene**. When canned or juiced, extremely ripe tomatoes are used, and the lycopene content is also concentrated by the processing. This guarantees the maximum intake of this unique nutrient that protects against prostate and breast cancers, heart disease and eye problems.

gingered-up beetroot

An extremely protective drink that sounds a bit bizarre. But before you turn the page, try it – you'll be pleasantly surprised. This is a blood and circulation mixture that **protects against fatigue**, loss of concentration and many forms of cancer.

400ml or 14 fl oz beetroot juice
4 drops ginger essence
100ml or 3½ fl oz ginger ale

In a medium saucepan, heat the beetroot juice until just boiling.

Pour into two mugs and add two drops of ginger essence to each.

Top up with ginger ale, and serve.

Serves 2

The red colouring in beetroot carries specific **anti-carcinogens** attached to its molecules, and it also more than doubles the amount of oxygen the body cells are able to absorb. This juice will boost natural resistance, protect convalescents from relapse and act as a valuable aid to good digestion. It's a mild liver stimulant, too.

aztec dream

Besides its wonderful taste, chocolate contains valuable antioxidant and protective substances. Combined with cardamom and star anise, it will also protect against **chest infections**, **sore throats** and **sinus problems**, while soya milk's natural plant hormones help strengthen bones.

300ml or 10 fl oz organic dark hot chocolate, prepared using half full-fat milk and half soya milk
4 cardamom seeds
a sprinkle of ground star anise
15g or ½ oz flaked almonds
1 generous handful fresh mint leaves
100g or 3½ oz fromage frais
2 sprigs mint, for garnish

Prepare the chocolate in a saucepan according to the directions on the packet, then add the cardamom seeds and star anise powder.

In a dry frying pan, gently heat the almonds until they start to brown and crisp.

Put the mint leaves and fromage frais into a blender and whizz until well combined.

Pour the hot chocolate into large mugs, top with the fromage frais, sprinkle with the almonds and add the sprigs of mint.

Serves 2

Besides the **B vitamins**, **minerals** and antioxidants in organic chocolate, there's calcium and **vitamin D** in full-fat milk. The natural bacteria and extra calcium from fromage frais, and peppermint oil from mint leaves, add extra nutrients and improve digestive absorption. Almonds are a rich source of protective **vitamin E**, zinc and selenium.

hot, hot chocolate

Isn't it great to know your favourite food is good for you? That's the case with chocolate, as long as you stick to modest quantities and use the best-possible quality. It contains chemicals that lift your mood, and it's also a rich source of antioxidants. So it's official: you can enjoy this **protective** drink with a clear conscience.

1 heaped tsp organic chocolate powder
300ml or 10 fl oz full-cream jersey milk
1cm or ½in cinnamon stick

In a mug, mix the chocolate powder with two teaspoons of the milk. Bring the rest of the milk to the boil in a saucepan.

Pour the milk into the mug containing the chocolate mixture.

Stir and serve with the cinnamon stick floating on top.

Serves 1

Quality chocolate with a minimum seventy per cent cocoa solids provides **iron** and **magnesium** as well as theobromine, the constituent that triggers the release of good-mood chemicals from the brain. Feeling happy and positive gives a substantial boost to the immune system and helps protect the body against infection and disease.

help, i'm a chocoholic!

We feel happy after eating chocolate, and being happy gives your **immune system** a **jump-start**. Yet chocolate is also a source of immune-boosting phytochemicals. Bananas, too, provide energy and essential nutrients, while the benefits of friendly bacteria, a good dose of calcium and the **mood-enhancing** benefits in nutmeg mean you'll soon be back for more of this one.

1 banana
400ml or 14 fl oz natural, live yogurt
1 heaped tbsp organic chocolate powder
2 small pinches of nutmeg

Peel and chop the banana.

Put the banana into a blender with the yogurt and chocolate powder.

Whizz until smooth.

Serve with the nutmeg sprinkled on top.

Serves 2

Theobromine from chocolate and **myristicine** from nutmeg are two plant chemicals that have mood-enhancing properties. Nutmeg also helps sleep and improves digestion, both of which are good for the immune system. Beneficial bacteria in live yogurt play a very important part in strengthening natural immunity. **Potassium** from the banana and **calcium** from the yogurt are just added bonuses.

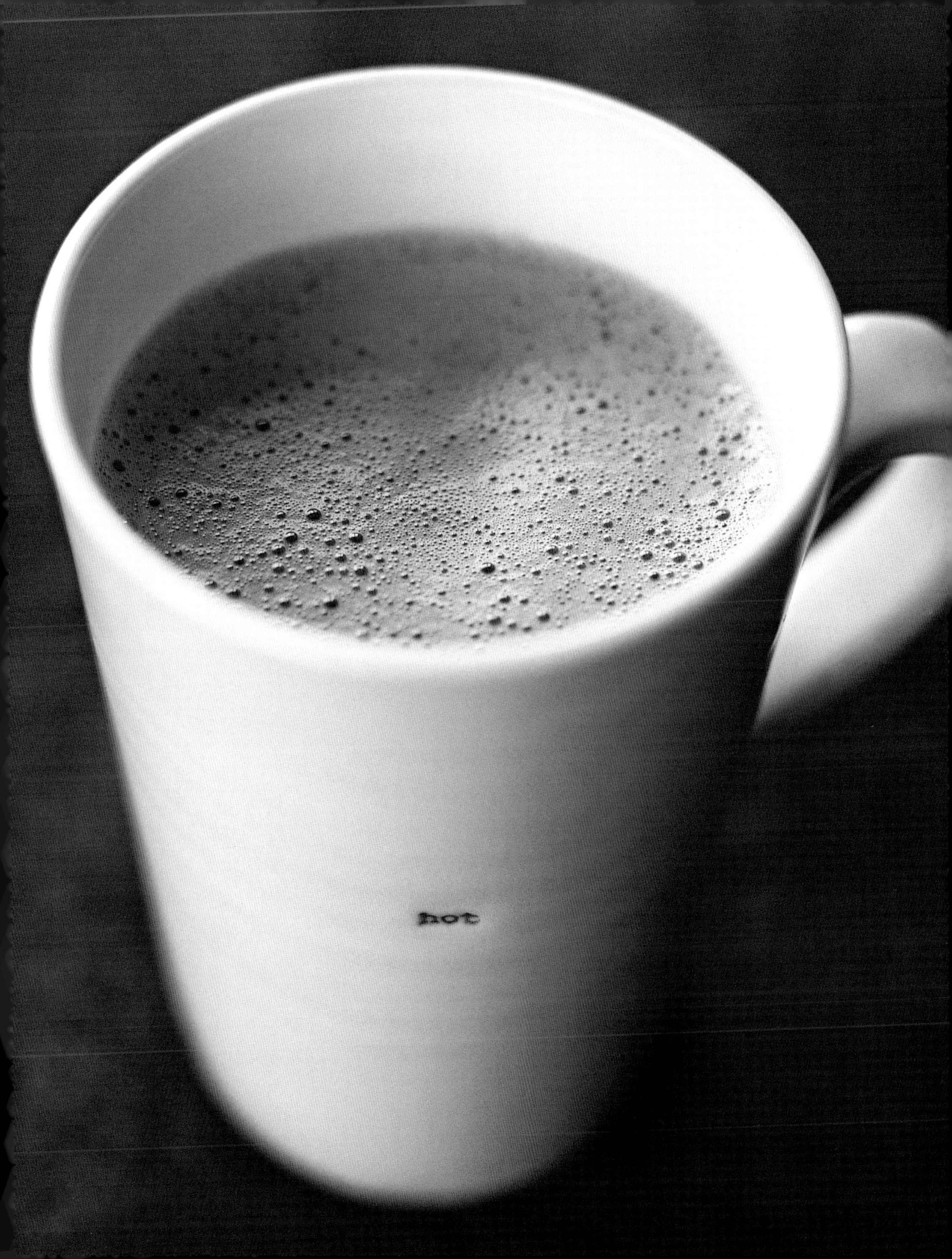
hot

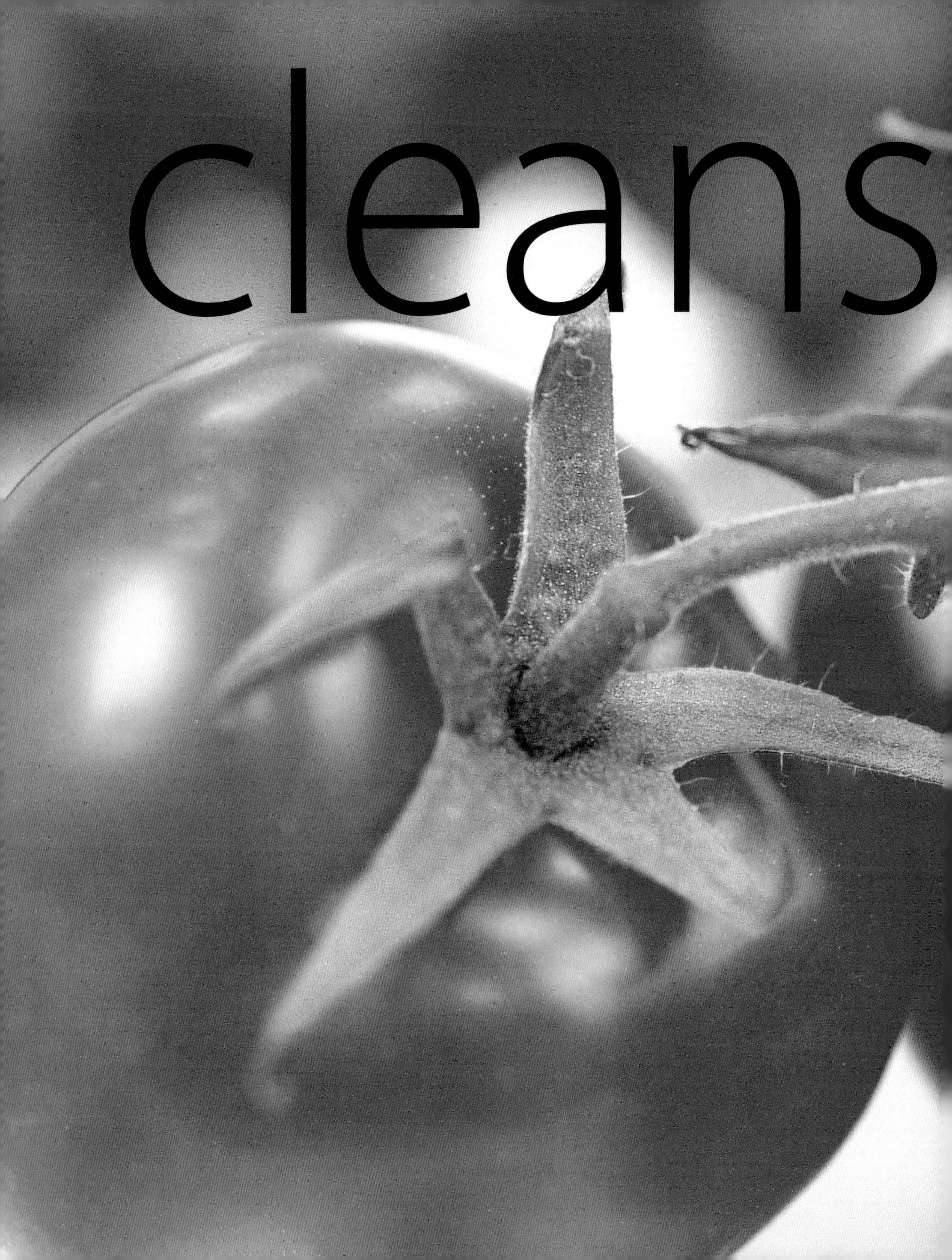
cleans

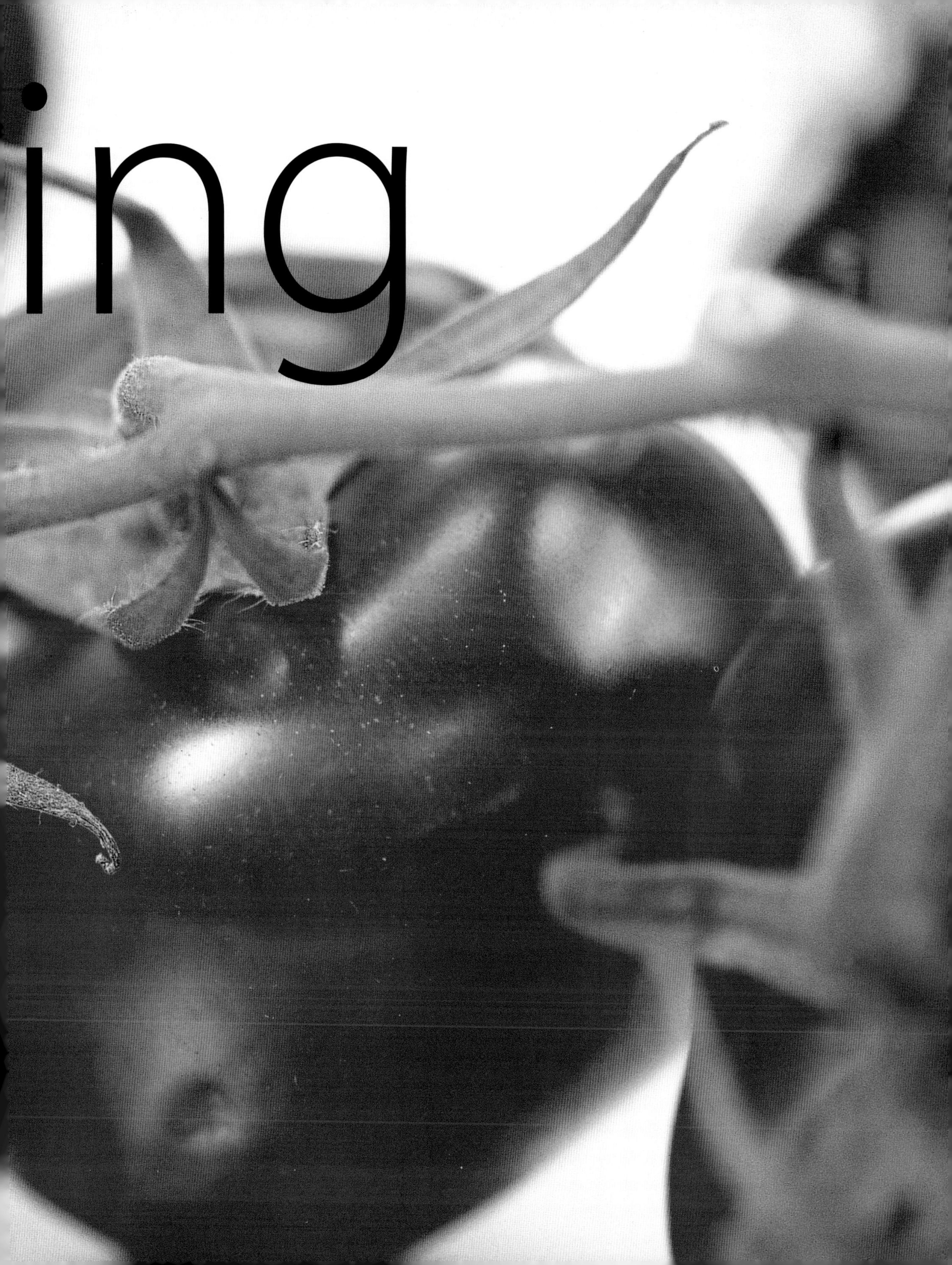

ing

The body has an amazing system for cleansing itself. The main organs involved are the liver and kidneys, so all cleansing regimes must focus on doing everything to improve their efficiency. Of course, the largest single organ in the body is the skin, and one of its major functions is also the elimination of waste products. All the dietary advice below applies in equal measure to a successful skin-cleansing regime. Yet there's no reason to become a food freak; after all, life is for enjoying. This means sharing a drink with friends, or indulging in the occasional "death by chocolate". The simple answer is to give your system an occasional rest and spring clean by using the recipes in this cleansing section and following the simple dietary advice below.

the kidneys

Some serious illnesses affect the kidneys' ability to do their cleaning-up job. High blood pressure, TB, repeated infections and kidney stones can all damage these complex and delicate organs. Severe injuries can also be a problem. As we age, the kidneys can become less efficient at getting rid of waste products, and this can be aggravated by the long-term use of many prescribed medicines. To stimulate kidney function, dandelion leaves, parsley, radishes, leeks and their cooking water, and parsley tea should be regulars in your diet. Most important of all is to drink plenty of water to reduce the risk of stones and infection.

Anyone with a tendency to kidney stones should avoid spinach, beetroot, rhubarb and chocolate, which all contain oxalic acid, as well as coffee, tea and cocoa, which contain irritating caffeine and large amounts of potassium.

The kidneys are amazingly efficient. Next time you eat asparagus, just see how long it takes before your urine develops the unmistakable and distinctive smell it produces. If your cleansing system is working properly, your urine should be a pale-straw colour, odourless, sterile and tasteless. If the colour starts to darken, you're not drinking enough, but if the urine remains dark even after a litre of water, see your doctor as this could be a sign of an underlying problem.

the liver

Think of the liver as the body's sewage plant: it's there to filter out all the unwanted and toxic rubbish and waste. But if you abuse your liver, or if, unfortunately, you develop some form of liver disease, it very soon becomes inefficient and unable to cope.

Keep a healthy liver by eating more globe artichokes for the liver-cleansing cynarin they contain; oily fish, rabbit and game, which are very low in saturated fat; Brussels sprouts, red cabbage and chickpeas for vitamin B_{12} and folic acid. The special fibre in oats is also very important to improve the elimination of fats that can damage the liver. You should also eat less red meat and fewer high-sugar foods, and drink fewer caffeine-containing drinks and sweet fizzy drinks. Avoid alcohol completely.

The huge increase of binge drinking among young people is a great concern, as this will inevitably lead to liver damage and a breakdown in the body's cleansing processes later in life. An early sign of liver malfunction is a yellowing, spotty skin, and I'm constantly amazed at how many young women who spend fortunes on clothes, make-up and hair are happy to spend even bigger fortunes every weekend on binge drinking, which is guaranteed to make them look prematurely old.

foods for thought

There are two more powerful weapons in your cleansing programme: juices and raw foods. You'll find lots of salads, herbal teas and juices in this chapter, as well as healthy recipes you'll be happy to serve to friends without them having any idea that they're eating a "cleansing" meal. Here you'll find some of the great old wives' favourites, such as French Onion Soup, traditionally enjoyed after a night on the tiles in Paris. There's even food for free, with a great soup made out of stinging nettles that helps to cleanse the kidneys, digestive system and the skin. Pick a few days each month to eat from this chapter – or why not do a whole week before you start the festive binge at Christmas?

cleansing checklist

- Eat more celery, parsley, watercress, fennel, dandelion, peppers, mint, citrus juices, fish, prunes, brown rice, wholegrain cereals, and drink more water.
- Eat fewer foods with E numbers, refined carbohydrates, less white bread, less of most commercial breakfast cereals, less animal protein, coffee, alcohol, sweets, chocolates and high-fat, -salt and -sugar snacks and convenience foods.

florence fennel salad

This salad is guaranteed to help any **cleansing** programme, thanks largely to the natural plant chemicals provided by fennel. Among others, this delicious bulb contains **essential oils** called anethole and fenchone, which are mildly diuretic and help the body get rid of excess fluid.

- 2 oranges, peeled and sliced
- 1 large bulb florence fennel, washed and finely sliced
- 1 large red onion, sliced
- juice of 1 orange
- 2 tsp balsamic vinegar
- a few sprigs fresh mint, to garnish

Put a layer of orange slices on to each of the four plates. Cover the oranges with the fennel. Sprinkle the onion on top of the fennel.

Mix the orange juice with the vinegar and drizzle the dressing over each plate. Garnish with the mint leaves.

Serves 4

The **fibre** and **vitamin C** in oranges, together with the red onion, improve digestive function and the elimination of cholesterol.

granny's cleanser

A tasty source of natural **fibre**. It's hardly surprising that a lot of old wives' tales turn out to be true. After all, many of them refer to practices that have been in use for hundreds of years, and if they didn't work at all, they wouldn't stand the test of time.

- 2 large granny smith apples, unpeeled
- juice of 1 lemon
- 2 celery sticks, preferably with leaves
- 2 tbsp seedless raisins
- 1 x 150g carton natural, live yogurt
- 1 tbsp cider vinegar
- 3 tbsp extra-virgin olive oil
- 1 tsp runny honey

Cut the apples into small wedges. Put them into a salad bowl, add half the lemon juice and mix thoroughly to prevent browning.

Scrub and slice the celery into 1cm or ½in chunks, chop the leaves and add to the apple pieces. Add the raisins.

Mix together the yogurt, vinegar, oil, honey and remaining lemon juice.

Add to the salad and toss lightly.

Serves 4

This recipe combines the traditional **cleansing properties** of apples with the gentle diuretic effect of celery and the high-fibre content of raisins. Add the natural bacteria in live yogurt, and you've got a salad that's not only rich in **iron, vitamin C,** pectin, potassium and cleansing essential oils, but is also bursting with flavour.

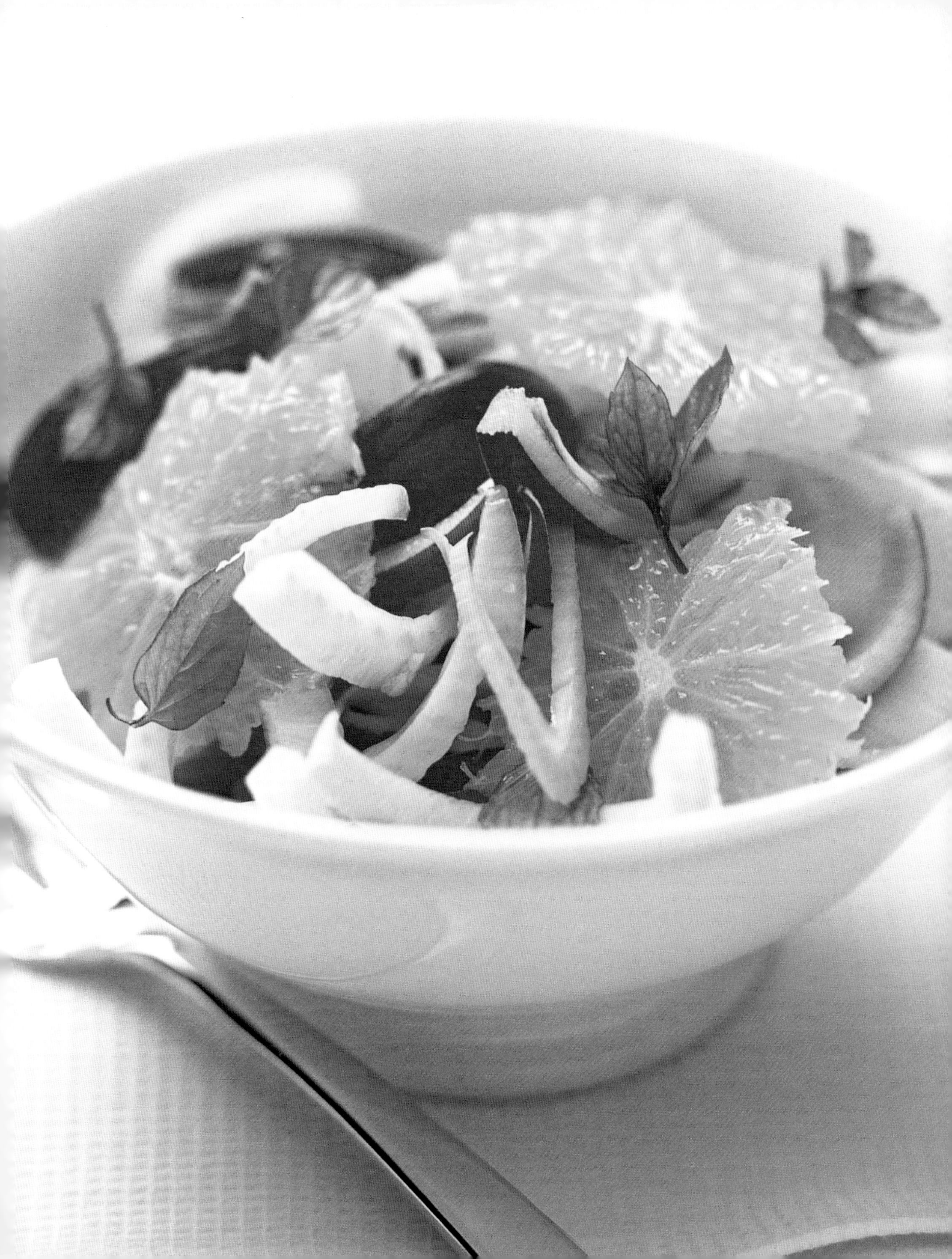

dandelion delight

Rich in iron – and effective for **fluid loss**. In the north of England, the country name for dandelion is "wet-the-bed", and in France it's called pis en lit – which means exactly the same thing. In most French street markets you can buy these delicious leaves alongside all the other salad ingredients.

1 generous bunch dandelion leaves
1 generous bunch lamb's lettuce
2 handfuls baby spinach leaves
2 tbsp extra-virgin olive oil
juice of 1/2 lemon

Thoroughly wash and dry all the leaves. Put them into a large salad bowl.

Pour on the oil and squeeze the lemon juice over the top.

Toss thoroughly so that every leaf is well coated.

Serves 4

Although the root of dandelion is the most powerful diuretic part of the plant, the leaves also increase water loss – hence their **cleansing action**. In addition, dandelion leaves are rich in iron, which you'll absorb better thanks to the **vitamin C** in the lemon juice.

bittersweet treat

Chicory and all curly endives are members of the same family of wonderful winter salad vegetables. They are descendants of wild chicory, which has a long history in traditional herbalism as a cleanser and **detoxifier**. In medieval times, it was used as an important late winter/early spring tonic plant.

juice of 1 lime
1 tbsp grapeseed oil
2 large oranges, peeled and finely sliced
2 heads curly endive, chopped into bite-sized pieces
1 large bunch watercress, washed
freshly ground black pepper, to taste

Whisk the lime juice into the grapeseed oil.

Lay the orange slices on a serving plate and cover with the endive leaves. Pile the watercress in the middle.

Drizzle with the grapeseed-oil dressing and season with pepper.

Serves 4

The **vitamin C** from the oranges improves the absorption of iron from the chicory and watercress, which is also a great source of **natural protective chemicals**. The peppery bite of watercress adds the digestive stimulation you need during those sluggish winter months.

waterfall salad

A strongly diuretic recipe that's great for women who suffer **fluid retention** and swelling around period time. This is also valuable for anyone suffering with **gout** or **arthritis**, as the celery and celery seed increase the elimination of uric acid, the chemical that aggravates inflamed joints.

2 sweet dessert apples, washed, cored and diced

1 tbsp raspberry vinegar

1 chunk watermelon, deseeded and cubed

1 chicory bulb

2 celery sticks, with leaves

1 tsp celery seed

1 tbsp walnut oil

Put the apples into a salad bowl, pour in the vinegar and mix well to avoid browning.

Deseed the watermelon and cut into cubes. Wash the chicory and slice into rounds. Wash and coarsely chop the celery and celery leaves.

Add everything to the bowl of apples, along with the celery seed, and mix gently. Pour in the walnut oil and mix again.

Serves 4

Apples are another **traditional remedy** for joint diseases, and watermelon is a traditional **cooling** fruit that also has mild eliminative benefits.

wonderful weed soup

A weed is just a plant growing where it's not wanted. In this recipe, you'll want as many edible weeds as you can find, because they're nutritious as well as having **therapeutic** and cleansing benefits. The same basic method will work for all delicate, leafy herbs, preserving their flavours as well as their colour.

85g or 3oz stemmed and well-washed mixed "weeds": dandelion, nettles, sorrel, rocket and salad burnet

45g or 1½oz unsalted butter

2 tbsp extra-virgin olive oil

1 small onion, chopped

175g or 6oz potatoes

1 litre or 34 fl oz vegetable stock (page 252)

225ml or 8 fl oz crème fraîche

Purée the weed leaves in a food processor. Add the butter and purée again; set aside.

Sweat the onion gently in the oil. Add the potatoes and cook gently until golden.

Add the stock and simmer until the potatoes are soft. Stir in the crème fraîche and purée again.

Just before serving, whisk in the leaves and butter.

Serves 4

Contains **iron**, potassium, **folic acid**, carotenoids and vitamin C. Dandelion is a powerful diuretic and a rich source of coumarins, relieving fluid retention and high blood pressure. Sorrel is a traditional herbalists' **detox plant**, whose tannins and volatile oils are good for the skin. Salad burnet **aids digestion**.

red, hot and healthy

Radishes are one of the great traditional foods for **stimulating the liver** and gall bladder. They increase the production of bile, which helps with the digestion of fat in the diet. They're also a great source of potassium, calcium and sulphur, making this salad one good, all-round, hot little number.

- 1 good-sized head radicchio, washed and separated into individual leaves
- 2 red peppers, sliced and seeds removed
- 4 small whole beetroot, cooked and cut into strips
- 12 medium radishes, quartered
- 4 tbsp standard salad dressing
- 1 bunch fresh chives, finely chopped

Arrange the radicchio leaves in a bowl.

Add the pepper slices, then the beetroot strips, then the radishes.

Drizzle with the dressing and sprinkle with the chives.

Serves 4

Stimulates cleansing organs and strengthens the blood. Red peppers are **rich in fibre**, beetroot is **good for the blood** and radicchio supplies some betacarotene. All in all, this is both a cleansing and immune-boosting recipe.

chervil courgette bake

Apart from its cleansing benefits, this dish is a truly tongue-tingling mixture of flavours, especially the delicate overtones of aniseed from the chervil. Chervil's **blood-purifying** properties are part of ancient herbal folklore; this herb has been regarded as a traditional spring tonic for centuries.

- 1 garlic clove
- 3 tbsp extra-virgin olive oil
- 4 tbsp succulent, chopped leaves of any fresh mixed herbs (coriander, chervil, chives, parsley, etc)
- 300g or 10½oz plump plum tomatoes, peeled and deseeded
- 8 small courgettes, cut lengthwise and deseeded
- ½ lemon, thinly sliced
- salt and freshly ground black pepper, to taste

Rub an ovenproof dish with the garlic, add the olive oil then stir in the chopped herbs and tomatoes.

Place the courgettes on top of the tomatoes and herbs, then cover with the lemon slices.

Season, cover with foil and bake in an oven preheated to 200°C (400°F/ gas mark 6) for about twenty minutes, until the courgettes are soft but not mushy.

Serves 4

Unpeeled courgettes are a valuable source of **betacarotene**, essential for the skin during any cleansing programme. Parsley provides **calcium** as well as diuretic volatile oils, which speed fluid elimination. Chives enjoy cleansing and detoxing properties.

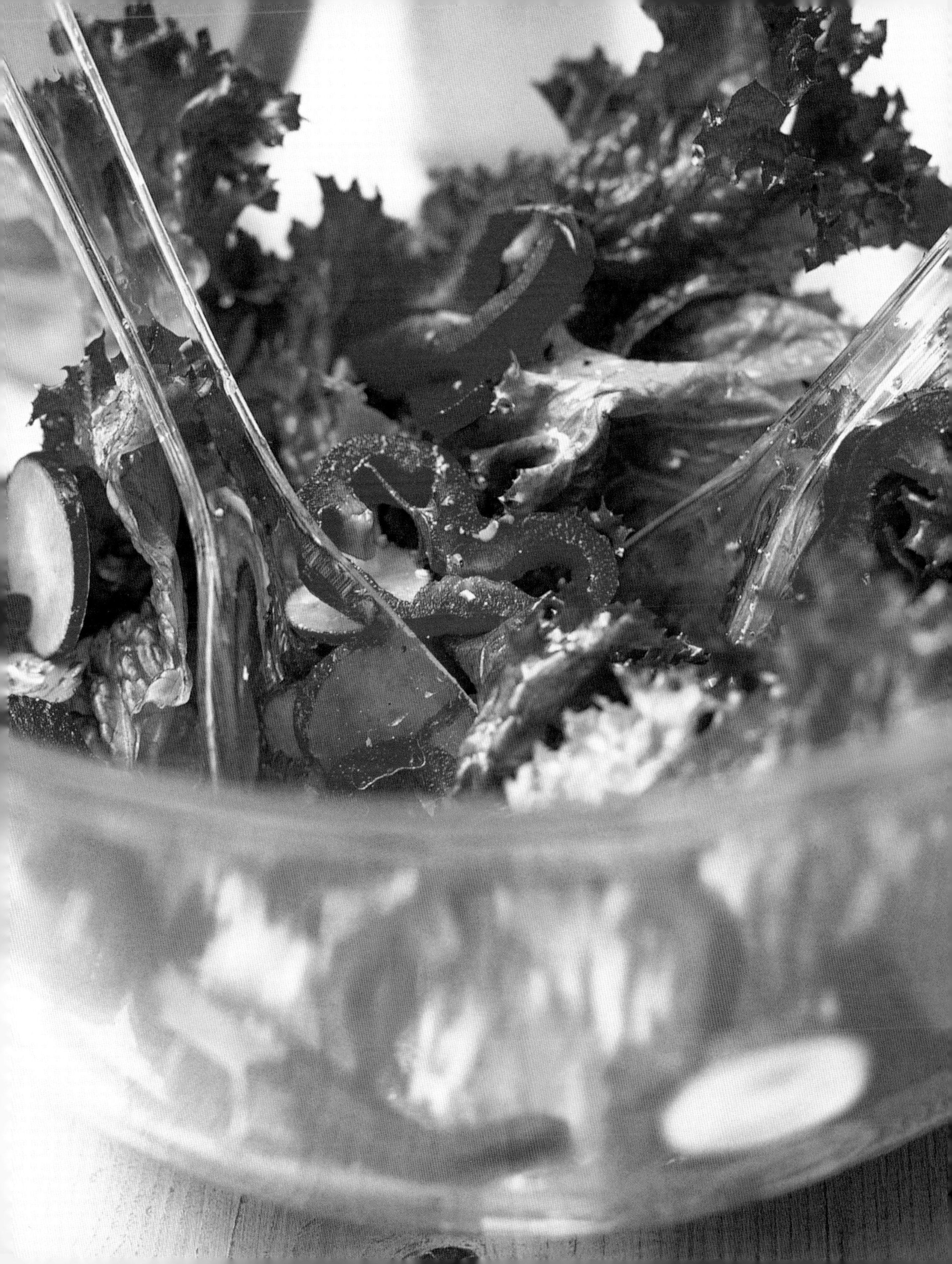

basil's brush

The complex flavours of basil, chives and garlic are perfect to bring out the taste of artichoke hearts in this **detoxing** dish. Unless you're an expert, preparing a pile of fresh artichoke hearts is a thankless task. Just this once, save yourself trouble by buying best-quality tinned ones.

2 x 350g can artichoke hearts
450ml or 16 fl oz white wine
6 garlic cloves, chopped
225g or 8oz parsley, chopped
125g or 4½oz chives, chopped
3 large plum tomatoes, chopped
125ml or 4 fl oz extra-virgin olive oil
5 tbsp basil leaves, snipped

Drain the artichoke hearts. In a large saucepan, boil the wine with the garlic for about three minutes. Add the artichokes, parsley, chives, tomatoes and oil to the pan and simmer until the artichokes are soft – about fifteen minutes.

Just before serving, stir in the basil leaves. Serve with some good, coarse bread for mopping up the sauce.

Serves 4

Cynarin from artichokes detoxifies the liver, while parsley has a diuretic effect. The purifying benefits of garlic, the slow-release sugar, **inulin** (also from artichokes) and the calming properties of basil give this dish additional health-enhancing qualities.

mushrooms with egg and buckwheat

Unlike other cereals, buckwheat doesn't contain gluten, the sticky proteins present in cereal grains. However, it is **rich** in rutin, a substance which strengthens the tiniest blood vessels in the circulatory system. This is a satisfying and **cleansing** dish, with the bonus of beneficial bacteria from the yogurt.

225g or 8oz wholegrain buckwheat
1 large free-range egg
60g or 2oz butter
450ml or 16 fl oz boiling water
1 large onion, finely chopped
1 tbsp extra-virgin olive oil
225g or 8oz mushrooms, thinly sliced
1 tbsp coriander leaves, chopped
1 pinch sea salt and freshly ground black pepper, to taste
1 x 125ml carton low-fat, natural, live yogurt

Boil the buckwheat for 15 minutes until soft. Beat the egg in a large bowl and add the buckwheat, stirring thoroughly. Put the mixture in a non-stick (but ungreased) pan and stir slowly over a low heat until toasted and dry.

Use a little of the butter to grease an ovenproof dish. Put in the buckwheat, the rest of the butter, a pinch of salt and the boiling water. Bake in an oven preheated to 180°C (350°F/gas mark 4) for twenty minutes.

While the buckwheat bakes, sweat the onions in the oil until they're soft, but not brown. Add the mushrooms and cook for another five minutes. Add the coriander and pepper, stirring constantly. When the buckwheat is done, stir in the onion and mushroom mixture, add the yogurt and serve hot.

Serves 4

Provides protein, lots of carbohydrates, fibre, plenty of **potassium** and valuable amounts of **iron**, **zinc**, copper, selenium, iodine, vitamin B_6, folic acid and vitamin A. This is a great detoxifier, as it stimulates digestive function as well as relieving varicose veins.

watercress soup

Like cabbage, broccoli and Brussels sprouts, watercress is a brassica, which means it contains **natural antibiotics** and cancer-fighting **phytochemicals**. It's also a great cleansing vegetable, protective against lung cancer. Besides tasting great hot, this recipe is equally delicious as a cold summer soup.

2 garlic cloves, finely chopped
1 tbsp extra-virgin olive oil
1 large onion, finely chopped
1 tsp curry powder
4 bunches watercress with stalks, well washed
900ml or 32 fl oz vegetable stock (page 252)
freshly ground black pepper, to taste
1 x 125ml carton low-fat, natural, live yogurt

Leave the chopped garlic to stand for ten minutes before cooking. In a large, heavy-bottomed saucepan, heat the oil and cook the onions on a moderate heat until soft and translucent (but not brown).

Add the garlic and cook for one minute. Add the curry powder, stirring continuously, and cook for another minute. Turn down the heat; add the watercress and stir and cook until wilted – around two to three minutes.

Add the stock and pepper, simmer for ten minutes, then liquidize. Pour into serving bowls and add a spoonful of yogurt to each.

Serves 4

Very low in fat, this soup provides ten per cent of the recommended daily **iron** intake, as well as modest amounts of iodine, selenium, folic acid and **vitamin A**.

aubergine and bulgur stir-fry

If you're trying to reduce your blood pressure, then aubergines are a must, as they reduce the amount of fat circulating in the arteries. Bulgur wheat, sometimes known as cracked wheat, is often used in place of rice in the Middle East. It's **highly nutritious** and has a unique **nutty** flavour.

250g or 9oz bulgur or cracked wheat
475ml or 17 fl oz water
6 tbsp extra-virgin olive oil
2 medium onions, finely sliced
2 large aubergines, cut into cubes
3 tsp ground coriander
3 tsp ground cumin
150g or 5½oz flaked almonds
100g raisins
sea salt and freshly ground black pepper, to taste

In a large saucepan, simmer the bulgur wheat covered in the water for ten minutes, or until most or all of the water has been absorbed and the grains are soft and tender. Drain if necessary.

Heat the oil and fry the onions until brown. Add the aubergines and, stirring frequently, sauté until brown (add extra oil if necessary since the aubergine acts like a sponge). Add the spices and cook for one minute, stirring constantly.

Lower the heat, add the flaked almonds and raisins and brown slightly. Stir the cooked bulgur wheat into the vegetables, add extra oil and sauté for one minute to heat through. Season to taste and serve immediately.

Serves 4

A good source of **protein**, fibre, **potassium**, iron, selenium and folic acid. Provides more than the daily requirement of **vitamin E** and modest amounts of vitamin A and C.

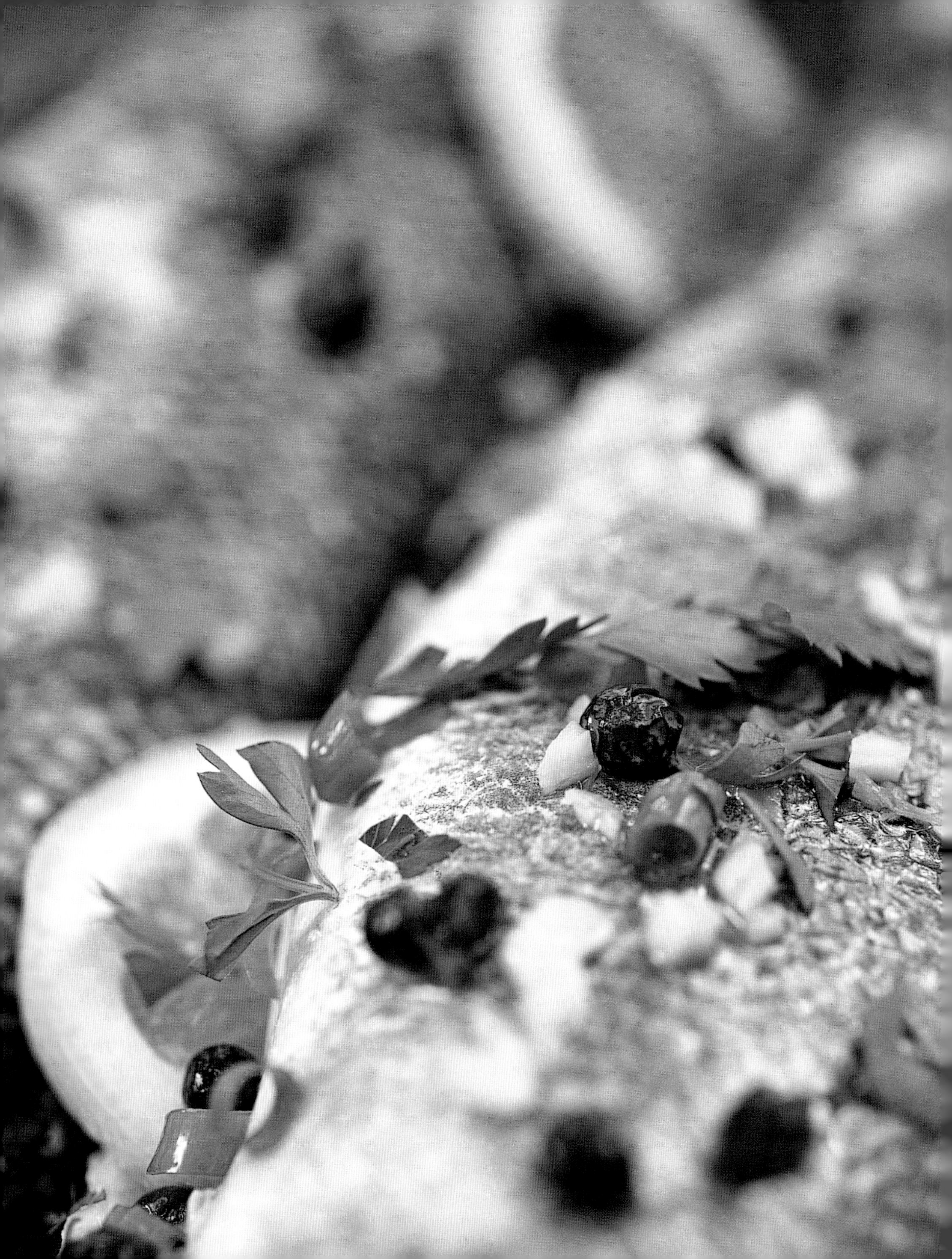

juniper fish

The use of juniper as a diuretic and **anti-inflammatory** is one reason for its inclusion here; its strong, tangy flavours are another. Together, these herbs complement the tender white flesh of the sea bass, making this a mouthwatering way to cleanse the system.

2 tbsp Welsh onion, finely chopped
3 garlic cloves, minced
1 tbsp juniper berries, crushed
2 tbsp parsley, chopped
675ml or 24 fl oz white wine
2 whole sea bass, scaled and gutted
extra-virgin olive oil
1 lemon, sliced

Mix the Welsh onions, garlic, herbs and wine.

Place the fish in a large baking dish and brush with olive oil.

Pour the wine and herb mixture over the fish.

Cover with sliced lemon.

Bake in a preheated oven at 220°C (425°F/gas mark 7) for about thirty minutes, basting frequently.

Serves 4

Fish provides **protein** and a rich supply of **minerals**, including **iodine**. Juniper is rich in the diuretic and anti-inflammatory **volatile oils** myrcene, sabinene, pinene and limonene. The sulphur compounds in garlic and Welsh onion fight bacteria and fungal diseases, while the diuretic benefits of parsley add to this dish's cleansing properties.

french onion soup

One of the most famous of all restorative soups, this traditional French onion recipe will fill your body with a sense of **well-being**. It's worth looking for some hard goat's cheese, preferably unpasteurized, as it's easy to digest and contains the beneficial natural bacteria used in the cheese-making process.

4 tbsp extra-virgin olive oil
50g or 2oz butter
4 large onions, very finely sliced
1.5 litres or 55fl oz vegetable stock (page 252)
1 large handful mixed parsley, sage and thyme leaves, finely chopped
100g or 3½oz hard goat's cheese, grated
4 slices cut off a wholemeal baguette

In a large saucepan, heat the olive oil and butter. Add the onions and sweat over a low heat until thoroughly softened – about fifteen minutes. Add the stock and herbs, reserving some of the sage. Simmer for about ten minutes.

Meanwhile, mix the goat's cheese with the reserved sage. Put the cheese mixture on to the bread and grill until the cheese is bubbling.

Serve the soup with the slices of bread, cheese and herbs floating on top.

Serves 4

To protect against infection and speed healing. Onions contain circulation-boosting **phytochemicals**. Thyme is rich in **thymol**, an antiseptic essential oil.

grilled paprika chicken

This is a super-easy and very quick recipe that exploits the wonderful texture and flavour of organic chicken. The detoxifying properties of garlic comibine with the **circulatory stimulus** of paprika and give this dish the unmistakable tang of Hungary.

2 tbsp extra-virgin olive oil
1 large lemon (juice and grated rind)
2 garlic cloves, smashed, not chopped
1 generous tsp paprika
freshly ground black pepper, to taste
4 medium organic chicken breasts, skinned and cut into large cubes

Combine the oil, lemon juice and zest, garlic, paprika and pepper in a shallow dish. Put the chicken cubes in the marinade and stir well to make sure they are all coated. Leave in the fridge for half an hour, but spoon the marinade over the chicken at least twice during that time.

Brush the rack of a grill pan with oil. Lift the chicken out of the marinade with a slotted spoon, place on the rack and grill on a high temperature for ten minutes, turning occasionally and basting with the marinade.

Serves 4

Providing large amounts of protein, **phosphorus**, potassium and lots of **selenium**, this low-fat, heart-friendly dish (only one gram of saturated fat per 100 grams) also stimulates the circulation and provides **slow-release energy**.

organic sicilian chicken

Here's a second quick recipe that **spares you** the **antibiotics** and **chemical residues** that will almost certainly be present in non-organic poultry.

3 tbsp wholemeal flour
2 tsp dried thyme
ground sea salt, to taste
freshly ground black pepper, to taste
8 medium organic chicken thighs
100ml or 3½ fl oz milk
4 tbsp extra-virgin olive oil
juice of 1 lemon

Mix together the flour, thyme and seasoning.

Dip the chicken pieces in milk, then coat thoroughly with the flour mixture; set aside.

Heat the oil in a frying pan, and fry the chicken on all sides until golden brown. Transfer to a wire tray placed over a baking sheet.

Pour the lemon juice over the chicken pieces and bake in an ovenproof dish in an oven preheated to 190°C (375°F/gas mark 5), for fifteen minutes. Can be served hot or cold.

Serves 4

The **antiseptic** properties of thyme and the cancer-fighting effects of **essential oils** in the lemon make this dish exceptionally healthy, as well as cleansing.

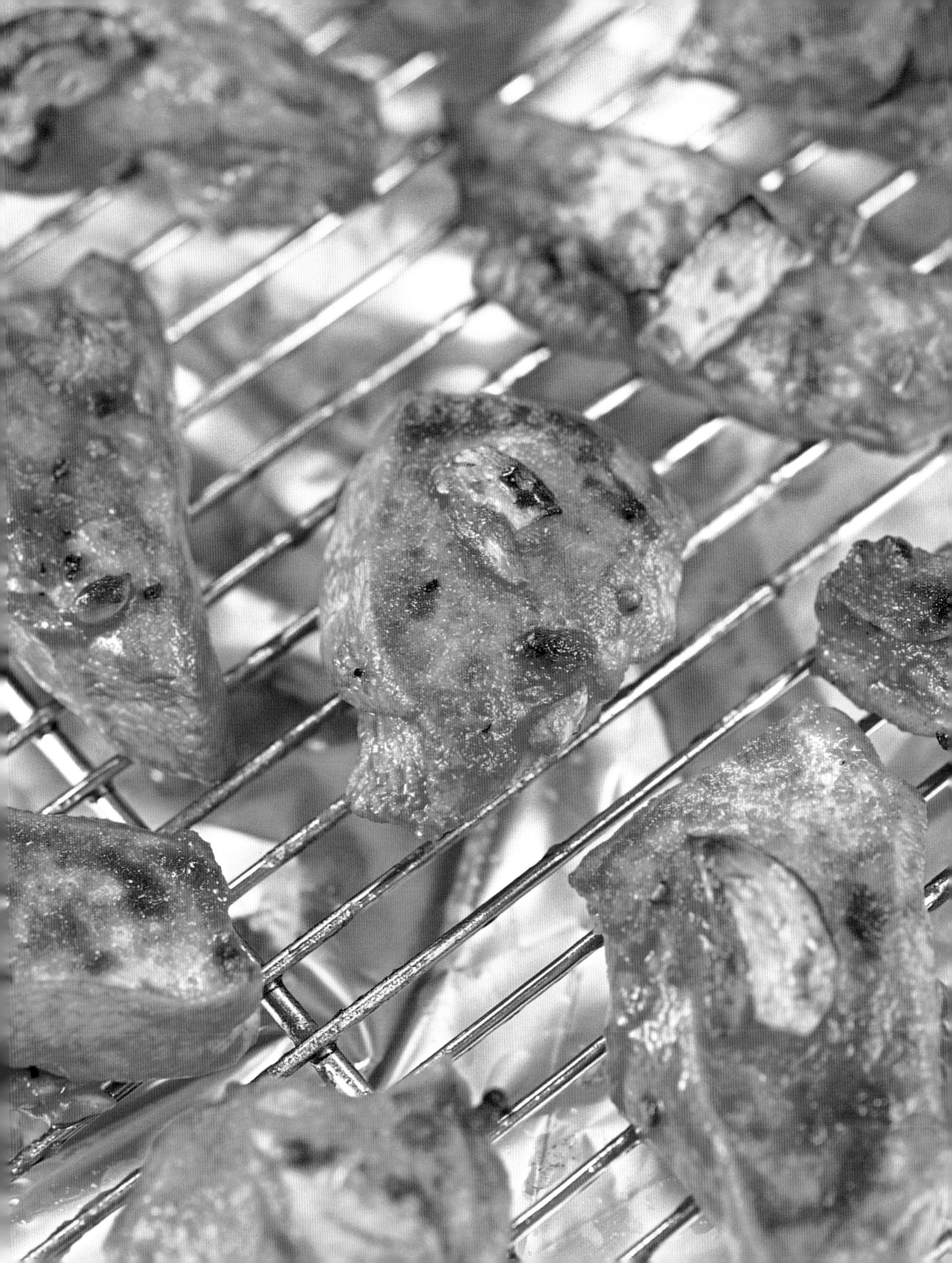

catmint chicken

One of the simplest main courses ever: all the vegetables cook with the meat, while the apples, cider and herbs give the most delicious flavour to the vegetables, particularly the potatoes. Catmint, also known as catnip, is rich in **purifying** volatile oils. As a cleansing herb for humans, it's definitely the cat's meow!

4 chicken portions, preferably free-range

450g or 1lb root vegetables (must include potatoes), cut into cubes

1 bramley cooking apple, peeled, cored and cubed

1 large sprig rosemary

3 large sprigs catmint

600ml or 20 fl oz cider

Wash and dry the chicken pieces.

Put all the ingredients together in a large casserole dish.

Cook in a preheated oven at 200°C (400°F/gas mark 6) for two hours – and enjoy!

Serves 4

A **protein-rich** cleansing dish that is also highly protective, thanks to the antioxidants in the root vegetables. Swedes and carrots are particularly rich in betacarotene, and the apple provides the cholesterol-lowering fibre **pectin**. Catmint offers **volatile oils** that stimulate sweating and help lower temperature.

nutty herb noodles

Simple, delicious and economical, this is a great supper dish at any time, in spite of its cleansing and detoxifying ingredients. You certainly don't have to be ill to enjoy it, but its **high energy** content also makes it a perfect food for convalescents.

450g or 1lb noodles

3 tbsp extra-virgin olive oil

225g or 8oz cooked chicken or ham, shredded

50g or 1¾oz pine nuts

2 tbsp mixed herbs (marjoram, basil, thyme, chives), finely chopped

3 tbsp parmesan, grated

Cook the noodles according to the directions on the packet.

Heat the olive oil; add the ham or chicken and sauté gently.

Toast the pine nuts in a dry frying pan for two minutes.

Add the noodles and the pine nuts to the meat mixture.

Stir in the herbs, and serve with parmesan.

Serves 4

The antiseptic and **antibacterial essential oils** thymol (from thyme) and linalool, terpinene and eugenol (from marjoram) combine with the **detoxing** properties of chives to make this a quick-and-easy inclusion in your cleansing regime.

fennel fillet

Low-fat, high-protein organic pork makes a healthy addition to your menu collection. Add the cholesterol-lowering and antibacterial effect of onions and the purifying properties of fennel, and you have a cleansing, **liver-stimulating** and **anti-inflammatory** meal that tastes terriffic.

1kg or 2lb 2oz lean organic pork fillets
3 tbsp extra-virgin olive oil
1 small onion, finely chopped
1 tbsp plain flour
150ml or 5 fl oz white wine
200ml or 7 fl oz yogurt or crème fraîche
1 tsp each fennel and savory, finely chopped

In a skillet, brown the pork fillets in the olive oil. Reduce the heat, cover and cook through, about twenty minutes. Remove the meat, keep warm and pour off all but three tablespoons of fat.

Add the onion and sweat gently. Blend in the flour and add the wine. Stir until thickened, add the yogurt or crème fraîche, then the herbs. Pour the mixture over the meat and serve.

Serves 4

Pork is an excellent source of protein, iron and **B vitamins**. Onions help lower cholesterol, while fennel's **volatile oils** stimulate the liver and the digestive tract. The pinenes, borneol and carvacrol in winter or summer savory help fight infections.

sorrel surprise

Organic veal is free from antibiotics, growth hormones and unwanted chemicals, but the delicate flavour of the escalope sitting on its bed of soft, green sorrel is reason enough to eat this dish. The bonus is that you can include it in any **cleansing** or **detox** regime.

4 veal escalopes, beaten thinly
6 tbsp olive oil
juice of 1 lime
2 tbsp oregano or chervil
salt and freshly ground black pepper, to taste
85g or 3oz unsalted butter
½ onion, very finely chopped
175g or 6oz sorrel, roughly torn
30ml or 1 fl oz natural, live yogurt

Marinate the escalopes in olive oil, lime juice, half the chervil or oregano and seasoning for at least two hours. Remove the veal from the marinade, and cook for about five minutes each side, under a medium-hot grill.

While the veal cooks, melt the butter in a saucepan, add the onion and cook gently until soft. Add the sorrel and the rest of the oregano or chervil. Cook until the sorrel is wilted – about four minutes.

Pour in the yogurt and heat gently. Put the sauce on to plates and top each with an escalope.

Serves 4

This low-fat, high-protein dish is a good source of **calcium** and **vitamin C**. The flavonoids and **anthraquinones** make sorrel a cleansing diuretic. Oregano is rich in carvacrol and thymol, making it antifungal and antibacterial. And if you use chervil, its volatile oils are diuretic and blood-purifying.

anise peaches

Few desserts can be enjoyed as part of a cleansing regime, but this one fits the bill, as its flavours are as good as its **cleansing** properties. The combination of catmint and anise brings out the subtle flavours of the peaches, resulting in a seemingly indulgent but nonetheless health-giving dish.

- 5 tbsp caster sugar
- 300ml or 10 fl oz water
- 3 star anise
- 4 large peaches, peeled and sliced
- 4 sprigs catmint

Heat the sugar with water over a low heat until dissolved. Add the star anise and simmer gently for seven minutes. Add the peaches and continue simmering for ten to twelve minutes.

Remove the fruit and place in a ceramic heatproof dish large enough to contain them in a single layer. Reduce the liquid by half. Pour over the fruit and serve garnished with sprigs of catmint.

Serves 4

Peaches are a rich source of **potassium**, **vitamin C** and protective flavonoids and carotenes. Anise contains anathole, coumarins and other useful volatile oils to aid digestion. This is a dessert recipe with flavours as good as its **cleansing properties**.

verbena delight

This exquisite variation on the classic Provençal clafouti is all the more delicious due to the combination of the slightly acidic cherries and the sweet, lemon-scented fragrance of verbena. This **digestion aiding** recipe works with any stone fruits, such as plums, peaches and apricots.

- 500g or approx. 1lb cherries, washed, stones removed
- 3 tbsp lemon verbena, finely chopped
- 4 free-range eggs
- 60g or 2oz caster sugar
- 50g or approx. 2oz flour
- 300ml or 10 fl oz crème fraîche or cream
- 3 tbsp brandy

Put the cherries in a buttered gratin dish. Sprinkle with the lemon verbena.

Whisk the eggs, stir in the sugar, then slowly mix in the flour.

Add the crème fraîche (or cream) and brandy; stir until well mixed.

Pour the egg mixture over the cherries and herbs and bake in an oven preheated to 180°C (350°F/gas mark 4) for thirty minutes.

Serves 4

Cherries are super-rich in **vitamin C**, potassium, **magnesium** and a host of cancer-fighting **phytochemicals**. When combined with lemon verbena's volatile oils, they make a valuable addition to any cleansing regime, gently calming the digestion and pepping up the nervous system.

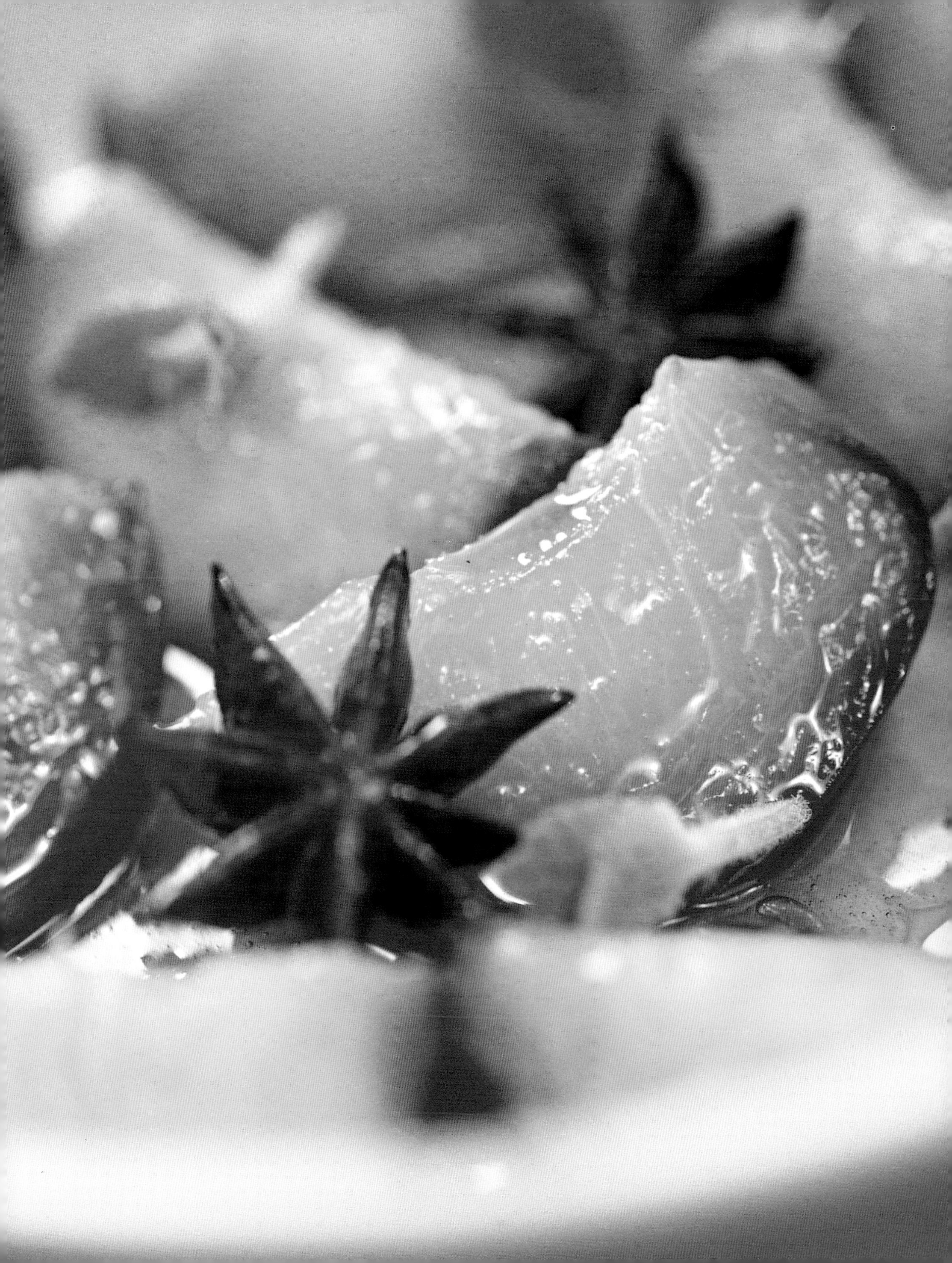

cucumber and mint slush

Cucumber isn't rich in nutrients as it's made up mostly of water, but it has long been used as a cleanser – externally and internally. It's really the mint that provides the major cleansing benefit here; because of its detoxing properties, it also helps **relieve headaches** and migraine.

1 large cucumber
4 large stalks mint
1 scant tsp natural sea salt
crushed ice
2 extra mint stalks, for garnish

Peel and deseed the cucumber.

Put into a blender or food processor with the mint and salt, and whizz until smooth, adding a little water if the consistency is too thick.

Chill thoroughly.

Serve poured over the crushed ice, with the extra mint stalks for garnish.

Serves 1–2

Cucumber provides a little **folic acid**, potassium and silica, but it's here mainly for its gentle diuretic effect. Mint provides **menthol** and menthone, natural phytochemicals that are antiseptic, cleansing and also act as a potent digestive. Sea salt means you get small quantities of iodine, which helps improve thyroid function. This, in turn, stimulates the whole metabolic process and increases eliminative functions.

fresh dill tea

The subtle flavours of dill combined with the clean, fresh taste of cucumber make a most refreshing cold drink. Dill is both cleansing and **mood-enhancing**, and it's an excellent remedy for all types of indigestion, especially colic in babies.

6 large stalks dill flowers
600ml or 20 fl oz water
½ cucumber

Reserving two of the most attractive dill tops, put the rest into a jug of boiling water. Leave for ten minutes. Strain, leave to cool, then chill in the fridge.

Meanwhile, strip the peel off the cucumber. Serve the tea with the reserved dill tops and cucumber peel floating on top.

Serves 1–2

Dill is a source of many **essential oils** and **phytochemicals**, the most important of which are carvone and eugenol. It contains myristicin, which is also found in nutmeg; that's why dill tea is not only cleansing but also mood-enhancing and stress-relieving.

fresh tomato juice

Commercial tomato juice nearly always has added salt and lacks the "sweet-and-sour" flavour of the freshly juiced fruits. The **acidity** of tomatoes is cleansing – even more so when combined with the diuretic properties of celery and the overall **detoxing power** of garlic.

10 ripe tomatoes
4 celery stalks, with leaves
1 small garlic clove, peeled
2 dashes worcestershire sauce

Put the tomatoes into a large bowl. Cover with boiling water and leave until cool enough to handle. Slip off the skins.

Wash and chop the celery roughly, reserving two sprigs of leaves.

Put all the ingredients through a juicer. Add the worcestershire sauce and stir. Chill in the fridge.

Serves 1–2

Ripe tomatoes are the richest source of the **carotenoid** lycopene which is highly protective against heart disease and prostate cancer. This drink also supplies **betacarotene** and lots of **potassium**, as well as vitamins C and E.

fantastic fennel

The liquorice-like taste of fennel imparts a deliciously unusual flavour to this drink. Fennel is a mild diuretic and a good digestive aid; it also balances female hormones. Apples are used by natural practitioners as a cleansing and detoxing food, as they have the ability to **remove toxic substances** from the system.

1 carrot, peeled and trimmed unless organic
2 large apples, unpeeled, uncored and quartered
2 pears
1 medium fennel bulb

Put all the ingredients through a juicer and mix well. Strain if necessary.

Serves 1–2

Fennel contains the **natural plant chemicals** anethole and fenchone. A traditional treatment for colic in children, fennel has a diuretic effect that makes it a useful cleanser. Apples and pears are rich in the **soluble fibre** pectin, which improves digestion. Apples are a rich source of ellagic acid, another cleansing phytochemical.

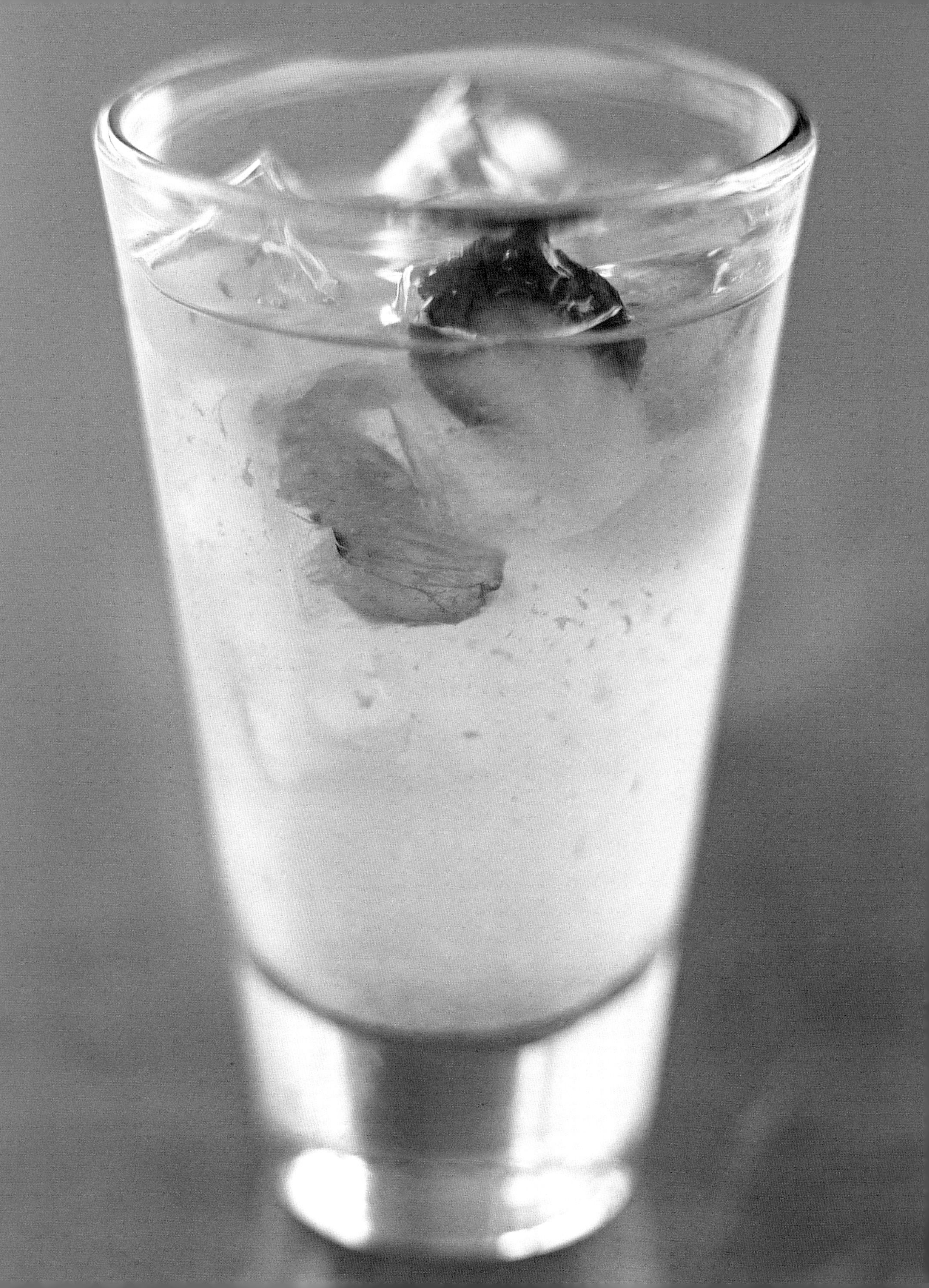

two-flower treat

Elderflowers contain cleansing natural chemicals such as tannins and rutin. Nasturtium flowers contain mustard oil, another **cleansing** and **antiseptic** chemical. Combined with ginger, one of the best **digestive** cleansers, and delicate lavender flowers, this makes a fabulous cooling, cleansing drink.

6 nasturtium flowers

crushed ice

2.5cm or 1in ginger root, peeled and grated

15ml or ½ fl oz pure rosehip syrup

750ml or 26 fl oz organic sparkling elderflower pressé

5g or ⅛oz lavender flowers, rubbed off the stalk

Put the nasturtium flowers into an ice-cube tray, fill with water and freeze. If you grow your own, it's worth making a supply, as they'll keep for at least three months. Fill a large glass tumbler a third full with crushed ice, add the ginger and rosehip syrup and stir well. Pour in the elderflower pressé and float the nasturtium ice cubes on the top. Sprinkle with lavender flowers.

Alternative method: Put all the ingredients except the nasturtium cubes in a cocktail shaker, shake vigorously and pour foaming into the glass, then add the nasturtium cubes and sprinkle with lavender flowers.

Serves 4–5

This drink is rich in **vitamin C**, most of which comes from the rosehip, but the elderflowers are a rich source, too. Nasturtiums are rich in the **essential oils** myrosin and spilanthol, that are cleansing and immune-boosting.

lady windermere's fan club

This recipe was given to us by my wife Sally's oldest friend, Diana, a keen golfer who spends her spare time at major golf tournaments. According to Diana, this drink is a favourite with lady golfers and female golf fans in the north of England. It's the ginger and the lemons that have the **cleansing** effect – and, of course, it tastes even better made with traditional ginger beer.

300ml or 10 fl oz chilled ginger beer

300ml or 10 fl oz chilled lemonade

2 shots angostura bitters

Just mix everything together and enjoy.

Serves 2–3

The natural constituents of ginger – gingerols and zingiberene – are **circulatory stimulants** and cleansers, while the **vitamin C** and citric acid from the lemons reinforce the cleansing properties of this drink.

lime concentrate

This delicious lime concentrate is very simple to make, and you get less than a teaspoon of sugar in a large glass of the drink, so the **wonderful tartness** of the lime juice is preserved. The gentle cleansing action of the citric acid and vitamin C is just what you need on a hot summer day.

7 limes
5 lemons
450g or 1lb caster sugar
450ml or 16 fl oz boiling water
25g or 1oz citric acid

Squeeze the juice from the limes and lemons. Mix the juices with all the other ingredients. Stir until the sugar has completely dissolved.

Place in airtight glass containers.

Use about two tablespoons to each glass of water. This concentrate keeps in the fridge for several weeks and can be frozen.

Makes about 1.7 litres or 60 fl oz

Lemons and limes are both rich in **bioflavonoids**, which protect the circulatory system. They also contain **potassium**, vitamin C and the essential oil limonene. This combination stimulates the kidneys, increases the flow of urine and has a gentle cleansing action.

popeye's secret

Popeye's belief that spinach is a great source of iron isn't true. There *is* lots of iron in spinach, but the body can extract little of it due to the oxalic acid also present in spinach leaves. However, it is a very **rich source** of nutrients that are **good for the eyes**. Mixed here with diuretic parsley, cleansing melon and antibacterial sage, spinach makes a cleansing and healing drink.

1 honeydew melon, peeled, deseeded and cubed
1 handful baby spinach leaves
4 sage leaves
2 stalks flat-leaf parsley, finely chopped and stalks discarded

Wash the spinach, sage and parsley.

Put the melon, spinach, and sage leaves into a blender or food processor and whizz until smooth. Scatter the chopped parsley over the juice to serve.

Serves 1–2

Melon provides **folic acid**, potassium and a little vitamin A, C and B, but it is renowned as a cleansing fruit. **Cancer-fighting phytochemicals**, large amounts of folic acid and eye-protective carotenoids lutein and xeaxanthine all come from spinach, while sage provides plant hormones and the **powerfully antiseptic** thujone.

prune and apricot smoothie

Prunes are an immensely effective cleanser due to their laxative effect, yet they are much more than that. Weight for weight, they're the most powerful protective food of all. Regular consumption of prunes really does protect you against **premature ageing**, heart disease, many forms of cancer and even wrinkles.

6 fresh apricots, washed and stones removed

250ml or 9 fl oz prune juice

Put the apricots into a blender or food processor with the prune juice and whizz until smooth.

Serves 1–2

Prune juice is rich in **betacarotene**, **iron**, B vitamins and potassium. Fresh apricots provide soluble fibre, some iron and lots more betacarotene. It's the way these two ingredients **stimulate bowel function** and improve digestion that produces the cleansing benefits.

the activator

Melon is regarded by naturopaths as a cooling cleanser, and in Indian Ayurvedic medicine it's used as a diuretic. It is also soothing to the digestion. The addition of watercress, broccoli and the tart apple make this "green juice" a **perfect cleanser**, as it's gently laxative and a powerful immune booster.

1 cooking apple, unpeeled, uncored and quartered

½ green melon, peeled and cut into chunks

85g or 3oz broccoli florets, without thick stalks

1 handful watercress

Put everything through a juicer, mix well and and serve.

Serves 1–2

Rich in **vitamins A, C** and **E**, this juice also contains folic acid, magnesium and potassium. It is particularly suitable for active men who enjoy regular sport (of course, women can take it, too). The **mineral content** will also replace losses experienced through sweating. Taken once or twice weekly, this cleansing juice ensures a substantial intake of **cancer-protective** nutrients thanks to the watercress and broccoli.

granny's lemon barley water

Lemon barley water has been a cleansing formula for hundreds of years. Particularly effective for **urinary problems**, it is also a great aid for most skin conditions, particularly **oily skins** and recurrent spots. Any of the three herbs enhance the cleansing abilities of this drink.

125g or 4½oz pot barley

55g or 2oz organic demerara sugar

2 organic unwaxed lemons

1.2 litres or 40 fl oz water

1 handful cowslip flowers, dandelion leaves or marjoram

ice cubes

Wash the barley and put it into a large jug. Put the sugar in a bowl. Scrub the lemons with warm water and grate the rind into the sugar; mix together and add to the barley.

Bring the water to the boil, pour over the barley, sugar and lemon rind, stir vigorously and leave to cool. Squeeze the juice from the lemons, add to the barley, stir again and strain through a fine sieve. If you have access to cowslip flowers or dandelion leaves, they make an unusual addition; if not, buy marjoram in the supermarket or grow your own. Serve over lots of ice cubes.

Serves 4

The naturally cleansing plant chemicals in cowslips, dandelions and marjoram give this drink a boost, though the very **high vitamin C** content is a major cleansing factor, too. There is also a rich content of cleansing and **protective bioflavonoids** from lemon peel, as well as the fibre from the barley. Modest amounts of B vitamins, some trace minerals and a small amount of protein are a bonus.

lemon express

Grapes are one of Nature's great cleansers; if you're cleansing your digestive system and reducing food consumption, their extra sugar will keep your **energy levels up**. The combination of grapes, soluble fibre in apples and the gentle diuretic effect of lemon makes this juice particularly effective.

3 apples, unpeeled, uncored and quartered

1 lemon, with peel if thin-skinned*

115g or 4oz white grapes

Put all the ingredients through a juicer, mix well and serve.

Serves 1–2

Rich in **vitamin C**, soluble fibre and natural sugars, this also contains **antioxidant bioflavonoids** and potassium. *Lemon pith is rich in **limonene**, now believed to have anti-cancer properties. For this reason, if you have to peel your lemon, it's best to peel it first, leaving on the white pith and then put it through your juicer.

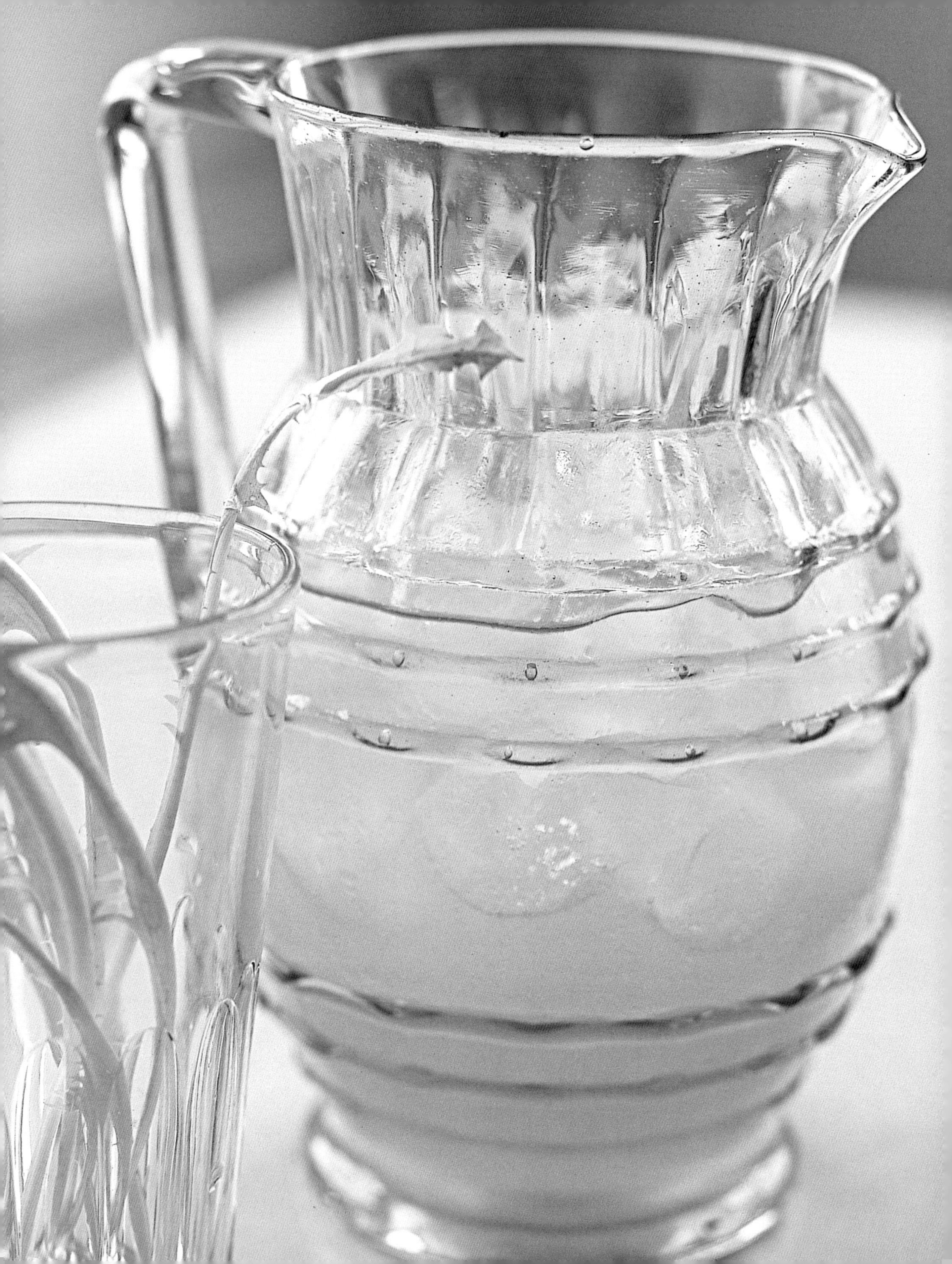

rainbow cocktail

This mixture of orange, pink, green and yellow-skinned citrus fruits is both a liver and **intestinal cleanser**. Its clean, tangy, wide-awake taste also makes it a favourite anytime drink. Use the Rainbow as an excellent start to a detox cleansing day.

2 oranges, peeled leaving pith behind
1 pink grapefruit, peeled leaving pith behind
1 lemon, with peel if thin-skinned
1 lime, peeled (unless it's a key lime)

Put all the ingredients through a juicer, mix well and serve.

Serves 1–2

Super-rich in **vitamin C**, and rich in vitamin A, this drink also contains a useful amount of potassium and calcium. The acidity of citrus juice helps remove unwanted bacteria from the digestive tract and encourages the growth of **beneficial probiotic bacteria**. A real digestive aid which should be drunk for two or three days after a course of antibiotics.

women's wonder

Women's Wonder is a powerful cleanser. In addition, thanks to the fennel, it contains phyto-oestrogens (plant hormones), which help **regulate periods** and bring some relief from PMS and menopausal symptoms. While this juice has been designed with women in mind, it's fine for men, too!

2 apples, unpeeled, uncored and quartered
2 carrots
1 chicory head, roughly chopped
½ bulb of fennel, roughly chopped

Put all the ingredients through a juicer, mix well, and serve.

Serves 1–2

Super-rich in vitamins A and C, rich in **folic acid** and **potassium**, this juice also contains a good amount of **iron**. Fennel and chicory exert a cleansing influence on liver and kidneys – perfect for easing the bloating that often accompanies periods. For women going through the menopause, this juice's **phyto-oestrogens** are a natural "hormone replacement therapy" to help prevent bone loss and subsequent osteoporosis.

ginger spice

This gentle cleanser benefits from the powerful volatile oils present in the ginger, as well as the **cleansing** and **digestive** benefits of carrot, apple and orange. This juice has **antiseptic** and **anti-inflammatory** benefits and is perfect to use at the onset of a cold or fever.

2 carrots, peeled and trimmed unless organic

1 apple, unpeeled, uncored and quartered

1 orange, peeled leaving pith behind

2.5cm or 1in ginger, peeled and sliced

Put all the ingredients through a juicer, mix well, and serve.

Serves 1–2

Rich in vitamins A and C and cleansing fibre from the apple. Ginger is one of the most **versatile** and **valuable** of all spices. In addition to its use for digestive problems, it also provides an **invigorating lift**.

minty morning

By combining the health-giving properties of oranges with the natural oils present in mint (the best digestive aid of all the herb family), this juice makes a powerful **digestive aid** and **cleanser** that gets to work right from the start.

4 large oranges

a generous sprig of mint

If you're making this juice in a citrus-fruit juicer, halve the oranges, juice them, finely chop the mint, and stir into the juice.

If using a regular juicer, peel the oranges, remove most of the pith and feed small bunches of mint leaves into the machine between each two or three pieces of orange.

Serves 1–2

Super-rich in **vitamin C**, this juice also contains **potassium**, **calcium**, folic acid and bioflavonoids. Oranges boost overall resistance and are good for the heart and circulatory system. In natural medicine, they are also considered beneficial to the intestines, as they make it difficult for unwanted bacteria to survive. They also help with unpleasant problems such as constipation and wind.

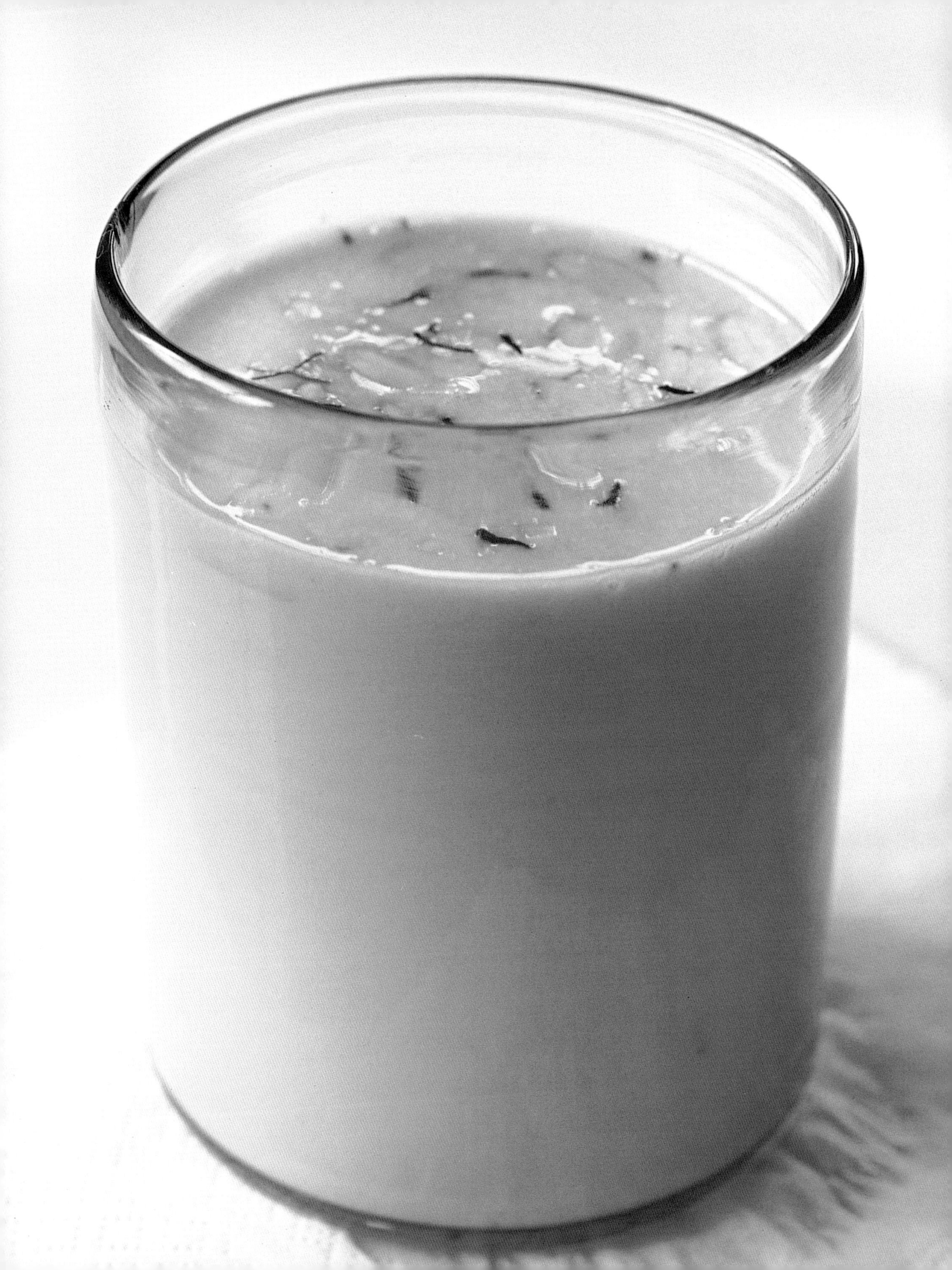

soya with saffron

Here's a smoothie simply bursting with nutritional value. Lots of protein, minerals, plant hormones and all the digestive protection of honey are present in this mixture. Saffron adds a wonderful colour, but it is also a **mood-enhancer** and helps **improve digestion**.

- 450ml or 16 fl oz soya milk
- 2 heaped tbsp runny honey
- 1 large pinch saffron
- 1 tbsp ground almonds
- 1 tsp slivered almonds

Put the first four ingredients into a blender.

Whizz until smooth.

Serve with the slivered almonds floating on top.

Serves 1–2

Saffron's main cleansing attribute helps to induce menstruation, preventing the build-up of waste products. The **phyto-oestrogens** in soya milk have a weak hormonal effect that is especially beneficial to women. Like all nuts, almonds provide a rich source of **vitamin E**, **essential fatty acids** and minerals.

waterfall

Another **powerful diuretic** juice. Waterfall's combination of celery and parsley will help ease even the most stubborn fluid retention. Although English curly parsley is fine for this recipe, the European flat-leafed variety has a richer, fuller and slightly smoother flavour, and if anything is an even better diuretic.

- 3 carrots, peeled and trimmed unless organic
- 2 apples, unpeeled, uncored and quartered
- 2 celery sticks, with leaves
- 1 handful of parsley, with stems

Put all the ingredients through a juicer, mix well, and serve.

Serves 1–2

Super-rich in vitamins A, C, E and **folic acid**, this juice is also rich in **potassium** and **magnesium**. As well having a strong diuretic effect, this superjuice will benefit the skin and is ideal for anyone with high blood pressure or heart disease, since it is very low in sodium. It also makes an excellent cleansing juice for use during pregnancy.

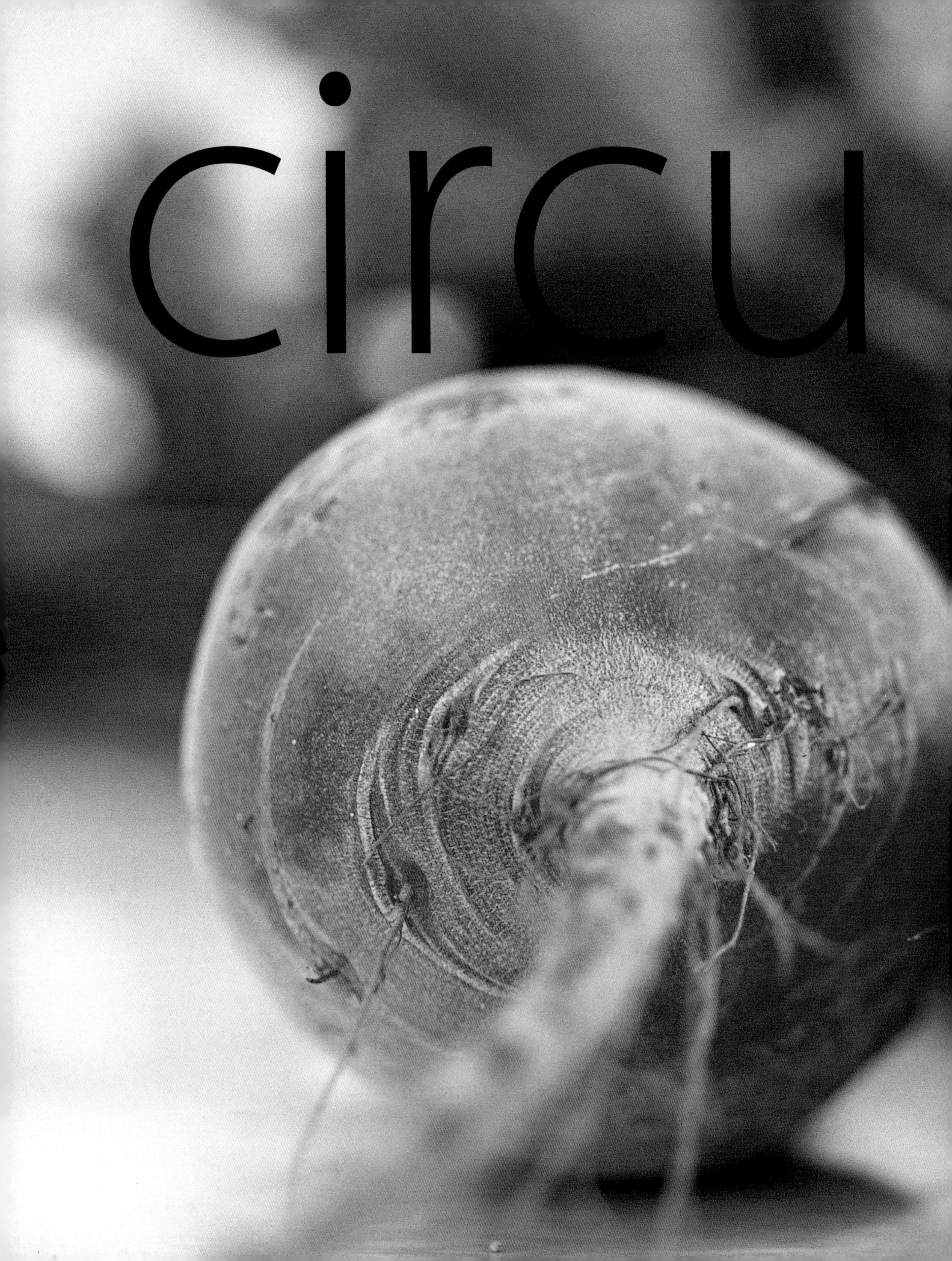
circu

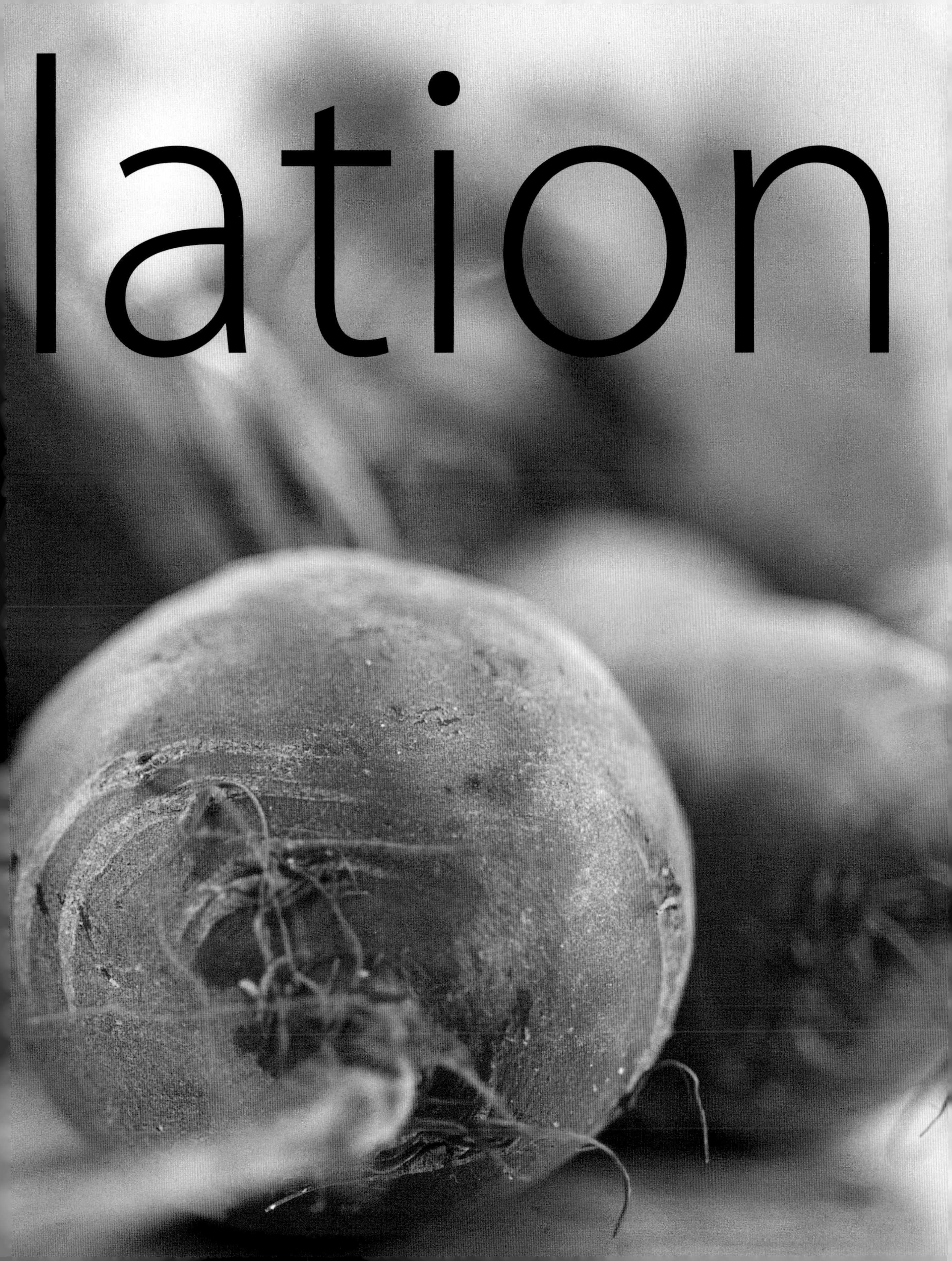
lation

Almost more than any other medical condition, circulatory problems are easier to prevent than to cure. Don't become a couch potato, don't put on too much weight and don't let your diet fall victim to burger chains, pizza parlours and convenience-food manufacturers. There's nothing wrong with an occasional treat, but as a staple diet they spell disaster.

One such circulatory disaster is high blood pressure. High blood pressure, or hypertension, is one of the most important factors in the cause of heart disease, which kills prematurely more people in the Western world than any other illness. It has no symptoms until the first stroke, kidney failure or heart attack. The good news is that you can reduce the chances of anyone in your family getting it. You can even do things to reduce blood pressure if it's already a problem by making simple changes.

Throughout daily life, the blood pressure varies considerably, depending on what is needed. Your brain must get a regular supply of 750cc each minute, and this is regardless of what the rest of your body is doing. If your arteries are narrowed, due to hardening, silting up with cholesterol or if they are constricted by nicotine, caffeine and excess alcohol, then the heart has to pump harder to push the blood around the system, and up goes the blood pressure.

It is at this point that self-help is the first and most important step. Treating high blood pressure with drugs is *not* a cure for the condition – it's merely a way of controlling the symptom. This may be a vital step when the pressure is much too high, but you can do things to help, even when medication is unavoidable. Many of my patients have been able to reduce the amount of medicine that they need to take, or even cut it out completely. (Never change your drug regime without your doctor's advice, however.) If you follow some simple suggestions for helping to reduce your blood pressure, your own GP will soon see when the readings start to fall, and he will want to reduce your drug intake. The three steps to reducing blood pressure are to change your diet, take regular exercise and learn some form of relaxation.

Other circulatory problems include coronary heart disease, angina, strokes, visual disturbances, senile memory loss, Raynaud's disease, intermittent claudication, chilblains and complications of diabetes. Whatever the specific problem or symptoms, however, the general food advice remains the same.

eating for good circulation

Herbs and spices have a part to play in treating most circulatory problems. Horseradish, ginger, cinnamon, cayenne, paprika and chillies are all circulatory stimulants and should feature prominently in your eating plan. But no matter how well you're eating, a healthy circulation needs regular exercise in order to stimulate the entire cardiovascular system. You don't have to become a fitness freak, a marathon runner or an aerobics addict; just half an hour's brisk walk three or four times a week, ten minutes of vigorous housework or gardening two or three times a day, playing your favourite sport, going for a swim or bicycling are all just fine. Exercise becomes even more vital for the elderly, the incapacitated and the disabled. Arm and hand movements, foot and ankle rotation, knee exercise, hip, thigh and even abdominal muscles can be exercised sitting in a chair, or lying in bed. No matter how little you think you can do, the more you do, the more you'll be able to do.

The recipes in this section are full of stimulating spices like ginger. You'll also find oatmeal to improve digestive function, prevent constipation and protect the heart and blood vessels; nuts for vitamin E; dates for fibre and extra iron; citrus fruits for bioflavonoids; and oily fish like salmon to protect the heart and blood vessels from inflammatory changes and help to maintain the elasticity of the larger arteries.

This is a cookbook, not a medical textbook, but you will find references to some of the specific circulatory problems in the introductions to the recipes that follow this introduction.

circulation checklist

- Eat more garlic, onions, oats, apples and pears for their cholesterol-lowering benefits; cabbage, carrots, broccoli and sweet peppers for betacarotene; blackcurrants, cherries and citrus fruits for vitamin C and bioflavonoids. Opt for buckwheat for its rutin; oily fish for omega-3 fatty acids; nuts, seeds, avocados and extra-virgin olive oil for vitamin E.
- Eat fewer of the saturated fats found in all meat and meat products – burgers, sausages, salamis, pâtés, meat pies – and fewer bakery goods such as Swiss rolls, Danish pastries, ice creams. Avoid all artificially hardened and hydrogenated fat, all trans fats and excess alcohol, and consume less caffeine, sugar and salt. Finally, of course, avoid smoking.

spiced lentil soup

In this soup, spices come into their own, working together to get your circulation buzzing. Add B vitamins and good fibre from the lentils, and calcium, phosphorus and magnesium from the coconut milk, and you have an effective, delicious and satisfying dish for **circulatory** health.

3 tbsp extra-virgin olive oil

1 onion, finely sliced

1 garlic clove, peeled and finely chopped

2.5cm or 1in fresh ginger root, peeled and finely grated

1 tbsp coriander seed, crushed well

1 tbsp allspice

1 tsp chilli powder

700ml or 25 fl oz vegetable stock (page 252)

1 x 400ml can coconut milk

150g or 5½oz green lentils

Heat the olive oil in a large saucepan. Stir in the onion and sweat gently for five minutes. Add the garlic and ginger and continue sweating them for four minutes.

Stir in the coriander, allspice and chilli powder. Cook, stirring continuously, for three minutes.

Add the stock and coconut milk and bring to a simmer. Stir in the lentils and continue to simmer for about thirty minutes.

Serves 4

A soup to spice up your blood flow. Ginger provides **gingeroles**, essential oils that dilate blood vessels, while chilli adds **capsaicin** for stimulating warmth.

curried parsnip and vegetable soup

Putting parsnips together with stimulating spices such as curry produces a soup that is seriously good for **circulation**. Adding beans and peas increases the fibre content and supplies beneficial protein, while the crème fraîche gives it a wonderfully creamy texture and supplies calcium, too.

4 tbsp extra-virgin olive oil

1 large onion, finely chopped

1 heaped tbsp curry powder

2 level tbsp flour

2 medium parsnips (about 500g or 1lb 2oz), washed, peeled and diced

1.2 litres or 40 fl oz vegetable stock (page 252)

200ml or 7 fl oz crème fraîche

100g or 3½oz French beans, trimmed and cut into 2.5cm or 1in fingers

100g or 3½oz peas, fresh or frozen

Heat the olive oil and gently sweat the onions for ten minutes. Remove from the heat and stir in the curry powder and flour.

Return to the heat and cook, stirring continuously, for three minutes. Add the diced parsnips and stir for two more minutes.

Pour in the stock and bring to the boil. Simmer for twenty minutes, or until the parsnips are tender. Liquidize the mixture, return to the pan and bring back to a simmer. Stir in the crème fraîche.

Add the beans and peas and cook for another seven minutes.

Serves 4

This one will keep your blood flowing freely. Parsnips are rich in **minerals** and **fibre**, and beans and peas supply beneficial **plant hormones**.

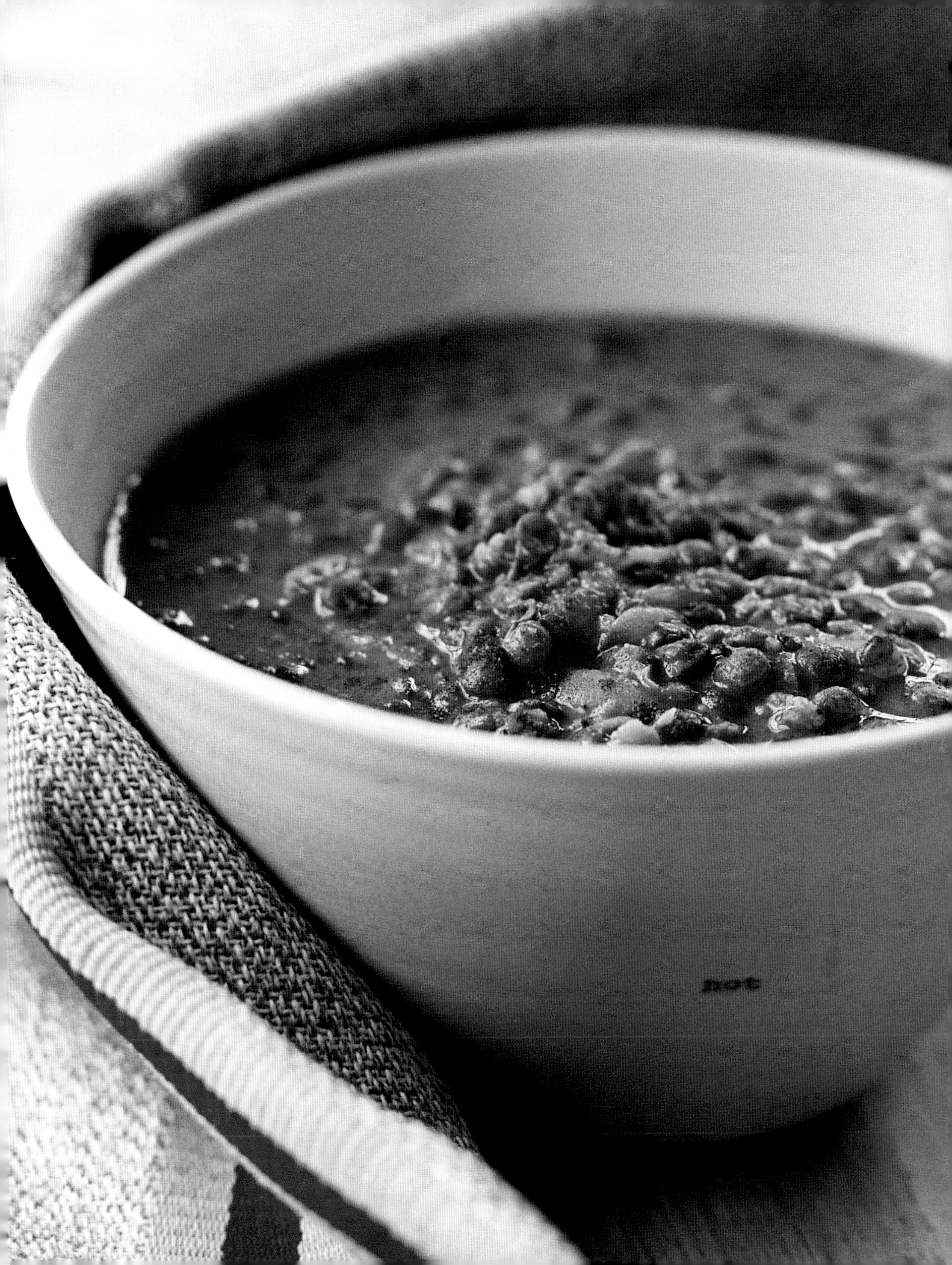
hot

ginger, leek and carrot soup

The leek is a member of the Allium genus of plants and, just like its onion and garlic relatives, it is a rich source of natural sulphur-based chemicals that improve the circulation. This recipe provides a triple boost from all three. As an extra **circulatory** bonus, there's plenty of ginger as well.

3 tbsp extra-virgin olive oil

1 red onion, finely sliced

3 plump garlic cloves, peeled and finely chopped

3 large leeks, trimmed and finely chopped

2.5cm or 1 inch fresh root ginger, peeled and grated

1kg or 2lb 4oz carrots, trimmed and peeled if not organic, finely diced

1.2 litres or 40 fl oz vegetable stock (page 252)

Heat the olive oil in a large saucepan. Add the onion, garlic, leeks and ginger and sweat gently for ten minutes. Drop in the carrot cubes and stir until covered with the oil mixture. Pour in the stock and bring to the boil.

Turn down the heat and simmer until the carrots are tender – about twenty minutes. Liquidize in a food processor or blender. Pour through a fine sieve, being careful to remove any unliquidized ginger.

Note: this soup is delicious hot or cold. This recipe makes enough to last two or three days.

Serves 4

Leeks contain **phytochemicals** that help lower cholesterol, which keeps blood-pressure levels down.

oatmeal and broccoli soup

As well as being a healthy breakfast food in the form of porridge, oats are a versatile ingredient and can be used to delicious advantage in many other ways. In this unusual soup, they're combined with broccoli to make a surprisingly light and delicate dish that offers **huge health benefits**.

2 tbsp extra-virgin olive oil

6 spring onions, finely chopped

600g or 1lb 5oz broccoli florets, washed, trimmed and halved if large

75g or 2¾oz oatmeal

750ml or 27 fl oz semi-skimmed milk

750ml or 27 fl oz vegetable stock (page 252)

sea salt and black pepper, to taste

4 tbsp natural, live yogurt

Heat the oil on a low heat and sweat the onions until soft – about five minutes. Add the broccoli and continue heating gently, stirring continuously, for three more minutes.

Mix in the oatmeal and continue cooking for four minutes, still stirring. Pour in the milk and stock, cover and simmer for ten minutes; season to taste.

Serve with a spoonful of yogurt in each bowl.

Serves 4

Oats are rich in **B vitamins** and **soluble fibre**, while broccoli supplies **vitamin C** and betacarotene, which protect the heart and help prevent cancer.

fennel, rocket and radish salad

A combination to help **regulate hormones** and boost sluggish blood. This salad uses the large white bulb of the Florence fennel. Its crunchy texture and unusual flavour of mild liquorice is beautifully complemented by the sharp bite of rocket and radishes.

- 1 large bulb florence fennel, sliced with green fronds set aside
- 12 radishes, trimmed and quartered
- 1 generous bunch rocket
- 3 tbsp standard salad dressing

Put all the ingredients except the green fennel fronds into a salad bowl. Add the dressing and toss lightly.

Sprinkle any fennel fronds over the top to serve.

Serves 4

Fennel has the specific effect of helping to regulate hormonal imbalances; this makes it an invaluable plant for women. Together with the circulatory stimulus of the **essential mustard oils** in radishes, as well as the **tannins** and other **volatile oils** in the rocket, the combination will give a quick boost to even the most sluggish of circulations.

citrus fig salad

A circulatory stimulant and energy-building combination. The earliest Olympic athletes were fed pounds of figs – with good reason. Figs are full of **blood-building** nutrients, and they contain the natural enzyme ficin, which improves the digestive absorption of the fruit's other constituents, especially the iron that is so vital for **healthy blood** and circulation.

- 8 ripe figs
- 1 generous bunch lamb's lettuce
- 2 tbsp fresh tarragon leaves, coarsely chopped
- juice of 1 lemon
- 1 tbsp extra-virgin olive oil

Wash, dry and quarter the figs. Wash and dry the lamb's lettuce.

Put the lamb's lettuce into a serving bowl with the tarragon.

Thoroughly mix the lemon juice with the olive oil. Add to the bowl and toss thoroughly to coat all the surfaces.

Arrange the figs over the top.

Serves 4

The added benefits of **essential oils** in tarragon and the generous amounts of **vitamin C** in the lemon juice make this salad a circulatory stimulant.

beetroot soup

Throughout Eastern Europe, beetroot is renowned for its **blood-** and **circulation-boosting** properties, and has been used to treat anaemia, poor circulation and even leukaemia. In this recipe, it is combined with carrots and lemon juice to provide a refreshing, nourishing soup for healthy blood.

1kg or 2lb 4oz fresh, raw beetroot (pickled ones are not suitable)

2 large carrots, trimmed and peeled if not organic

1 medium white onion, peeled

1 clove garlic, peeled

5 tbsp extra-virgin olive oil

1.5 litres or 55 fl oz vegetable stock (page 252)

juice of 1 lemon

400ml or 14 fl oz natural, live yogurt

Grate the beetroot, carrots, onion and garlic, or chop them in a food processor. Heat the oil in a large saucepan. Add the vegetables and sweat gently for ten minutes.

Add the stock, cover, and simmer for forty minutes. Strain into a clean saucepan and bring back to a simmer. Stir the lemon juice into the yogurt.

Serve the soup with a swirl of the yogurt and lemon mixture on top. Alternatively, serve cold, substituting white seedless grapes for the yogurt and lemon mixture.

Serves 4

Beetroot is rich in **iron**, which helps prevent anaemia. Carrots supply betacarotene to **protect capillaries**. Vitamin C in lemons prevents damage to artery walls.

nutty dates and grapes

Here's a rich source of vitamin E for a healthy heart and circulatory system. An unusual mixture of bean sprouts from the culinary traditions of the Far East, almonds and dates from the Middle East, and grapes from southern Europe makes this a **super circulation booster**.

1 bag bean sprouts

20 seedless black and white grapes, halved

12 fresh dates, halved and stones removed

1 tbsp walnut oil

1 tsp sesame oil

1 tsp balsamic vinegar

1 tsp light soy sauce

2 tbsp blanched almond halves

freshly ground black pepper, to taste

Arrange the salad in four serving bowls, putting the bean sprouts in the bottom and sprinkling the other ingredients on top.

Whisk together the oils, vinegar and soy sauce. Drizzle each bowl with a little dressing – but don't toss. Scatter over the almonds and season with black pepper.

Serves 4

Dates are an excellent source of iron. Almonds provide **essential fatty acids** and protein, while grapes contain circulation-protecting **antioxidants** and vitamin C.

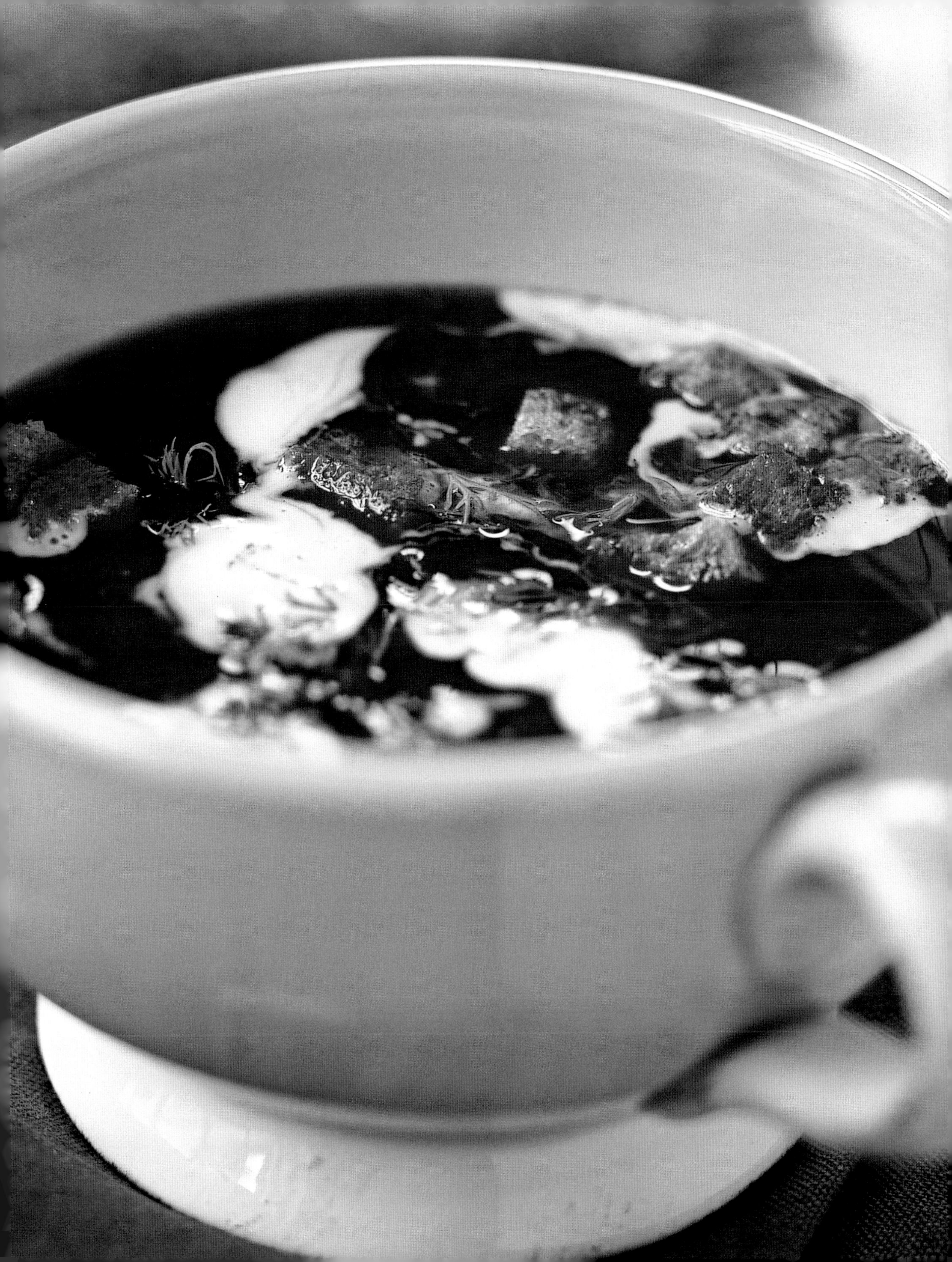

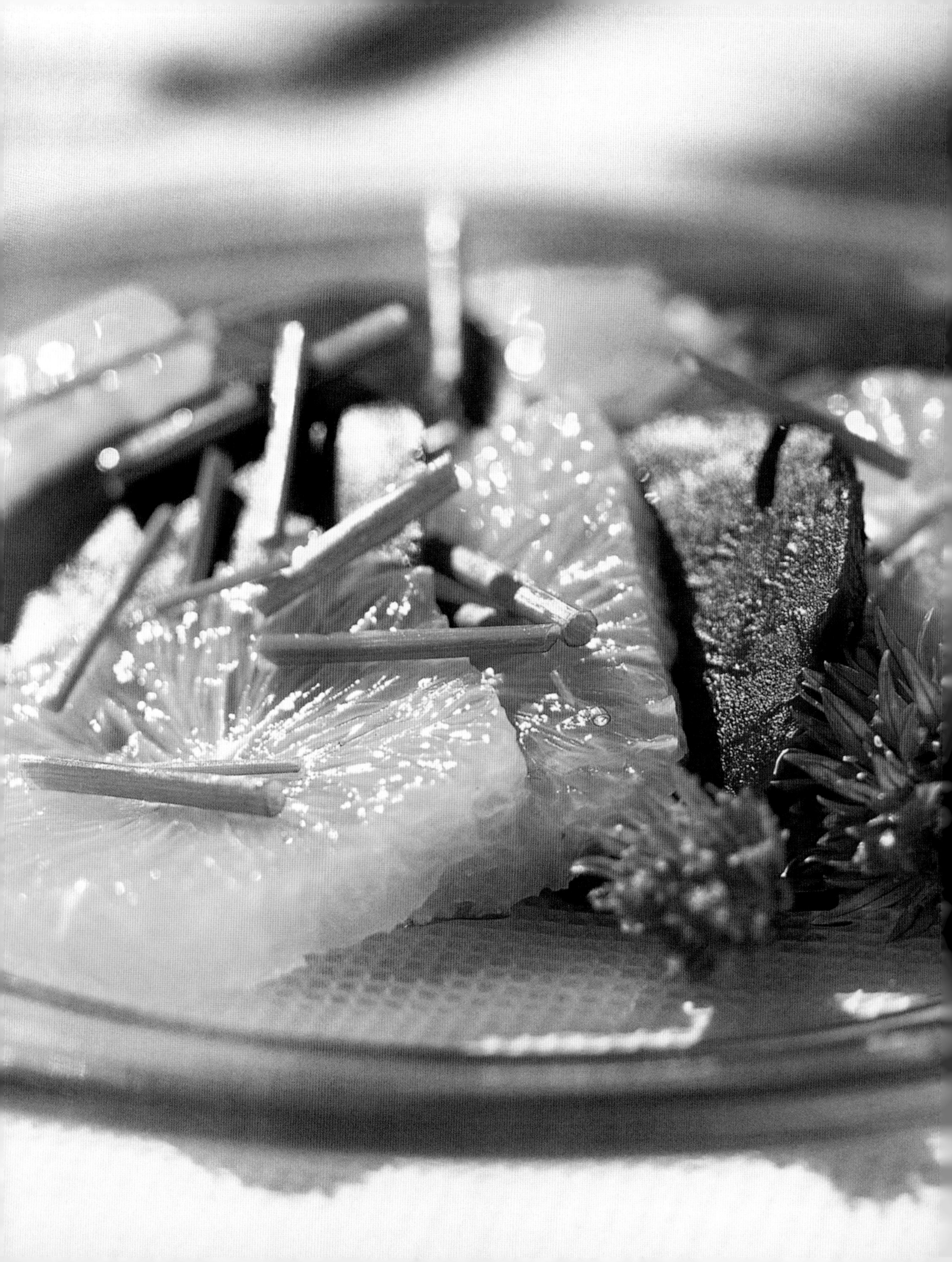

beetroot and orange with chives

A light but effective **blood-builder**. Throughout Eastern Europe, beetroot has been a traditional remedy for blood and **circulatory disorders** for centuries; in fact, the juice is given to anyone suffering from leukaemia.

3 large cooked whole beetroot, thickly sliced

2 large oranges, peeled, sliced and pith removed

1 bunch fresh chives

6 chive flowers (optional)

3 tbsp standard salad dressing

Arrange alternate slices of beetroot and orange on one large platter or four individual plates.

Scatter the whole chives over the top. Decorate with the chive flowers, if desired; they are edible and taste delicious.

Drizzle with the dressing and serve.

Serves 4

Combined here with slices of fresh orange, this salad is rich in protective **vitamin C** and **bioflavonoids**, and the heart and circulatory benefits of chives.

shades of salmon red

Heart-protective and **packed with antioxidants**. With a slice of good, crusty wholemeal bread, this salad makes a meal for four. All oily fish are good for the circulation, and salmon is one of the best. Although more expensive, it's worth choosing wild salmon.

675g or 1½lb fresh wild salmon

2 bay leaves

6 peppercorns

1 sprig fresh dill

1 garlic clove, peeled and chopped

1 small fresh green chilli, deseeded and finely sliced

1 large red pepper, deseeded and cubed

7.5cm or 3in chunk of cucumber, peeled and chopped

1 x 150g or 5½oz carton low-fat, natural, live yogurt

1 head radicchio, separated into leaves

Put the salmon into a large pan of cold water with the bay leaves, peppercorns and dill. Bring slowly to the boil, turn off the heat and leave to cool. Remove the skin from the fish and flake into a bowl.

Stir the garlic, chilli, pepper and cucumber into the yogurt, pour over the flaked salmon and stir gently. Arrange the radicchio leaves on top and serve.

Serves 4

The **omega-3 fatty acids** in fish protect both heart and arteries, and help prevent the build-up of plaque inside blood vessels. Red peppers add betacarotene and vitamin C for more protection while the **capsaicin** in the chillies dilates tiny capillaries.

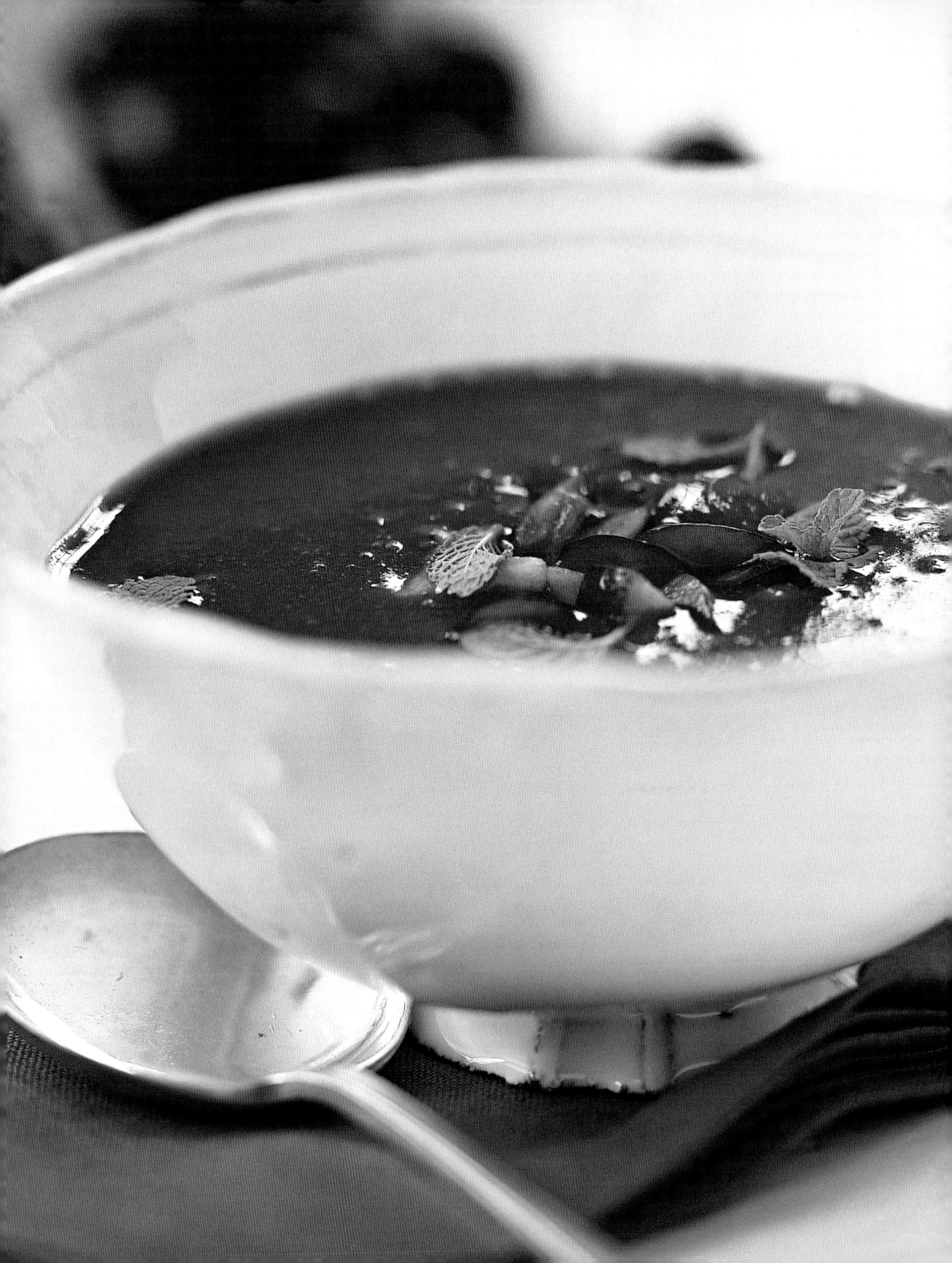

sweet cherry soup

It's easy to think of cherries as a delicious summer treat, but they're much more than that. Ripe, plump cherries are a storehouse of **circulation-boosting** nutrients. Combined with an extra dose of vitamin C from the cranberry juice, this soup will benefit anyone's circulatory system.

- 1kg or 2lb 4oz cherries, stoned (weight when stoned)
- 250ml or 9 fl oz cranberry juice
- 500ml or 18 fl oz water
- 1 glass sweet white wine, such as Muscat de Beaumes-de-Venise or the less expensive Monbazillac
- 1 level tbsp arrowroot
- 4 sprigs mint

Blend the cherries in a food processor or blender and sieve to remove the skins. Put the pulp into a large pan with the cranberry juice, water and wine and bring slowly to the boil, stirring well.

Stir the arrowroot into two more tablespoons of water and mix thoroughly. Pour the arrowroot mixture into the fruit stock and stir continuously until slightly thickened.

Serve garnished with the sprigs of mint. It's delicious warm or cold. Substitute the wine with extra fruit juice if you're serving children.

Serves 4

For a circulatory boost. Cherries are rich in **bioflavonoids** and **vitamin C**, both of which support healthy blood.

ginger and lemon zizz

A hot drink when you're freezing has about the same effect on your body temperature as a pint of boiling water does to an ice-cold bath. The difference here is that this drink really does "ginger you up" and gets those **blood corpuscles** fairly **whizzing round your veins** and arteries.

- 2.5cm or 1 inch root ginger
- 200ml or 7 fl oz water
- ½ lemon

Peel and grate the ginger. Put into an infuser or mug.

Boil the water and add it to the mug. Cover and leave for ten minutes.

Juice the lemon half, reserving two slices. Strain the ginger tea into a mug and add the lemon juice. Serve with the lemon slices on top.

Serves 1

The pungent shogaols and the stimulating **gingerols** and **zingiberene** in ginger have a dramatic effect on blood circulation, making this root a great remedy for poor circulation, chilblains and Raynaud's disease. The bioflavonoids in lemon help by strengthening blood-vessel walls.

hot chilli mango

The hot chilli sauce will get the blood whirring around your **circulatory system**, and the taste is less fiery than you'd expect, thanks to the soothing sweetness of the mango. The perfect drink when you come in from a brisk winter's walk, or a cold morning on a sports field.

500ml or 18 fl oz home-pressed mango juice (or a good commercial variety)

2 tsp hot chilli sauce

Put both ingredients into a saucepan.

Heat until just boiling.

Serve immediately in mugs or heatproof glasses.

Serves 2

Mango contains masses of **vitamins A, C** and **E**, together with potassium and iron, making it a super protector of the heart and circulatory system. Chillies contain the circulatory stimulant capsaicin. Within moments of enjoying this drink, the tiny blood vessels dilate, your skin flushes and you're suffused with warmth and comfort.

beetroot bopper

Beetroot is reputed to improve the **oxygen-carrying capacity** of blood, making the **circulation** more efficient. The combination of beetroot and horseradish is widely used as a pickle-type condiment in Eastern Europe, and the flavours are just brilliant together.

1 tsp freshly grated horseradish (or use a strong commercial variety)

500ml or 18 fl oz beetroot juice

Whizz the horseradish in a blender with 125ml or 4 fl oz of the beetroot juice. Put the rest of the juice into a saucepan.

Add the blended horseradish and stir until well combined.

Heat gently until just boiling.

Pour into mugs and serve.

Serves 2

Beetroot contains specific cancer-fighting chemicals, so we should all be eating it on a regular basis. Horseradish is one of the great circulatory stimulants, containing a chemical called **sinigrin**, which not only speeds up the circulation, but when crushed is converted into a powerful antibacterial called allylisothiocyanate.

hot banana smoothie

There's something very comforting about this combination of bananas, milk and cocoa, that gets its hidden punch from the added cinnamon. This drink not only helps **improve circulation**, it also protects against **heart disease** and high blood pressure, and will even relieve the distress of **PMS**.

2 small bananas, peeled
300ml or 10 fl oz milk
125ml or 4 fl oz natural, live yogurt
1 heaped tsp mixed cocoa powder and ground cinnamon

Put the first three ingredients into a blender and whizz until very smooth.

Pour into a saucepan and heat gently until just simmering.

Use a cappuccino wand or whisk to stir up a froth.

Pour into two mugs or heatproof glasses and serve with the cocoa powder scattered on top.

Serves 2

Bananas are rich in potassium – important for normal heart function and for the prevention of high blood pressure. Thanks to their **vitamin** B_6 content and their ability to prevent fluid retention, they also reduce the symptoms of PMS. Add the cocoa's theobromine, and **volatile oils** from the cinnamon, and it won't be long before you're glowing.

slemp

A favourite from Holland, this is drunk by everyone who manages to get their skates on and go for a stimulating winter race along the frozen canals. They return with **cheeks aglow**, healthily out of puff and ready for this drink to get them warm and add to the **circulation boost** of the exercise.

4cm or 1½in cinnamon stick
2 strands saffron
3 cloves
1 nutmeg, cut in half
1 tbsp dried green tea
850ml or 30 fl oz milk
peel of 1 unwaxed lemon, finely grated
¼ tsp salt
sugar (preferably golden caster sugar), to taste

Tie the spices and tea in a piece of muslin. Put the milk into a saucepan and add the muslin bag.

Add the lemon peel to the pan, along with the salt.

Simmer gently for one hour. Remove the spice bag.

Pour into mugs and sweeten to taste.

Serves 6

Essential oils such as saffronal and crocins from saffron, myristicin from nutmeg, cinnamaldehyde from cinnamon and eugenol from cloves are all circulation stimulants, and the **antioxidants** in green tea make this drink powerfully protective.

oranges and lemons

All citrus-fruit juices protect and improve the circulation, thanks to their exceptionally high vitamin C content. Adding the rind helps protect the integrity and **strength** of the **walls of** both **arteries** and **veins**. There is an additional benefit in the enormous increase in natural immune resistance.

4 unwaxed oranges

1 unwaxed large lemon

30ml or 1 fl oz orange-flower water

Juice the oranges and lemon and take two curls of both orange and lemon rind.

Mix the juices together and heat gently in a saucepan until just simmering.

Pour into two heatproof glasses.

Divide the orange-flower water and rind curls between the glasses to serve.

Serves 2

Vitamin C helps protect individual cells from damage, making it vital for the protection of the entire circulatory system. The **bioflavonoids** in the peel and pith improve your absorption of vitamin C and have their own strengthening effect on blood-vessel walls.

sorrel tea

This tea is one of the favourite tonics of the herbalist. The earliest Roman physicians knew that sorrel helped the body get rid of surplus fluid. In the time of Henry VIII, it was a highly prized vegetable that the king adored, and his doctors used it as one of the earliest spring **blood tonics**.

1 large handful fresh sorrel leaves, roughly torn

250ml or 9 fl oz water

runny honey

Put the sorrel in a mug or infuser.

Boil the water, add to the mug, cover and leave for ten minutes.

Strain and sweeten with honey.

Serves 1

Sorrel is believed by herbalists to both improve and cleanse the circulating blood. Its **natural phytochemicals**, including **flavonoids** and anthraquinones, are the active ingredients. It can be costly, but it will grow brilliantly in a decent-sized pot. As well as this tea, use it just like spinach in cooking and salads.

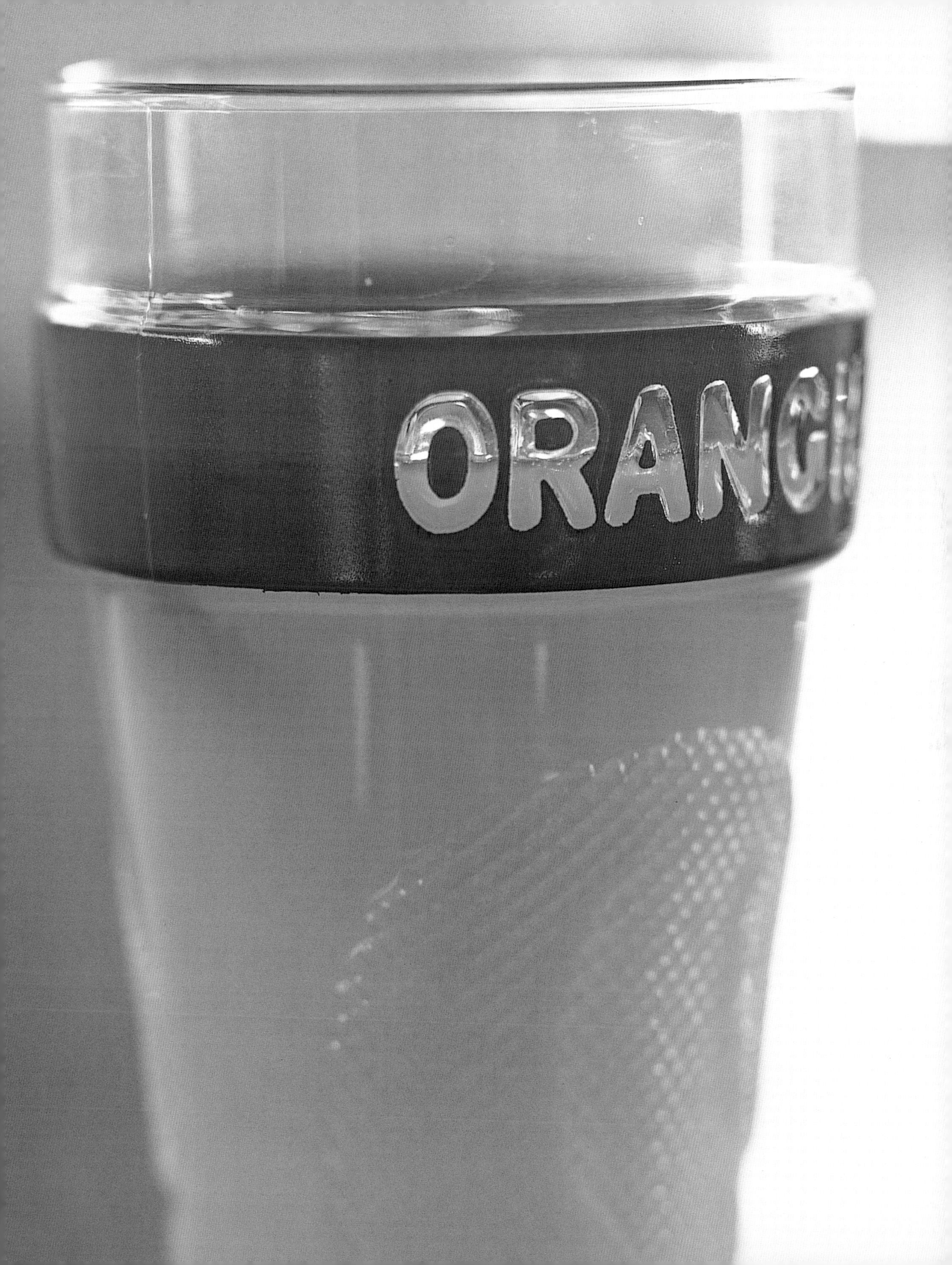
ORANG

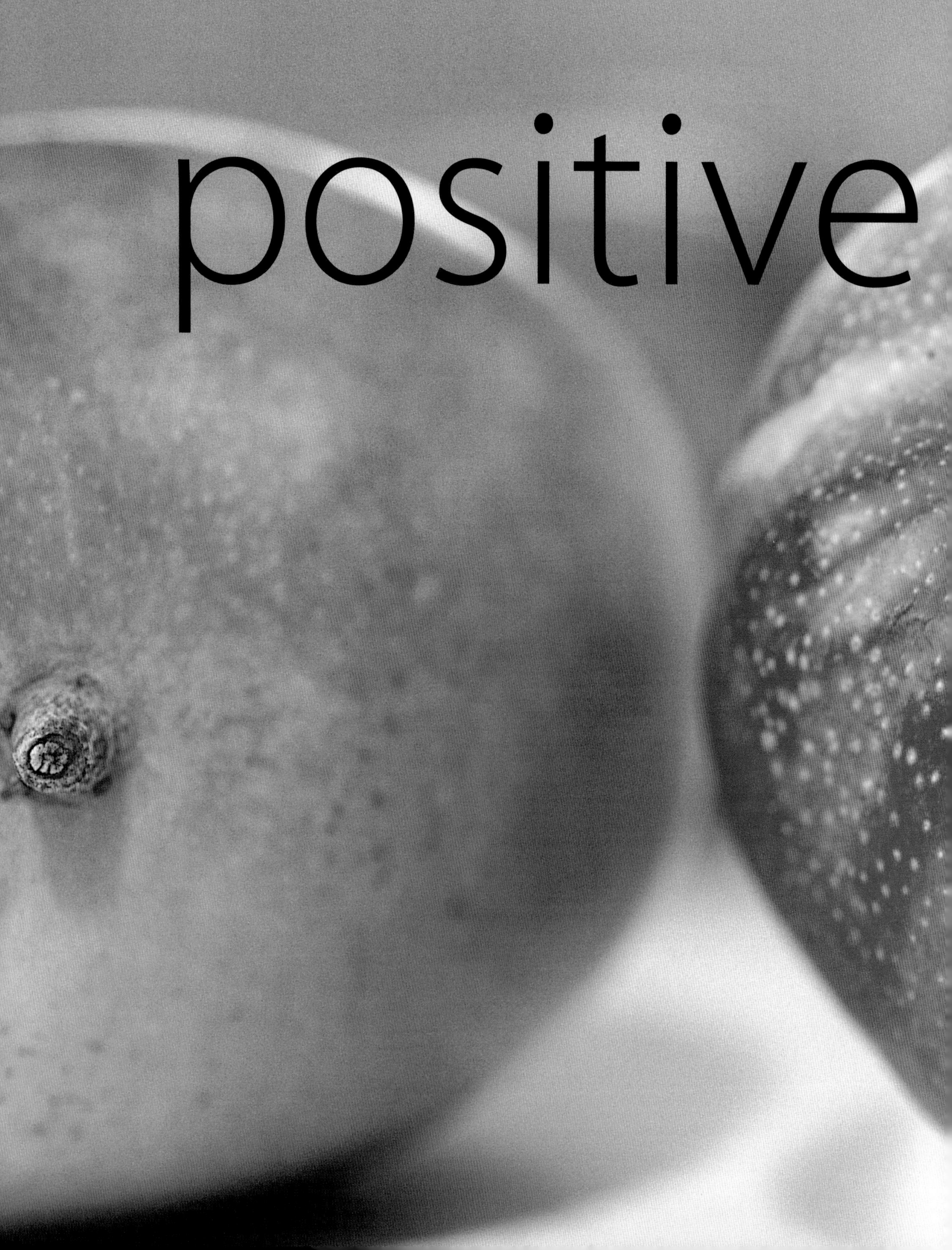
positive

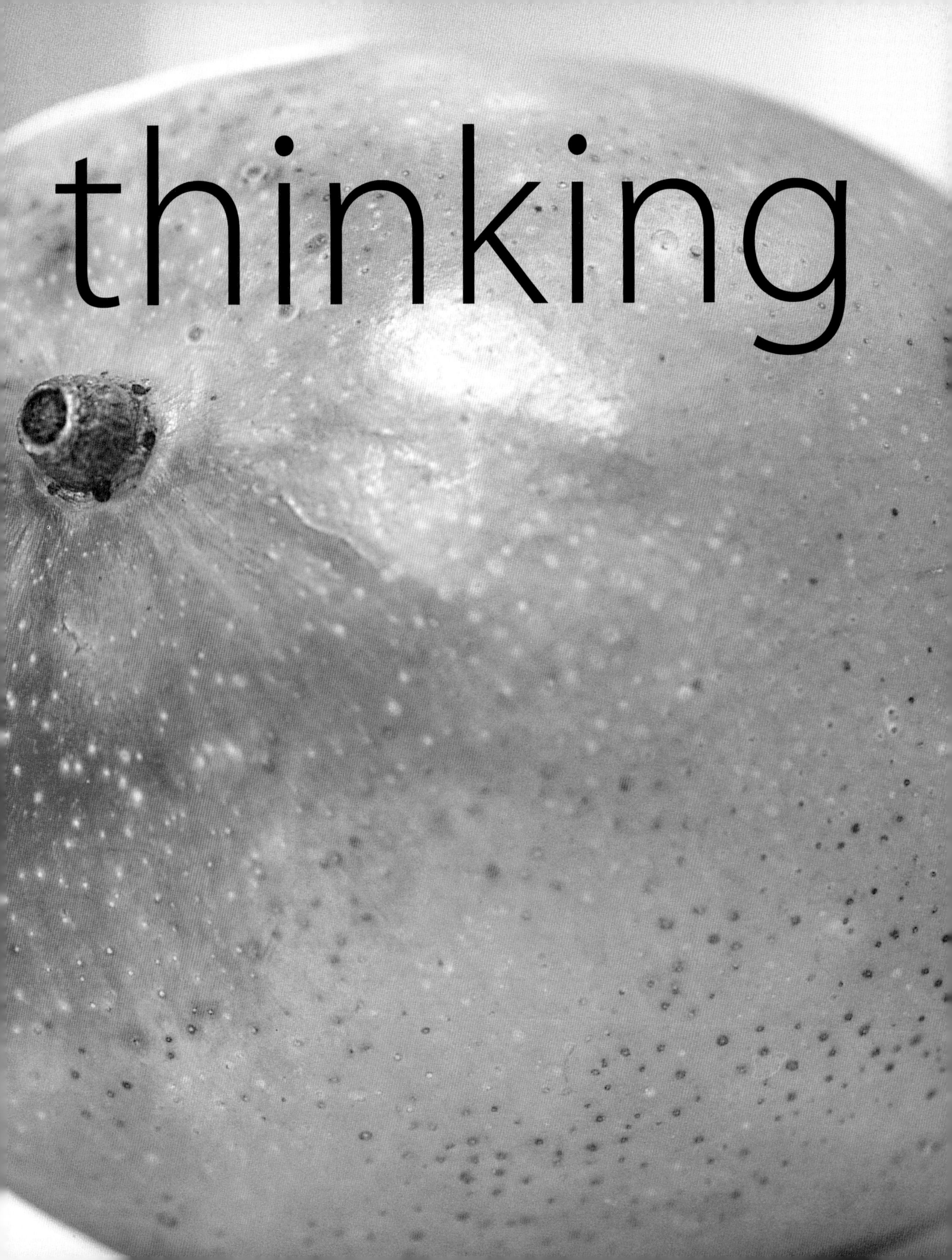
thinking

When granny said, "eat your fish, it will make you brainy", she wasn't far off the mark. All oily fish contains essential fatty acids, which makes it a vital food for any woman planning to have a baby, or who's pregnant or breast-feeding. Fatty acids form a major part of a developing baby's brain tissue, and there's now substantial evidence that women whose diets are very low in fish oils have children who tend to be slower at mental development.

But it's not just oily fish that make good brain food; the protein in all fish provides some of the slow-release energy that helps keep a constant supply of blood sugar flowing to the brain. This is exactly what our brain needs to function consistently. While all forms of protein are good brain nourishment, it's important to avoid the negative effects of animal protein, which contains large amounts of saturated fat. Poultry, game, and lean free-range beef are ideal, especially if you remove all visible fat and avoid eating the skin on chicken, duck or turkey.

Saturated fat can lead to raised cholesterol, which consists of fatty deposits in the arteries and narrowing of the blood vessels that supply the brain. This is often the first step towards declining brain function. For the same reasons, wholegrain cereals, all beans, garlic, leeks and onions should be regular ingredients in your cerebral eating plan. All of these foods help the body to get rid of cholesterol and so work towards keeping the levels of this damaging deposit healthily low, ensuring the maintenance of an adequate and continuous blood supply which carries essential nutrients to every cell in the brain.

Modest amounts of alcohol are good for your brain, too. The high levels of antioxidants that prevent brain-cell damage are a major component of red wines, so a couple of glasses a day are a great ally in the maintenance of good mental function and the power of positive thought. Alcohol itself is also valuable, whether it comes from white wine, beer, spirits or liqueurs; in small amounts, it has the effect of opening up the tiniest blood vessels at the end of the circulatory system and improving blood flow to the brain.

That's the good news, and it holds true if you consume two or three glasses of wine, two or three pub measures of spirits or up to two pints of beer a day. The bad news is that once you start to exceed these quantities, alcohol has exactly the opposite effect and makes these minute vessels contract, depriving the brain of blood and leading to rapid deterioration in mental ability and decision-making. Thoughts become negative. Depression is the hallmark of those abusing alcohol.

the role of herbs and spices

Herbs and spices have a vital role as brain foods. Some, like basil, nutmeg, lemon balm and coriander, have an effect on mood and emotion. Others have a more direct impact on mental function; the two most powerful of these are sage, synonymous with wisdom, and rosemary, which has been linked with improved memory since the times of the ancient Greeks.

The most important of the spices is chilli, which has an almost immediate effect on the circulation, opening up the tiniest blood vessels and leading to an almost instant rush of blood to the head. This accounts for the beads of sweat on the forehead within seconds of your first mouthful of a strong chilli con carne. Ginger comes a pretty close second and will also provide really quick brain stimulation, whether taken as tea, a sprinkle of powder on your melon or fresh in a stir-fry.

As we live in an age of an ever-growing older population, the maintenance of good brain function assumes even greater significance. By accentuating all the positive aspects of diet and eliminating the negatives, you dramatically increase your chances of maintaining the ability to think positively, as well as mental agility, well into old age. But food alone isn't enough. The brain is like any muscular part of the body: if you don't use it, you lose it. Keep it active by reading, conversation, crossword puzzles, learning a few lines of poetry and memory games. Most important of all is the process of calculation; following these recipes and working out the quantities is a start. So, for your brain's sake, get cooking!

positive thinking checklist

- Eat more oily fish, white fish, poultry, game, lean, free-range beef for protein and the iron needed to carry oxygen in the blood to the brain. Avoid narrowing of the brain's blood vessels by eating wholegrain cereals, beans, garlic, leeks and onions. Modest quantities of alcohol, sage and chilli are excellent brain boosters and a top aid to positive thinking.
- Eat less saturated fat in manufactured meat products; and avoid excessive quantities of alcohol and foods with a high refined sugar content, which can lead to fluctuating blood sugar levels and an inability to concentrate and focus mental energy.

spicy parsnip soup

Parsnips, turnips and swedes are rich sources of slow-release energy, which helps keep the blood-sugar level on an even keel, **preventing mood swings**. This soup also provides a form of instant energy in the honey, making it the perfect meal to take to work for a hot, **sustaining** lunch.

- 50g or 1¾oz unsalted butter
- 1 large onion, finely sliced
- 600g or 1lb 5oz mixed parsnips, turnips, celeriac, swede and potatoes, peeled and cubed
- 3 tbsp runny honey
- 1.5 litres or 55 fl oz vegetable stock (page 252)
- 150ml or 5 fl oz natural, live yogurt
- 2 tsp garam masala

In a large saucepan, melt the butter over a low heat. Add the onion and heat gently for five minutes. Add the vegetables and stir to coat well in the butter. Remove from the heat and drizzle in the honey, stirring to coat all the vegetables.

Pour in the stock and bring to a boil. Simmer until the vegetables are tender – about twenty minutes.

Liquidize in a food processor or blender. Return to the heat. Stir in the yogurt and garam masala and heat through.

Serves 4

A soup designed to provide therapeutic energy to feed positive thoughts. The root vegetables provide slow-release energy, while garam masala supplies mood-elevating spices.

spicy spinach soup

Here is a nutritious soup that also promotes a good mood. Spinach mixed with lots of chilli (a mood stimulant) and coriander – essential oils that have **enhanced moods** for centuries – turns this soup into a **nutritional powerhouse**, providing vitamins that help keep both mind and body healthy.

- 4 tbsp extra-virgin olive oil
- 2 red onions, finely chopped
- 3 garlic cloves, peeled and finely sliced
- 1 tsp chopped fresh chilli, deseeded
- ½ handful each freshly chopped parsley, mint and coriander leaves
- 600g or 1lb 5oz washed spinach (no need to remove stalks)
- 1.5 litres or 55 fl oz vegetable stock (page 252)
- 200ml or 7 fl oz crème fraîche

In a large saucepan, sweat the onions in the oil for two minutes. Add the garlic and continue heating for two more minutes. Stir in the chilli, parsley, mint and coriander, and heat for a further two minutes.

Finely chop the spinach, add to the pan with about three tablespoons of the stock, and heat for another two minutes, stirring continuously.

Add the rest of the stock and simmer for about ten minutes.

Stir in the crème fraîche and serve.

Serves 4

A bowlful of this soup is guaranteed to lift the spirits. Spinach is a rich source of **folic acid**, one of the essential **B vitamins**.

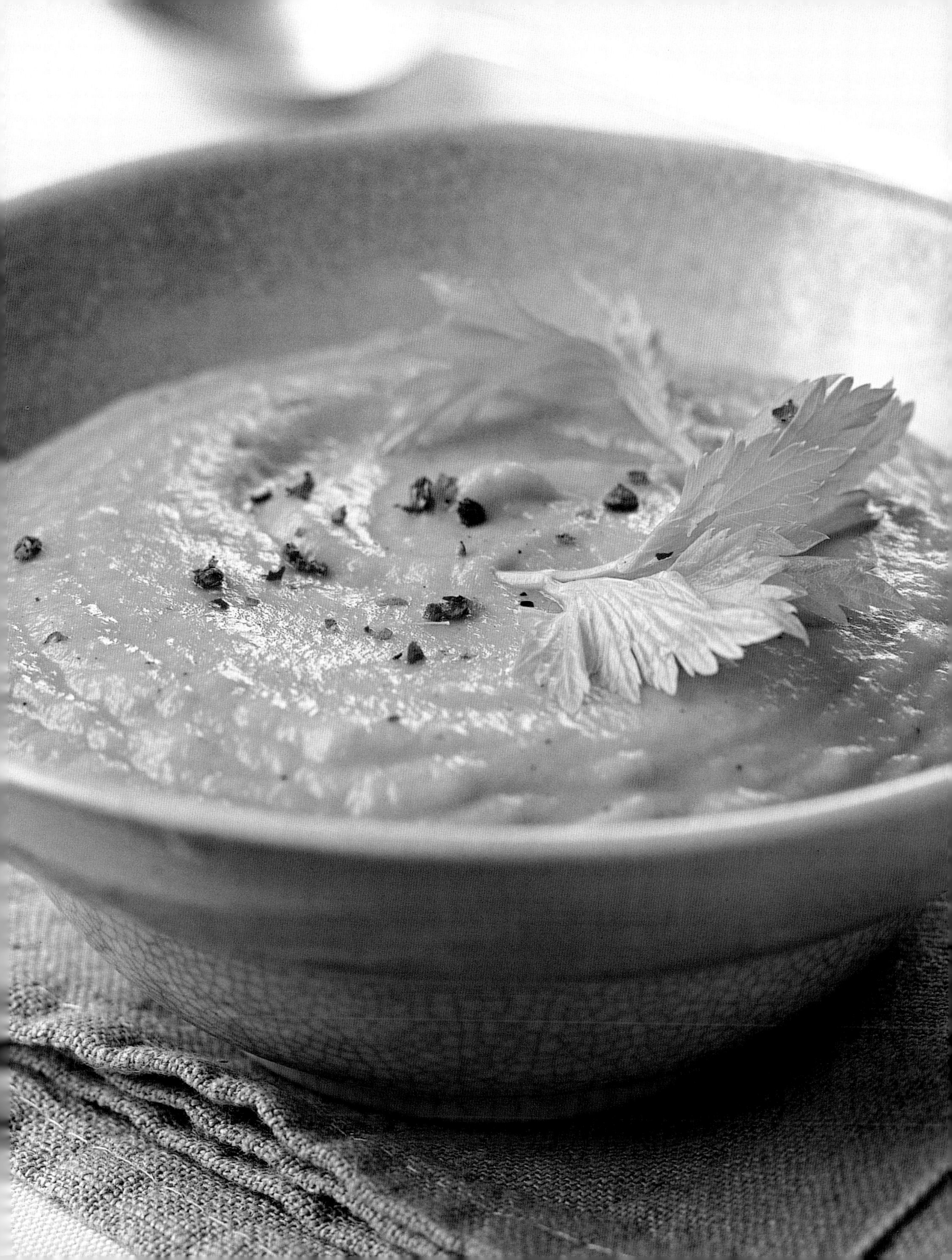

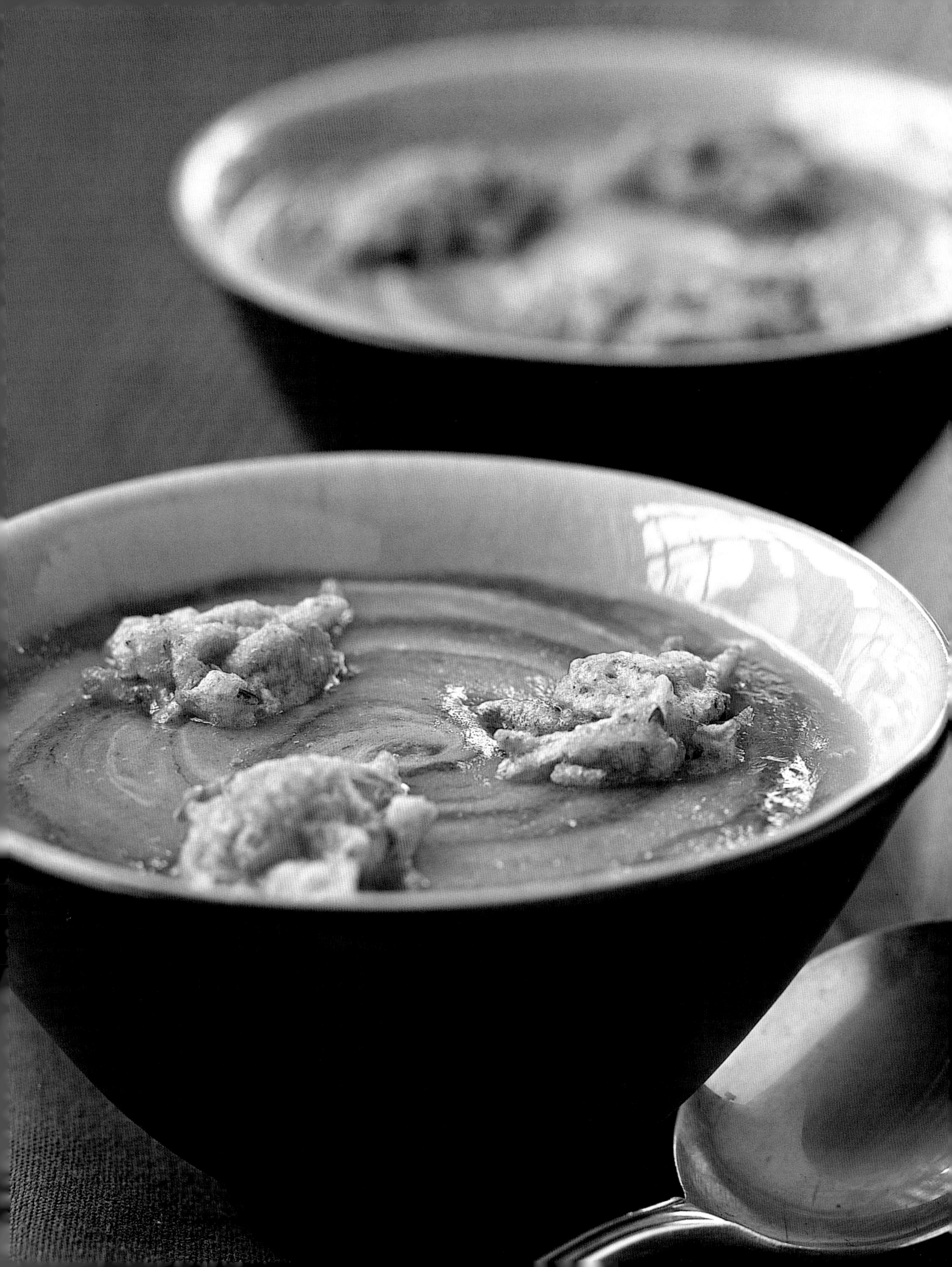

hot tommy

Packed with **vitality**, **energy** and valuable nutrients, this tomato-based, almost soup-like beverage is like an instant shot in the arm. Easily digested and with a savoury tang to please even the most jaded of palates, it will soon be on your list of favourites.

300ml or 10 fl oz vegetable stock (page 252)
200ml or 7 fl oz milk
1 x 400g can tinned, crushed tomatoes
1 large onion, finely grated
20g or 3/4 oz sago

Put all the ingredients into a large pot or saucepan, and simmer for one hour. Strain and serve in mugs.

Serves 4

Tomatoes are the richest sources of the nutrient **lycopene**. This member of the **carotenoid** family is one of the most protective of all the phytochemicals and will quickly boost your lowered vitality. Sago is a quickly digested **energy source**, providing the healthiest form of carbohydrates.

carrotiander soup

A variation on a traditional soup recipe. The combined flavours of basil and coriander, and the calcium-rich smoothness provided by the crème fraîche give this easily digestible soup a completely new dimension. It's a calming and effective **feel-good dish** that tastes great, too.

1 medium onion, finely chopped
2 tbsp extra-virgin olive oil
900g or 2lb carrots, finely cubed
½ tsp dried basil, plus 10 large fresh leaves, roughly torn, for garnish
½ tsp dried coriander, plus 5 fresh leaves, roughly torn, for garnish
1 litre or 35 fl oz vegetable stock (page 252)
250ml or 8 fl oz carton crème fraîche

Sweat the onion gently in the oil for five minutes. Add the carrots and dried herbs, stir thoroughly, and continue sweating for fifteen minutes, stirring occasionally.

Pour in the stock, bring back to the boil and simmer until the carrots are soft but not mushy. Liquidize using a mouli or blender, or cool slightly, put through the food processor, and gently reheat.

Serve with a dollop of crème fraîche and garnish with fresh herbs.

Serves 4

Enormously rich in **betacarotenes**, this dish is a valuable protector against heart and circulatory disease and some cancers. Its mood-enhancing properties come from the eugenol in basil and the **coriandrol** from coriander.

good-mood green salad

A soothing salad that gently lifts the spirits and clears the mind. With parsley, sage, rosemary and thyme – sounds like a folk song, but our ancient forebears knew plenty about the **mood-boosting** benefits of these extraordinary herbs. They weren't used for flavour alone but for their medicinal properties as well.

a good selection of mixed green salad leaves

1 handful each fresh basil, chives, parsley, mint, sage and thyme

2 tbsp extra-virgin olive oil

juice of ½ lemon

Wash and thoroughly dry all the leaves. Remove the leaves from the herbs, then wash and dry. Tear the basil into small pieces. Snip the chives with scissors. Chop the parsley, mint and sage. Mix the thyme leaves with all the other herbs.

Mix together the olive oil and lemon juice. Add the herbs to the leaves and combine thoroughly. Add the dressing and toss very lightly – just enough to coat the leaves.

Serves 4

The calming power of basil, the soothing effects of all types of lettuce and the mind-clearing power of mint, combined with the memory-boosting benefits of sage, make this beautifully light salad a mental marvel.

traditional tabbouleh

Keep blood-sugar levels on course for a **calm**, assured day. This staple salad comes from Lebanon, although there are many variations throughout the Middle East. You can vary this recipe to suit your personal tastes. The basic ingredient is bulgur wheat, sometimes known as burghul or cracked wheat.

150g or 5½ oz bulgur wheat

2 garlic cloves, peeled and finely chopped

6 tbsp extra-virgin olive oil

juice of 1 lemon

2 ripe plum tomatoes, coarsely chopped

½ cucumber, peeled and chopped

4 spring onions, finely sliced

4 tbsp chopped flat-leaf parsley

4 tbsp chopped fresh mint

freshly ground black pepper

Stand the bulgur wheat in a bowl of cold water for half an hour. Mix the garlic with the olive oil and lemon juice, and leave to marinate while you prepare the rest of the salad.

Strain the bulgur wheat, getting it as dry as possible, then put into a serving bowl. Add the tomato, cucumber, spring onions, parsley and mint.

Add the garlic dressing and stir thoroughly. Season with plenty of freshly ground black pepper. Cover tightly with cling film. It will taste good in an hour or two, but fantastic if you leave it until the next day.

Serves 4

Bulgur wheat has a delicious nutty flavour and is rich in **protein** and **B vitamins**. What's more, it is a good source of slow-release energy, which will keep your blood sugar – and your moods – on an even keel.

protein plus

A delicious, quick-and-easy salad that **boosts brain function** with plenty of good protein and vital essential minerals.

300g or 10½oz full-fat cottage cheese, preferably organic

freshly ground black pepper

1 large stick celery, with leaves if possible, thinly sliced

10 radishes, quartered

½ green pepper, deseeded and cubed

100g or 3½oz chopped walnuts

Put the cottage cheese into a large bowl and season with black pepper.

Add the celery, radishes and pepper to the cottage cheese, mix together, then sprinkle the walnuts on top.

Serves 4

Cottage cheese is rich in **protein** – important for brain function – and easily digested. Add it to the walnuts for more protein, **minerals** and **essential fats**, and the celery for its cleansing action, and you couldn't find a quicker or easier mood booster.

upbeet herbal salad

An unusual salad, with **mood-enhancing** properties. This creamy pink mixture brings a blaze of colour as an unusual starter, a light lunch with wholemeal bread, a side dish or an accompaniment to a barbecue. It has the added piquancy of horseradish, a popular combination in Eastern Europe.

700g or 1lb 8oz cooked beetroot, preferably baby bulbs

grated zest and juice of ½ lemon

1 tsp fresh horseradish, grated (or 2 tsp ready-made sauce)

1 heaped tbsp chives, finely snipped

1 tsp tarragon, finely chopped

1 tsp lemon balm, finely chopped

1 x 250ml or 8 fl oz carton natural, live yogurt

Cut the beetroot into chunks – or slice it, if it's large enough.

Sprinkle with the lemon juice and stir in the zest.

Stir the horseradish and herbs into the yogurt and pour this mixture over the beetroot.

Leave for one hour to allow the flavours to combine.

Serves 4

Lemon balm is a traditional antidepressant and heart tonic, and the **phytochemicals** in tarragon are calming and sleep-inducing. The blood-building benefits of beetroot and **probiotic bacteria** in the yogurt give this recipe health-promoting properties.

aromatherapy salad

A **calming combination** that benefits the senses. After all, aromatherapy doesn't just mean a special type of massage…

6 ripe organic tomatoes, thinly sliced
1 large red onion, thinly sliced
4 tbsp extra-virgin olive oil
1 generous bunch fresh basil
freshly ground black pepper
chunks of crusty organic wholemeal bread

Layer the tomato and onion in a fairly large shallow dish. Pour on the olive oil. Tear the basil into small pieces and sprinkle over the top. Season with the pepper.

Serve with the bread, making sure you leave a bit left over to mop up the succulent mixture of oil and tomato juices.

Serves 4

The benefits of this wonderful treatment come from a combination of touch and smell. This mood-boosting salad assaults your olfactory senses with the pungency of onion and the heavy, sweet scent of basil. You'll hardly have to eat it to feel better.

old wives' salad

A **mood-booster** for the brain, filled with slow-release energy. As usual, the old wives are right as far as this tale is concerned: fish really is good for your brain. In this salad, it's even more beneficial, due to all the B vitamins and slow-release energy of oatmeal.

6 tbsp fine oatmeal
750g or 1lb 10oz fresh whitebait
1 good head lollo rosso
½ iceberg lettuce, shredded
rapeseed (canola) oil, enough for deep frying
3 tbsp chilli oil
1 tbsp real malt vinegar
2 tsp runny honey

Put the oatmeal into a large plastic bag. Add the whitebait and shake vigorously until all the fish are well coated.

Spread the leaves of the lollo rosso over the bottom of a serving dish, and pile the iceberg on top.

In a deep frying pan, heat the rapeseed oil, add a handful of whitebait and cook until crisp – approximately two to three minutes. Drain on kitchen paper. Repeat until all the fish are cooked.

Pile the whitebait on top of the lettuce. Mix together the chilli oil, vinegar and honey, and pour over the salad.

Serves 4

Using chilli oil provides an enormous boost to the circulation, thanks to the **capsaicin** that chillies contain, so the brain is guaranteed all the blood it needs to keep it – and you – happy.

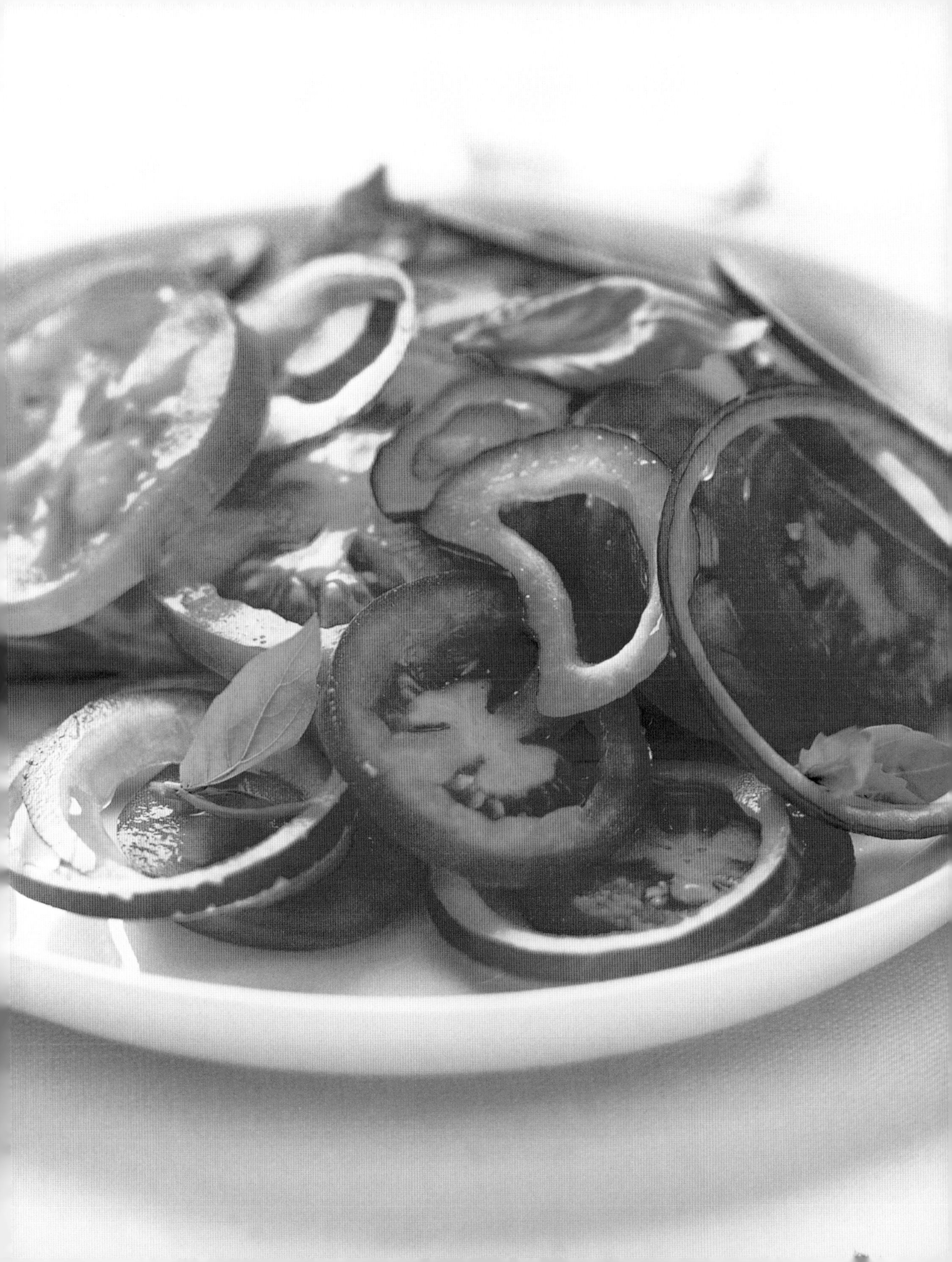

smokie soup

This unusual combination of porridge and smoked mackerel gives a **massive mood boost**. In addition to the slow-release energy from the porridge oats and the protein content of the fish, the garlic, leeks and onion add flavour and loads of protective phytochemicals.

4 tbsp extra-virgin olive oil
2 onions, finely chopped
2 leeks, washed and finely chopped
1 garlic clove, peeled and finely chopped
1 large carrot, trimmed and peeled if not organic, grated
1 large potato, peeled and grated
500ml or 18 fl oz each fish stock (page 253) and water
4 smoked mackerel fillets, skinned
55g or 2oz unsalted butter
100g or 3½oz fine porridge oats
4 tbsp double cream

In a large saucepan, sweat the vegetables gently in the oil until soft – about ten to fifteen minutes. Add the stock and water mixture and simmer for fifteen minutes.

Poach the mackerel fillets with the butter and just enough water to cover them for about six minutes. Pour the poaching liquid into the stock.

Flake the fish, add to the soup and stir in the oats. Remove from the heat, cover and leave to stand for ten minutes.

Serve with one spoonful of cream in each bowl.

Serves 4

To boost energy and mood. Mackerel provides **essential fatty acids**, while porridge oats are rich in **B vitamins** and soluble fibre. Olive oil provides **vitamin E**.

rosemary salmon

The essential fatty acids in oily fish are vital for brain development, and since the time of ancient Greece, rosemary has been used as an all-round mental tonic. Besides **aiding memory**, it also helps **lift depressive moods**. Food for thought, indeed!

4 salmon steaks
2 tbsp rosemary oil
8 lemons, thinly sliced
4 generous sprigs dried rosemary
1 medium onion, thinly sliced
2 tbsp dry white wine

Rub both sides of the fish with rosemary oil. Place in a baking tray lined with a piece of foil large enough to fold over the top of the fish. Put two slices of lemon and a sprig of rosemary on each steak. Drizzle with a little more oil, surround the fish with the sliced onion and sprinkle with white wine.

Seal the foil parcel loosely and place in an oven preheated to 190°C (375°F/gas mark 5) for twenty minutes.

Serves 4

The **volatile oils** in the rosemary act specifically on the brain, clearing muddled or tired heads. This recipe is also ideal for anyone with arthritis, gout or rheumatism, as it's rich in **essential fatty acids** that have natural anti-inflammatory properties.

canard aux herbes

The unusual combination of saffron and anise is a perfect complement to the rich, meaty duck. The **memory-enhancing** benefits of rosemary, the increased libido generated by anise and the general **mood-improving** properties of saffron make this the perfect meal to mend lovers' quarrels.

4 duck breasts, skinned, preferably organic
150ml or 5 fl oz extra-virgin olive oil
4 tbsp white wine or sherry vinegar
4 large sprigs oregano
2 large sprigs rosemary
4 anise seeds, crushed
1 pinch saffron

Remove any tendons from the duck breasts.

Mix together the rest of the ingredients and pour over the duck breasts. Leave to marinate for at least two hours.

Cook the duck breasts under a grill preheated to high for seven minutes each side, basting frequently with the marinade.

Serves 4

High in protein and low in fat, duck is a good source of **iron** and **B vitamins**. Rosemary's **volatile oils** enhance memory, anise provides aphrodisiac properties, and saffron and oregano contains substances to lift the spirits.

hearty herring

Traditional herring with lemon, olive oil and fennel leaves is given an interesting twist in this recipe by the addition of curry-plant and bay leaves. Due to its **spirit-lifting** effects, this makes a perfect meal if you're feeling a bit blue, but its nutritional value makes it equally good during pregnancy.

6 tbsp extra-virgin olive oil
3 tbsp white-wine vinegar
1 lemon, sliced
1 bunch fennel fronds
6 curry-plant leaves
2 bay leaves
4 herrings, filleted
2 tsp herb mustard, tarragon-flavoured

Mix together the oil, vinegar, lemon, fennel, curry-plant and bay leaves. Season the fish fillets to taste, then pour the oil mixture over them. Cover and marinate in the fridge for at least three hours.

Drain the fish, wipe dry and shallow-fry in olive oil for about four minutes each side.

Strain the marinade and heat through. Add the mustard to the marinade and pour over the fish to serve.

Serves 4

Bay's volatile oil laurenolide is a powerful mood-lifter. The **fenchone** in fennel helps regulate women's hormone levels, preventing mood swings. The combination of herbs with the herring's **essential fatty acids** makes this a perfect dish for affairs of the heart.

fruity duck salad

Packed with protein and energy for **good concentration**, this salad is substantial enough to be a meal, and the bit of extra work involved in making it is honestly worth the effort.

- 4 duck breasts, skin removed
- 300g or 10½oz chinese noodles
- 1 large ripe pawpaw, deseeded and sliced
- 2 ripe kiwi fruit, peeled and sliced
- 1 bag mixed salad leaves
- 3 tbsp peanut, rapeseed or safflower oil
- 1 tbsp rice vinegar
- 1 tsp light soy sauce

Put a large pan of water on to boil.

Bash the duck breasts gently to flatten them. Cook under a grill preheated to high for about three minutes each side, until they're just pink in the middle.

Meanwhile, put the noodles into the water. Cover a serving plate with the salad leave.

Strain the noodles and toss with the oil, vinegar and soy sauce. Pile the noodles on top of the leaves, then arrange the duck breasts on top of the noodles. Arrange the fruit around the plate, and enjoy!

Serves 4

The perfect combination of brain-activating **protein**, slow-release energy for extended concentration, **enzymes** to improve digestion and gently calming **phytochemicals**. This is the perfect lunch to prepare ahead of an afternoon of mental exertion.

minty lamb meatballs

The traditional Greek way of cooking with lamb, herbs and spices creates an amalgam of wonderful flavours as well as a unique and mind-altering aroma.

- 700g or 1lb 4oz lean lamb, minced
- 1 onion, large, very finely chopped
- 2 garlic cloves, very finely chopped
- 1 tsp oregano, dried
- 3 tbsp finely torn fresh mint leaves
- 3 tbsp flat-leaf parsley, chopped
- 1 tsp cumin
- 2 small eggs

In a large bowl, combine the lamb, onion and garlic until thoroughly mixed. Season to taste.

Combine the oregano, mint, parsley and cumin and blend into the lamb mixture. Beat the eggs and mix into the meat and herbs. Form the mixture into walnut-sized balls (makes approximately twenty) and refrigerate for one hour.

Transfer the meatballs into a greased baking dish. Cover with foil and cook in an oven preheated to 180°C (350°F/gas mark 4) for forty-five minutes. Remove the foil. Turn up the heat and cook for another ten minutes, shaking the dish until the meatballs are slightly crisp.

Serves 4

Rich in **protein** and **B vitamins** and a good source of **iron**, this recipe combines all the protective benefits of onions and garlic with the mood-enhancing **essential oils** of oregano and the mind-stimulating properties of mint.

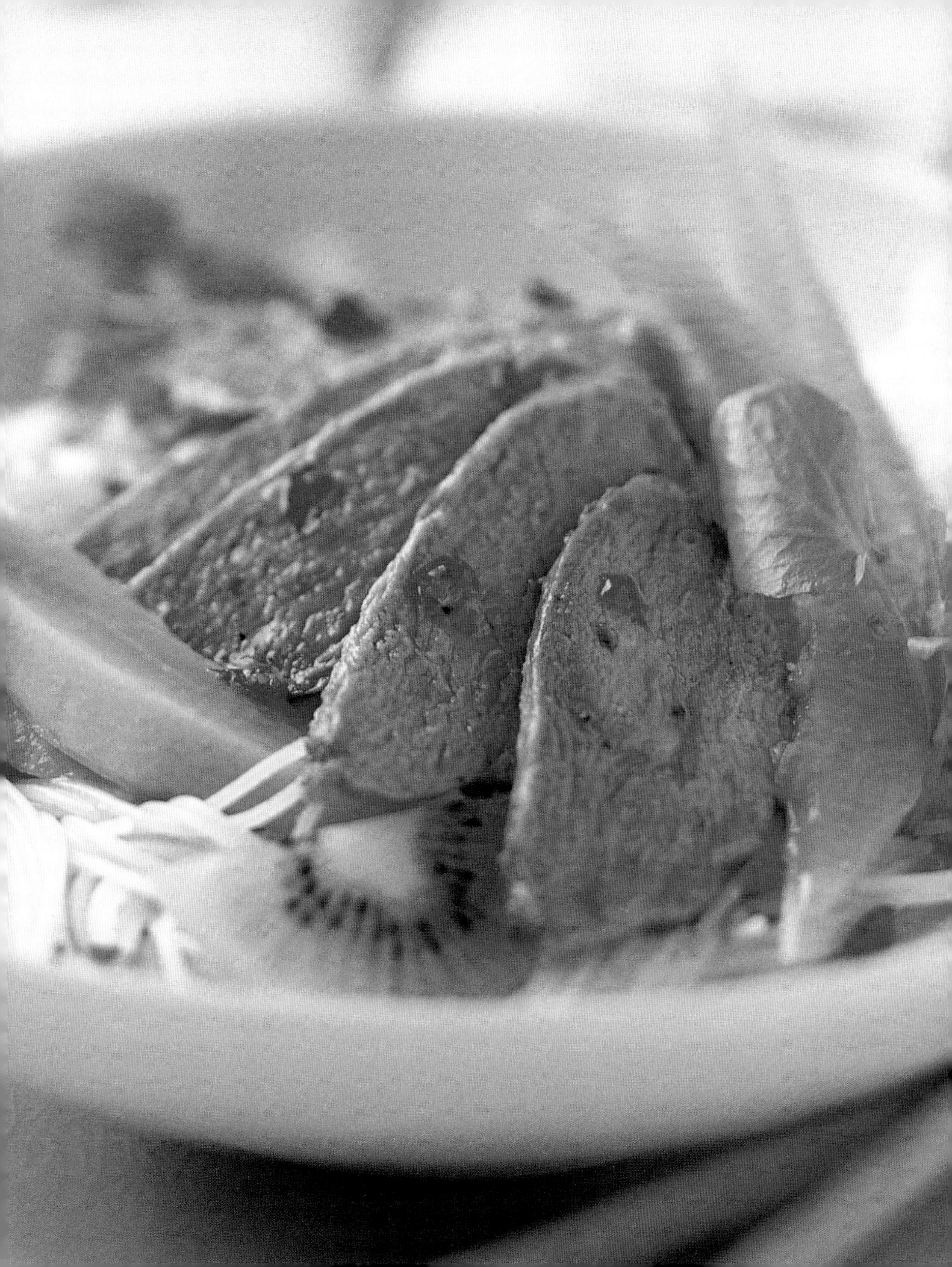

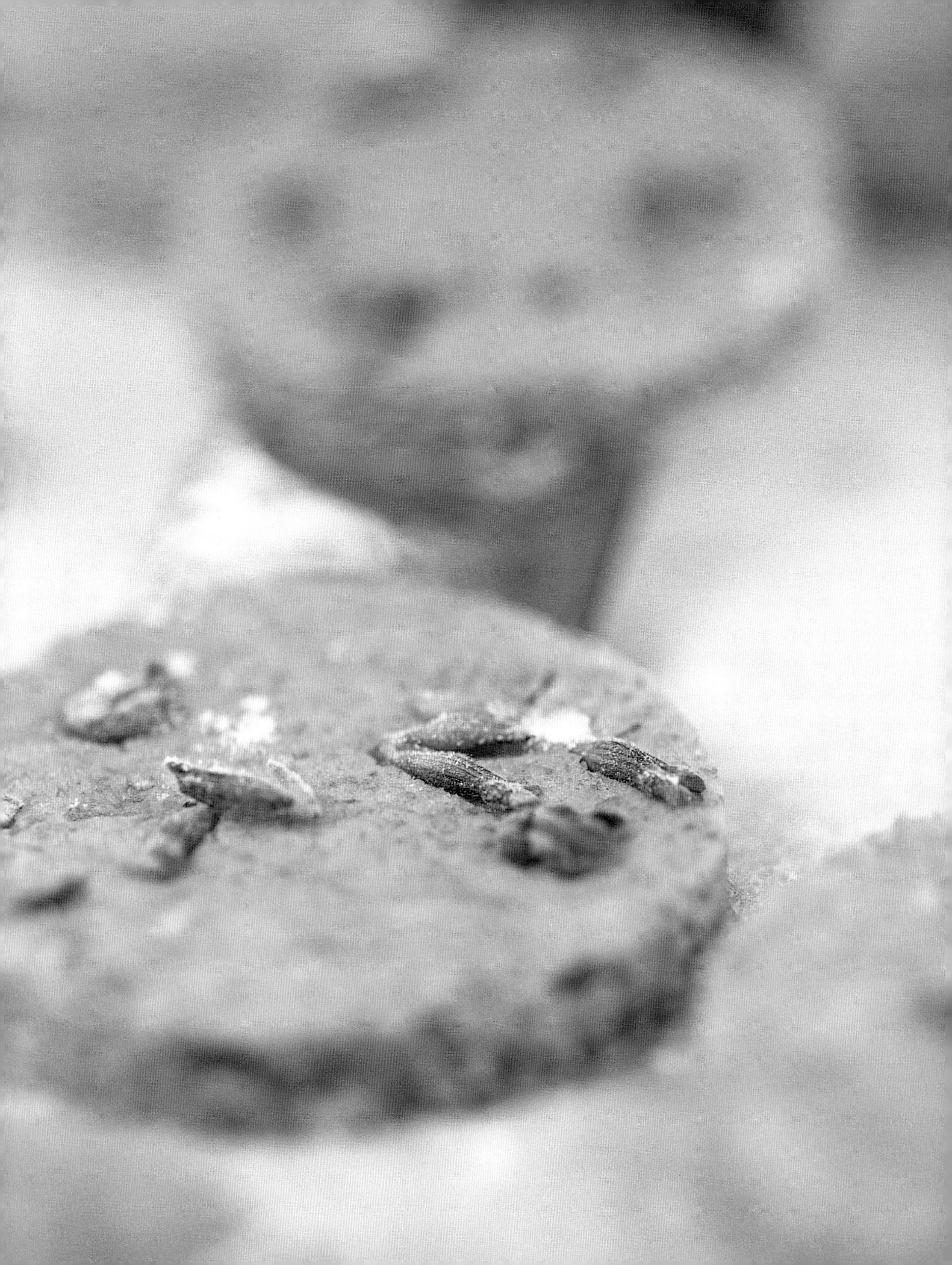

pancetta, onion and green lentil soup

Like all the legumes, lentils are rich in nutrients that fuel and maintain an even metabolism, which in turn promotes a **sense** of **well-being**. These components, together with exceptionally high levels of B vitamins and minerals from the other ingredients, make this a rich, filling and satisfying soup.

- 4 tbsp extra-virgin olive oil
- 1 large onion, very finely diced
- 1.2 litres or 40 fl oz chicken stock (page 253)
- 300g or 10½oz green lentils, preferably puy
- 250g or 9oz pancetta (or unsmoked bacon) cut in one piece, rind removed, finely cubed

In a large saucepan, sweat the onion gently in three tablespoons of the oil. Add the stock and bring to the boil. Pour in the lentils, rinsed if necessary.

Simmer until tender – about fifteen to twenty-five minutes, depending on the variety of lentils.

About five minutes before the soup is ready, fry the pancetta in the remaining oil until crisp and cooked through. Drain on kitchen paper. Serve the soup scattered with the pancetta cubes.

Serves 4

For good general nutrition. Lentils are an excellent source of **protein** and **complex carbohydrates**, both of which are necessary for good brain function.

lavender biscuits

Most people associate its sweet aroma with the garden, but lavender is also a great herb to use for flavouring food. Its ability to calm the **nervous**, relax the **stressed** and grant sleep to **insomniacs** is legendary. Once you've tried these, you'll never want to eat bought biscuits again!

- 115g or 4oz butter
- 55g or 2oz caster sugar
- 175g or 6oz 75% wholemeal self-raising flour
- 2 tbsp lavender leaves, freshly chopped
- 1 tsp lavender flowers, removed from the stems

Cream the butter and sugar. Add the flour and lavender leaves and knead into a dough.

Roll onto a floured board, sprinkle with the flowers and press them into the dough with the rolling pin.

Cut into shapes and bake on a greased baking sheet in an oven preheated to 230°C (450°F/gas mark 8) for about ten minutes.

Makes a good dozen

The **protein**, **vitamins** and **fibre** in the flour, and the tremendous calming effects of lavender make them a far better (and more enjoyable) alternative to sleeping pills or tranquillizers. Lavender oil is also a traditional remedy for the relief of headaches.

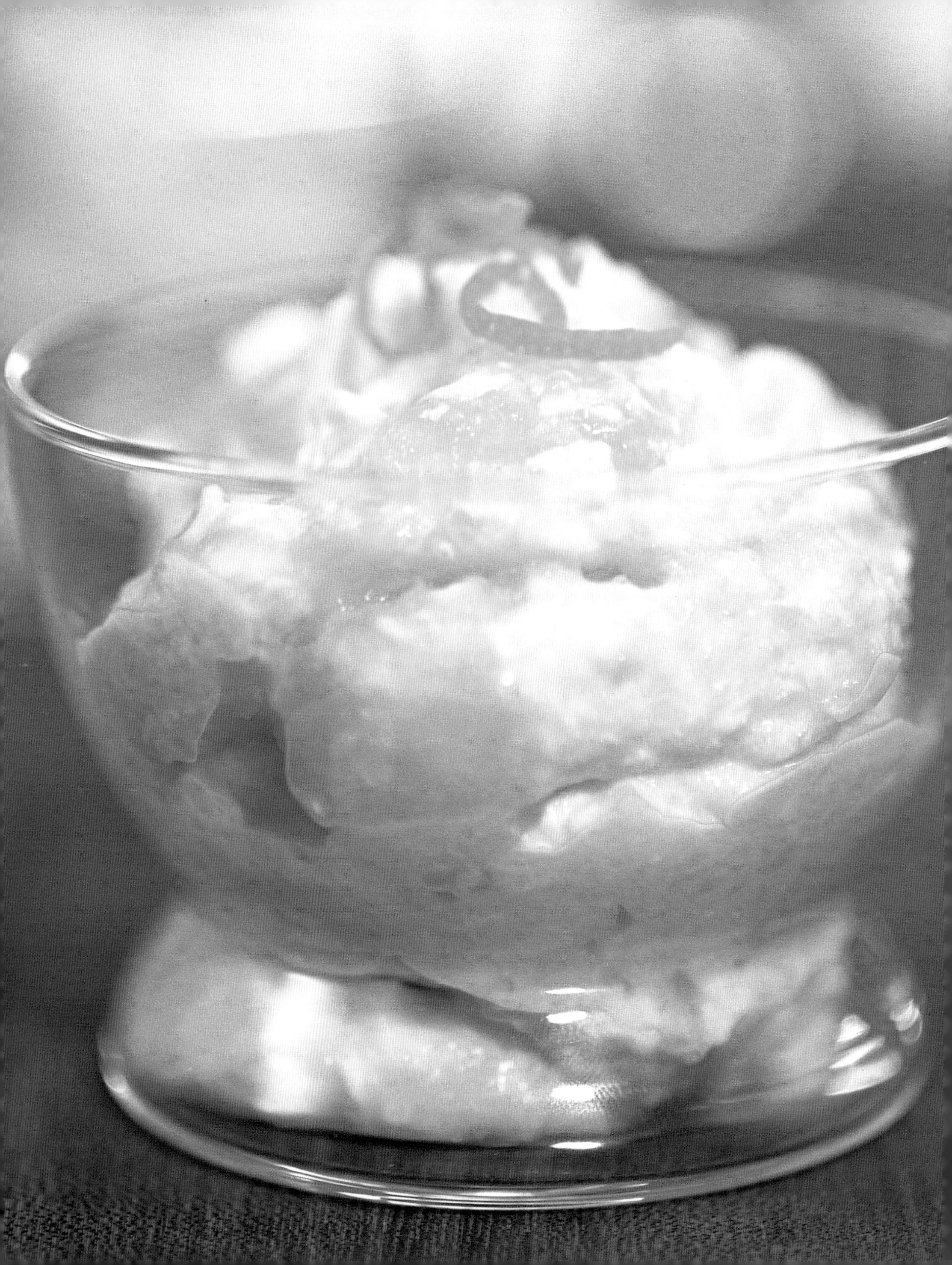

aromatic apples

The tartness of the Bramley cooking apple is unique to the British Isles, and it is this acidity that mixes so well with the Mediterranean flavours of hyssop, scented geranium and smooth mascarpone cheese. This recipe makes a great breakfast dish, as well as being an ideal source of easily digestible nutrients.

100ml or 4 fl oz water
60g or 2oz caster sugar
1 sprig hyssop
900g or 2lb peeled bramley apples, cored and sliced
500g or approx. 1lb mascarpone cheese
2 tsp scented geranium leaves, chopped

Pour the water into a saucepan. Add the sugar and hyssop and boil gently until the sugar is dissolved.

Remove the hyssop. Add the apples to the sugar mixture, cooking very gently over a low heat. When cooked to a smooth purée, fold in the mascarpone.

Place the mixture in individual dishes, sprinkle with geranium leaves and leave in the fridge to chill before serving.

Serves 4

The **aromatic oils** in apples contain substances that, when inhaled, act directly on the brain. Just smelling an apple can relieve migraines and lower blood pressure, so this combination is ideal to elevate your mood at the end of a meal. Hyssop is calming.

life saver

Just the juice to revive that sinking feeling! Of all lettuces, iceberg probably has the least amount of nutrients. However, it will keep well for two weeks if wrapped in clingfilm. It has a much sweeter flavour than other lettuces and contains the highest levels of **natural calming** substances.

3 apples, unpeeled, uncored and quartered
2 oranges, peeled leaving pith behind
1 lemon, unpeeled if thin-skinned
2 handfuls iceberg lettuce

Put all the ingredients through a juicer, mix well and serve.

Serves 1–2

Super-rich in **vitamin C** and **folic acid**, this juice also contains **vitamin A**, iron, calcium and masses of potassium. It is also a good source of protective flavonoids. Lettuce contains substances known as lactones, and was used by the ancient Assyrians as a mild sedative.

lemon and ginger tea

When you're feeling a bit low or run down, here's a quick fix that I really do recommend. The cleansing citrus flavour of lemon is an ideal combination with the tropical heat of ginger. Together they provide an almost **instant mood boost**, raising energy and **gingering up** the **circulation**.

2.5cm or 1in fresh ginger root, peeled and grated
600ml or 20 fl oz boiling water
1 lemon

Cover the grated ginger with the boiling water.

Add the juice of half the lemon and leave to cool.

Put in the fridge to chill.

Strain and serve with slices taken from the other lemon half.

Serves 2–3

Lemons provide more than **vitamin C**; they're also a rich source of **natural bioflavonoids**, which help strengthen and protect the walls of blood vessels. Add ginger's **essential natural oils**, and you'll benefit from one of the most effective stimulants in the herbal repertoire.

rosemary milk

Most people don't automatically associate milk with rosemary. After all, they don't fit together in the same way as, say, fish and chips or bread and jam. But when you're feeling low, getting over an illness or just under the weather, this drink will provide comfort, calmness and a **feeling** of **mental alertness**.

1 x 15cm or 6in stem rosemary
250ml or 9 fl oz milk

Break the rosemary into four pieces.

Put three of the pieces into a saucepan and add the milk.

Bring slowly to the boil and simmer for five minutes.

Press the rosemary against the side of the pan to extract the juices, then discard.

Serve with the reserved rosemary floating on top.

Serves 1

Rosemary is known as the herb of remembrance – and that's no coincidence. Its **natural chemicals** act as stimulants to the areas of the brain that control your memory, a fact well known to the ancient Greeks and Romans. The herb is also mood-enhancing, anti-inflammatory, antibacterial and stimulating.

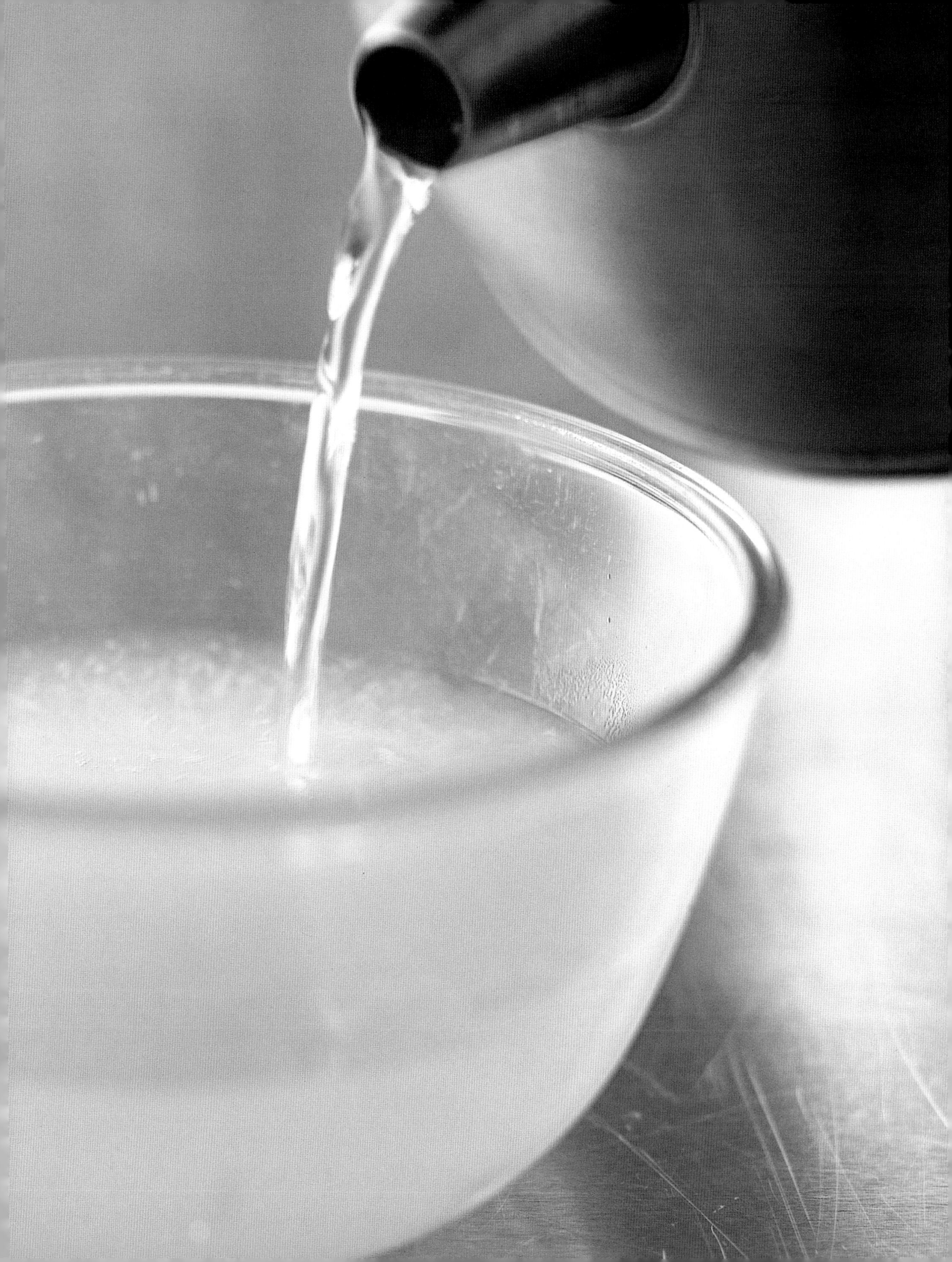

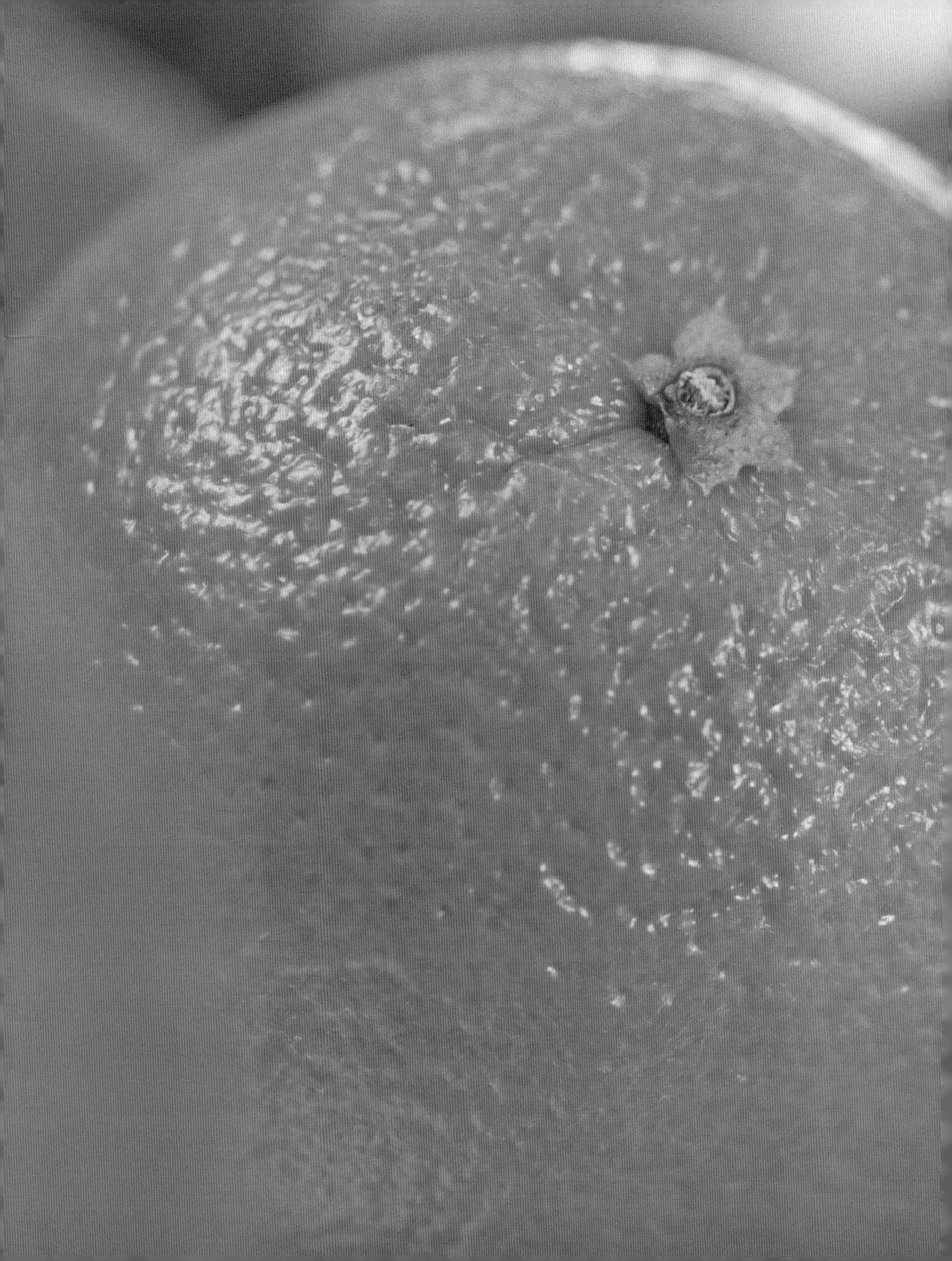

healing

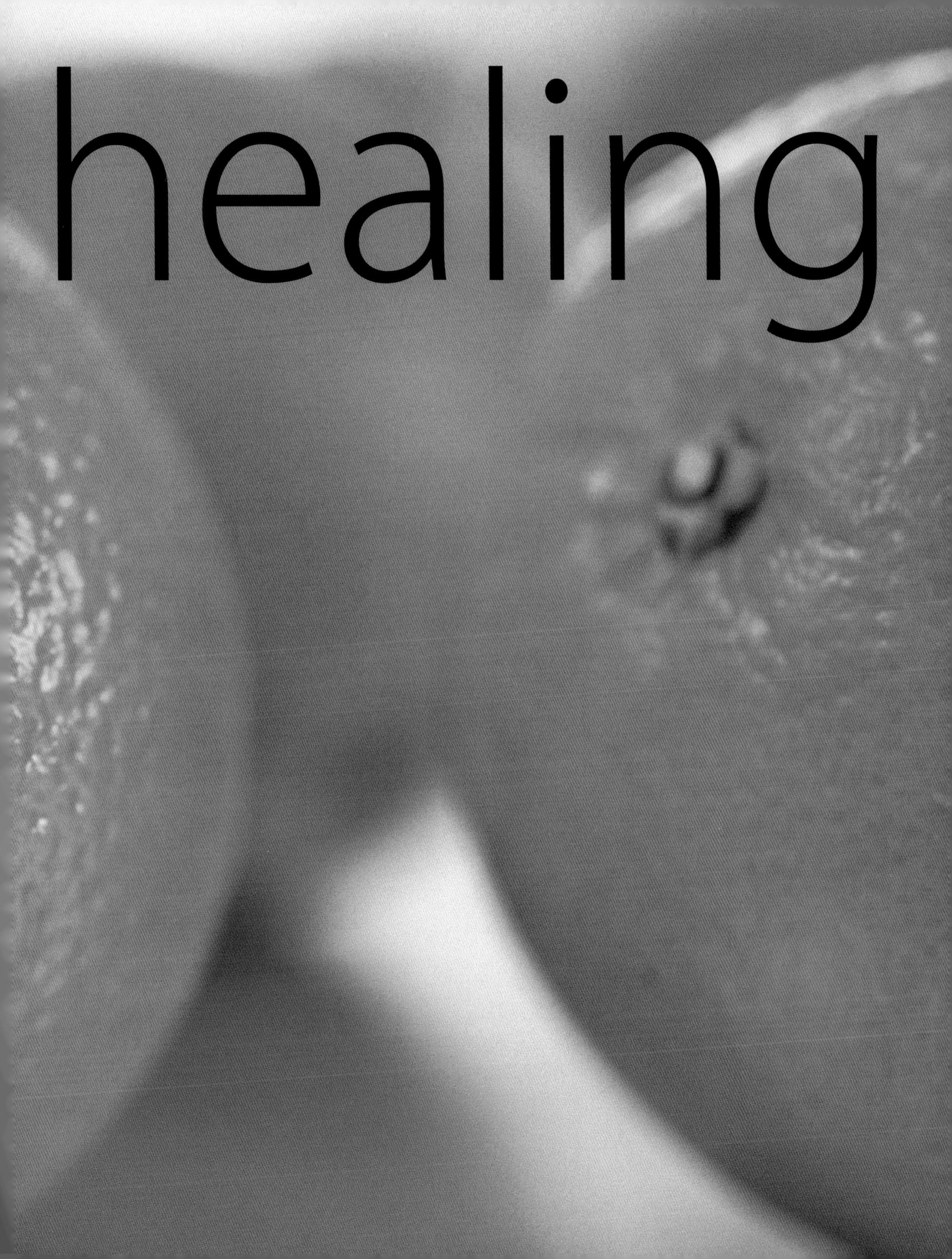

The human body has the most amazing ability to heal itself, yet it needs the right tools to do the job. Prevention is always better and easier than cure, but if your regular diet is rich in healing superfoods, then your chance of avoiding serious illness is greatly increased. This is particularly true in respect of the diseases of Western civilization: heart disease, high blood pressure, stroke, diabetes and many types of cancer, including lung, prostate and colon. In terms of healthy eating, it's what you do most of the time that really matters; the occasional treat, binge or gourmet holiday isn't going to do you any harm at all.

There's never a time when it's sensible to ignore the principles of following a diet made up predominantly of healing foods, because you never know when illness or accident might happen. A hospital bed is not the best place to get the wake-up call about your junk-food-eating habits. If your immune system is working well and you have a healthy level of the protective and healing foods in your system, then you are consuming a diet that increases your chances of a speedy recovery.

Convalescence used to be an integral part of all medical treatment. A period of time that allows recovery from illness or operation should still be considered an essential part of any cure. Nutritional needs depend on the type of illness, but the general principle is to include healing foods that are easily digestible, nutrient-rich, appetizing and easy to eat. The antioxidant vitamins A, C and E, protective minerals like zinc and a high intake of iron to ensure good haemoglobin are also essential.

Hospital diets are notoriously poor, especially in Britain. Virtually no fresh fruit; unappetizing, wilted salads, and overcooked vegetables kept warm for hours result in severe depletion of vitamin C. This in turn makes the patient more liable to infection, slower wound healing and the development of bed sores. A study by Professor John Garrow published in the *British Medical Journal* shows that the poor quality of hospital food doubles the number of days spent in hospital by elderly patients recovering from hip fractures. Observations on well-nourished older patients demonstrate that giving them a simple vitamin and mineral supplement daily shortens the time it takes for them to recover from infectious illnesses.

Traditionally, all cookery books used to contain a section on convalescent and invalid cookery, with recipes that included healing foods. It saddens me that this is no longer the case. So, unless you've got some of your grandmother's old cookery books, here are some ideas.

food to aid recovery

Breakfasts should include porridge, yogurt with honey and pine kernels, melon, soaked dried fruits with yogurt and cinnamon, wholemeal toast, boiled, poached or scrambled eggs. Lunches: white fish, oily fish, broccoli, spinach, carrots, free-range chicken, rosemary, thyme, garlic and sage. Evening meals: light salads; soups made with root vegetables, barley, and millet; fruit salads with almonds; low-fat cheeses and avocados. Extras: fresh fruit, especially grapes, dates, kiwi fruit, citrus fruits and berries, unsweetened fresh fruit juices, vegetable juices, dried fruit, fresh nuts, and seeds.

This is also the place for the wonders of "Jewish penicillin": chicken soup. That great antiviral, antibacterial, body-and-soul-healing recipe that's been passed from generation to generation really is a cure for colds, flu, chest infections and probably many other ailments. Made with real chicken, real vegetables, real herbs and, most of all, real *love*, it is a powerful healing food as confirmed by scientific studies.

healing foods checklist

• Eat more blackcurrants, berries, citrus fruits and kiwi fruit – rich in vitamin C and bioflavonoids; cabbage and all its relatives for the antibacterial sulphur and cancer-protective phytochemicals they contain; apples for their ability to help the body eliminate cholesterol and toxic residues. Opt for live yogurt for the immunity-boosting benefits of probiotic bacteria; dates for iron and easily converted calories; oats for protein, B vitamins, calcium, potassium and magnesium; fish for easily digested protein and minerals. Choose root vegetables, broccoli and carrots for betacarotene, dried fruits for energy and garlic, cinnamon, sage, rosemary and thyme for their antiseptic and circulation-stimulating properties.

• Eat fewer refined carbohydrates, less sugar and alcohol, and fewer high-bran foods, animal fats and red meat. Avoid convenience food, instant "just add water" products and nutritionally poor takeaways.

brussels sprout and stilton soup

A cornucopia of revitalizing, re-energizing and **restorative** nutrients! In addition to the benefits of the sprouts, onions and garlic, this soup contains a gentle cleansing action from the parsley, and lots of bone- and body-building calcium from the Stilton. By the way, it tastes absolutely fabulous, too.

4 tbsp extra-virgin olive oil

1 red onion, finely chopped

2 garlic cloves, peeled and chopped

2 celery stalks, finely chopped

1.3 litres or 45 fl oz vegetable stock (page 252)

500g or 1lb 2oz brussels sprouts, cleaned and peeled

300g or 10½oz stilton, rind removed and cubed

1 handful chopped parsley

In a large saucepan, heat the olive oil over a low heat. Add the onions, garlic and celery, and sweat gently for five minutes.

Add the stock and Brussels sprouts and simmer until the vegetables are tender – about fifteen minutes. Liquidize or blend until smooth.

Add the stilton, return to a simmer and cook until the cheese has melted. Serve immediately, with the parsley scattered on top.

Serves 4

A soup to revitalize the system. Brussels sprouts are rich in cancer-fighting **phytochemicals**. Garlic and onions are heart-protective and infection-fighting.

ajo blanco

This traditional garlic soup of southern Spain provides the **extreme healing** properties of garlic's sulphur compounds, combined here with the instant energy derived from natural grape sugars and the extra protein from the almonds. The result is a super-restorative bowl of strengthening nutrients.

170g or 6oz ground almonds

3 tbsp extra-virgin olive oil

4 garlic cloves, peeled and very finely chopped

100g or 3½oz white breadcrumbs

700ml or 25 fl oz water

250ml or 9 fl oz grape juice

100ml or 3½ fl oz natural, live yogurt

400g or 14oz seedless white grapes, halved and peeled

Mix together the almonds, oil and garlic thoroughly. Put into a food processor or blender and add half the breadcrumbs, half the water and half the grape juice. Whizz until completely combined. Pour into a clean bowl.

Put the rest of the water and grape juice into the processor or blender – no need to rinse it out. Add the yogurt, and pulse about five times until combined. Pour the yogurt mixture into the breadcrumb mixture and stir thoroughly. Leave in the fridge to cool for about an hour.

Serve garnished with halved grapes.

Serves 4

Serve this one for a speedy recovery. Garlic is antibacterial and antifungal. Live yogurt provides **probiotic bacteria** that help restore the immune system.

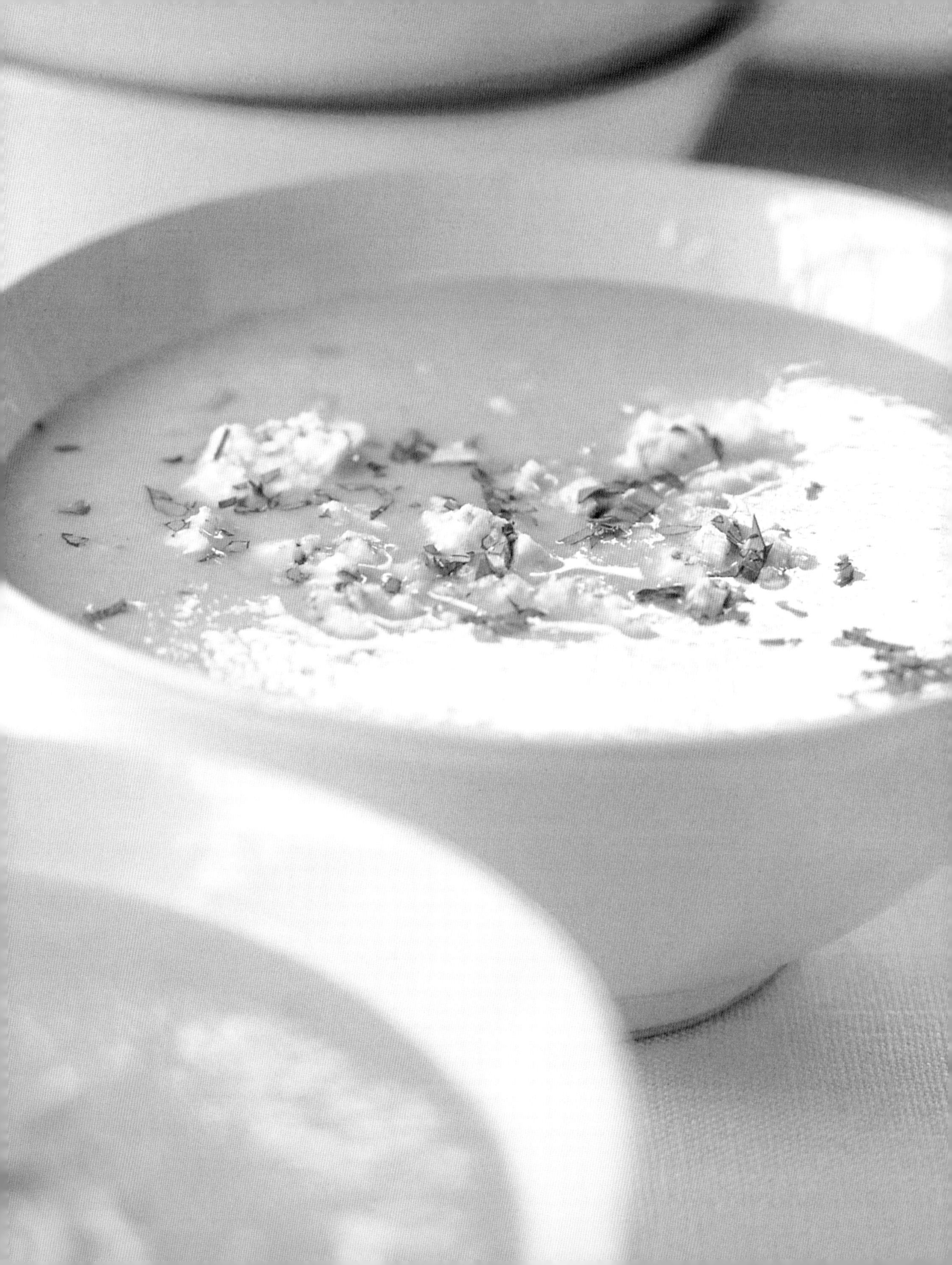

hauser broth

Back in the 1960s I met a fascinating man called Gaylord Hauser, an early pioneer of natural medicine and healthy eating in America. He created this recipe as part of his fasting regime, basing it on the **cleansing alkaline** soups that were part of the traditional European natural-health movement.

125g or 4½oz carrot, grated

125g or 4½oz celery, with leaves, all finely chopped

50g or 2oz spinach, shredded

1 litre or 35 fl oz water or vegetable stock (page 252)

125ml or 4 fl oz tomato juice

1 tsp honey

1 small handful chopped parsley or snipped chives, or a mixture of both

Simmer the vegetables in the water or stock for thirty minutes.

Add the tomato juice and honey and cook for five more minutes.

Liquidize or blend until smooth.

Serve garnished with the parsley or chives.

Serves 4

A soup to cleanse and heal the system. Celery and parsley are effective diuretics. Carrots contain healing **betacarotene**. Tomatoes are rich in **protective** lycopene.

butterbean, parsley and garlic soup

Butterbeans are a favourite of middle and southern Europe, as well as the southern United States. This soup is especially good when made with chicken stock, as this adds more **healing** enzymes. The vegetable option is almost as effective – it will provide more **skin-restoring** betacarotene.

4 tbsp extra-virgin olive oil

1 onion, finely chopped

2 garlic cloves, peeled and chopped

1.5 litres or 55 fl oz chicken or vegetable stock (pages 252–3)

2 x 400g cans butterbeans, thoroughly rinsed

2 large handfuls parsley, very coarsely chopped

In a large saucepan, heat the oil over a low heat. Add the onions and garlic and sweat gently until softened.

Add the rest of the ingredients. Simmer until the beans are slightly tender – about fifteen minutes.

Serves 4

This soup provides a welcome boost of slow-release energy. Butterbeans are rich in **protein**, **fibre**, slow-release energy, **B vitamins** and natural plant hormones that are a valuable aid to women. Parsley is gently diuretic.

mushroom and bean broth

When your body or mind – or worse, both – have been through the mill, there's no food quite so physically and emotionally **restorative** as this interesting broth. The subtle flavour and **immunity-boosting** benefits of mushrooms mix with the kidney beans to help kick-start the body's regulatory mechanisms.

- 25g or 1oz dried porcini mushrooms
- 2 stalks celery, roughly chopped
- 2 large leeks, trimmed, washed and chopped
- 1 large sprig sage
- 3 bay leaves
- 1 x 400g can kidney beans, thoroughly rinsed
- 200g or 7oz natural, live yogurt

Soak the mushrooms in 1.5 litres or 55 fl oz freshly boiled water for fifteen minutes. Strain them, reserving the liquid, and chop them coarsely. Pour the liquid into a large saucepan and bring back to a simmer.

Add the celery, leeks, sage and bay leaves. Simmer for another fifteen minutes. Strain again and reserve the liquid.

Add the kidney beans and chopped mushrooms and heat for ten minutes.

Stir in the yogurt and serve.

Serves 4

To soothe both mind and body. Kidney beans are a source of **protein**, restorative energy and **natural plant hormones**. Sage contains **essential oils** that ease digestion and help regulate moods.

leek and lentil soup

Like all members of the *Allium* genus of plants, leeks have a long and effective history in the folklore of **healing** foods. They've been used as a medicinal food since the time of the ancient Romans, and are valued just as much today. If you're recovering from a cold, flu or bronchitis, then this is the soup to choose.

- 1.5 litres or 55 fl oz vegetable stock (page 252)
- 200g or 7oz puy lentils
- 1 tbsp extra-virgin olive oil
- 200g or 7oz organic back bacon, cut into thin shreds
- 3 large leeks, trimmed, washed and very finely chopped
- 2 garlic cloves, peeled and chopped
- matzo dumplings (page 162)

In a large saucepan, heat the vegetable stock, then pour in the lentils. Leave them to cook for about twenty minutes.

Meanwhile, in a separate pan, gently heat the olive oil and sweat the bacon for five minutes. Add the leeks and garlic. Heat very gently until softened.

Once the lentils are tender, add the vegetables and bacon to the stock. Add the matzo dumplings and simmer for fifteen minutes.

Serves 4

Make this soup to heal throat and chest infections. Leeks contain **antibacterial phytochemicals**, while lentils supply easily digested protein and the essential trace minerals **zinc** and **selenium**.

broad bean, tomato and sage salad

A bundle of nutrients for a **natural lift**. Throughout the Mediterranean, broad beans are known as fava beans, and many imaginative recipes use them fresh, raw, cooked and dried to provide a huge source of nature's nutrients.

400g or 14oz shelled broad (fava) beans, fresh or frozen

10 sun-dried tomatoes

10 fresh purple sage leaves

1 handful sage flowers (optional)

2 tbsp pumpkin seeds

3 tbsp standard salad dressing

Cook the beans in unsalted boiling water until just tender. Plunge them into ice-water to cool and freshen. Chop the sun-dried tomatoes coarsely. Wash and dry the sage and tear into small pieces. Mix together all the above ingredients in a shallow dish.

If you're lucky enough to grow your own sage, sprinkle the flowers on top. Add the pumpkin seeds. Add the dressing and leave to marinate for at least one hour before serving.

Serves 4

As well as fibre, fava beans are rich in **protein**, they contain no fat, offer loads of **potassium** and they're a good source of **selenium**, **zinc** and **iron**. In this dish, you'll also get mind-improving **volatile oils** in sage, and lycopene from the sun-dried tomatoes.

bean sprout booster

Bean sprouts and seeds of all types should be high on your list of favourites if you're in need of a **quick burst** of restoration. All sprouts are a wonderful source of vitamins and minerals.

1 bag of bean sprouts

1 bunch of watercress

200g or 7oz shelled walnuts, coarsely chopped

2 white onions, coarsely chopped

½ ripe avocado, peeled and stone removed

2 tbsp walnut oil

1 tbsp rice vinegar

1 tsp light soy sauce

Freshly ground black pepper, to taste

Place the bean sprouts, watercress, walnuts and onions in a bowl.

Mash the avocado together with the walnut oil, vinegar and soy sauce, add the dressing to the bowl.

Toss well and season with black pepper to taste.

Serves 4

The **enzymes** contained in seeds and sprouts help to enhance the body's absorption of essential substances. Adding walnuts increases the amount of **B vitamins** provided by this salad, as well as offering the extra benefits of **essential fatty acids** and protein.

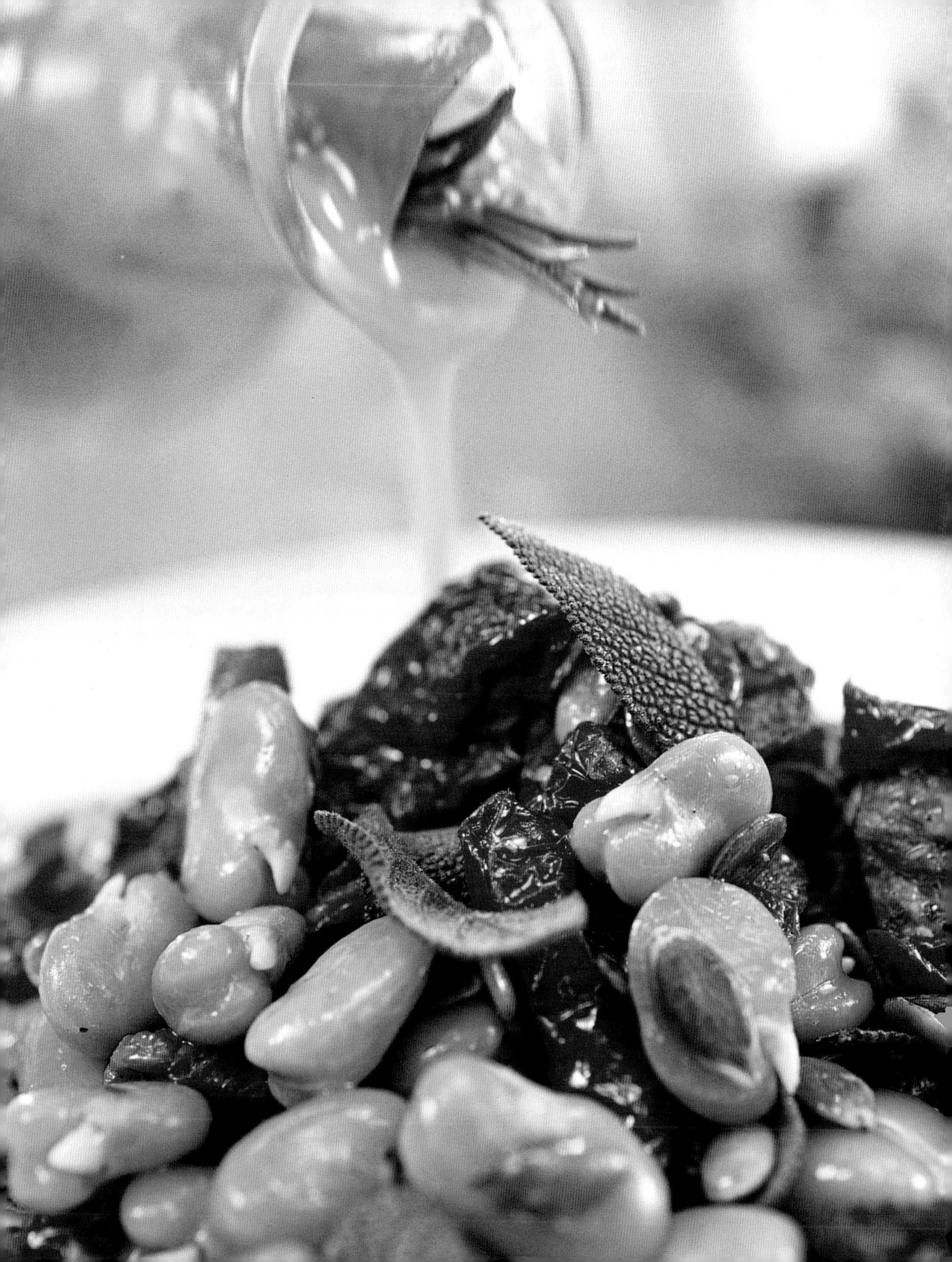

chicken soup with matzo dumplings

There cannot be a more renowned natural "kitchen medicine" than this traditional Jewish chicken soup. Used as the key to **recovery** by generations of mothers and grandmothers, it is surprisingly easy to make, and its soothing flavour makes it ideal as a first choice for any recovery programme.

- 100g or 3½oz unsalted butter
- 2 organic eggs, beaten
- 4 tsp parsley and mint, chopped
- 90g or 3¼oz matzo meal
- 4 tbsp warm water
- 2 litres or 40 fl oz chicken stock (page 253)

Mix all the ingredients, except the stock, thoroughly. Leave covered in the fridge for about two hours. Bring the stock to a gentle simmer.

Roll the refrigerated mix into eight balls – and don't worry if they're very moist. Drop them into the stock.

Bring back to a simmer. Leave to simmer for about fifteen minutes.

Serves 4

A great recovery soup. Chicken provides **healing enzymes**, **B vitamins** and minerals. Eggs are rich in restorative vitamin E.

luscious mulligatawny

Like many dishes inherited from the days of the Raj, this soup is not only hot, spicy and **warming**, but nutritionally valuable as well.

- 4 tbsp extra-virgin olive oil
- 500g or 1lb 2oz mixed carrots, leeks, celery and parsnips, very finely diced
- 4 plump spring onions
- 2 large garlic cloves, peeled and finely chopped
- 4 tsp green curry paste
- 1.2 litres or 40 fl oz chicken stock (page 253)
- 1 mango, juiced, or 100ml or 3½ fl oz mango juice

Coat the vegetables and garlic in the oil and sweat them in a large, covered saucepan for ten minutes.

Add the curry paste and continue cooking for another ten minutes, stirring occasionally. Pour in the stock and simmer until the vegetables are tender.

Add the mango juice and heat through.

Serves 4

To warm and fortify the constitution. Leeks, garlic and onions supply protective **phytochemicals**. Carrots and mango juice provide vital betacarotene.

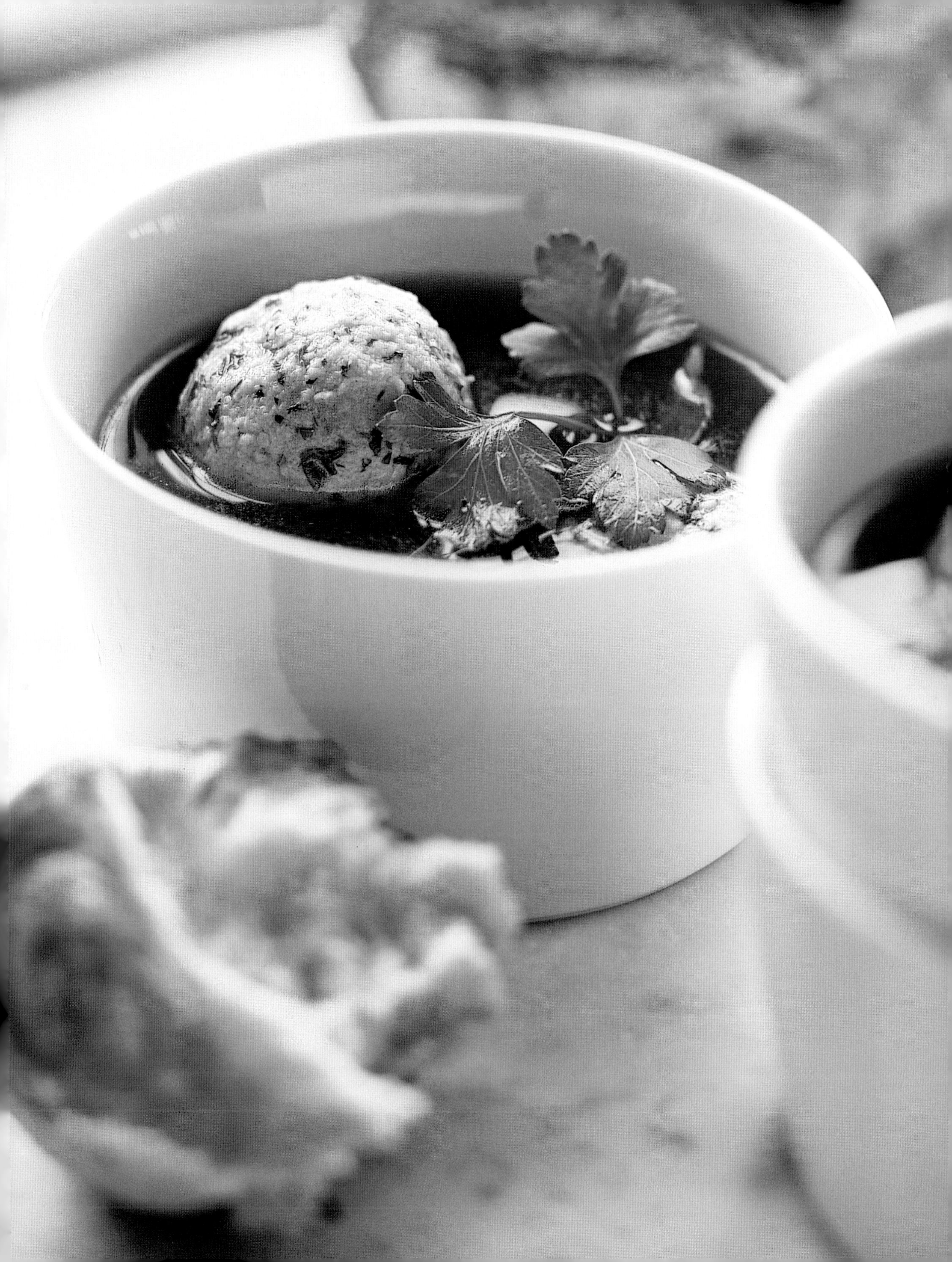

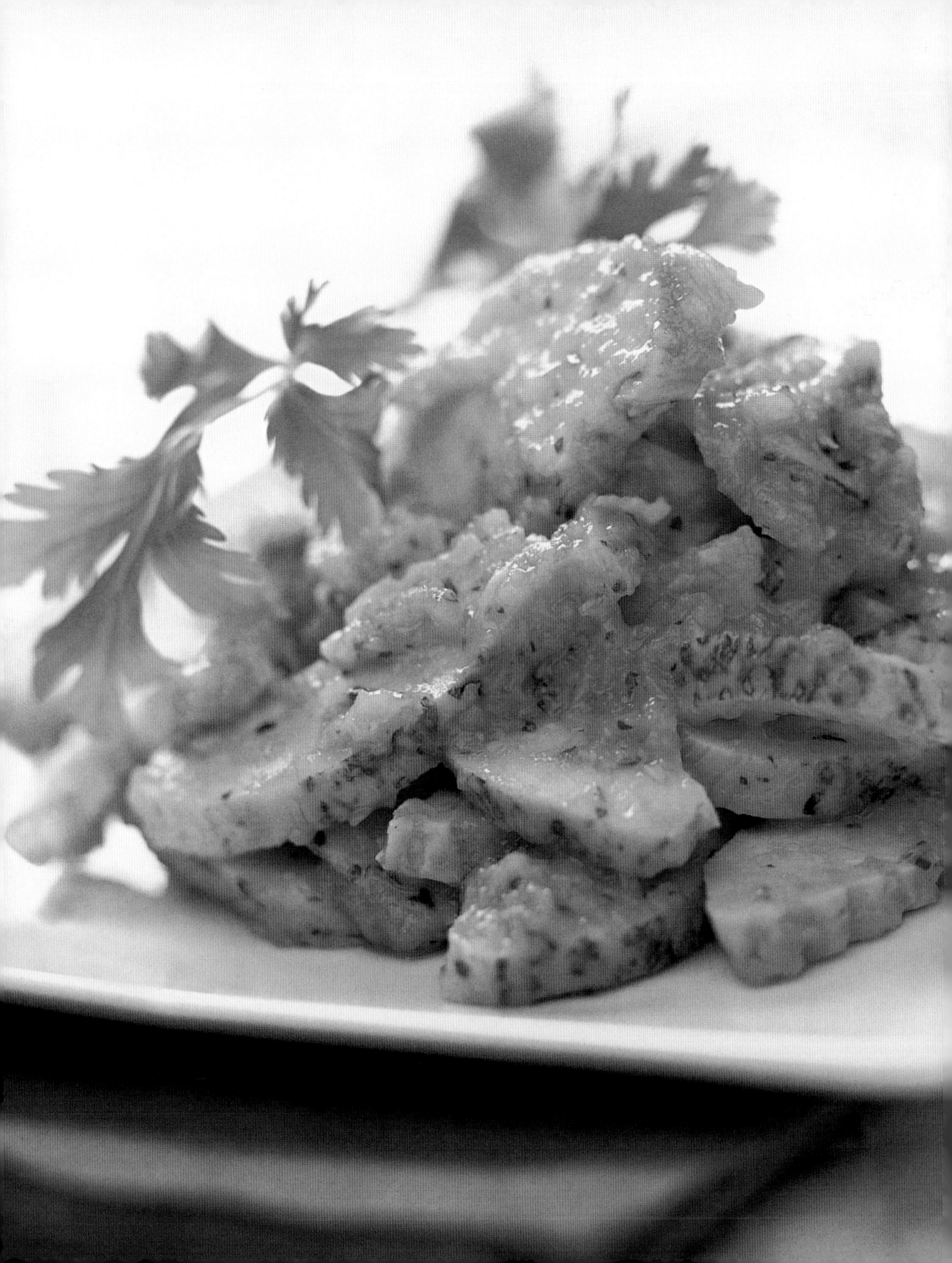

chicken and mango tango

Gives a **gentle boost** to the **brain** and **nervous system**. This is a special dish for me. Our friend Caroline made it for us when my wife, Sally, and I got married. Sally now makes it often, and it's a particular favourite for friends who were at our wedding and are now so welcome in our home.

1 large (or two small) ripe mangoes, peeled and stone removed

2 sticks celery, roughly chopped

2 limes, juiced

4 large spring onions, trimmed (leaving succulent green tips) and chopped

150ml or 5 fl oz extra-virgin olive oil

1 large bunch fresh coriander, washed and roughly chopped

1 medium-sized cooked chicken (or use the leftovers from yesterday's roast)

4 large leaves iceberg lettuce, washed

½ cucumber, peeled, halved, deseeded and diced

Put the mango, celery, lime juice and spring onions into a food processor or blender. Blend or process on a moderate speed. Add the olive oil gradually. Add half the coriander to the dressing without whizzing any further.

Remove all the white meat from the chicken (use the rest to make super-immune-boosting chicken soup) and take off any skin and extra fat.

Arrange the lettuce leaves on a plate. Sprinkle the cucumber pieces over the lettuce. Pile the chicken on top and pour on the dressing. Garnish with the rest of the coriander leaves.

Serves 4

Chicken is the perfect restorative food for the brain and nervous system, as it contains **B vitamins** as well as protein. Mangoes are a terrific source of betacarotenes, which are not only **protective antioxidants** but also converted by the body into **vitamin A**.

sauerkraut and caraway salad

Long before freezing, shredded cabbage was preserved with salt and fermentation to provide vitamin C during winter months. The beneficial bacteria that live in the **digestive** system are encouraged by the lactic acid formed during fermentation, increasing the amount of nutrients absorbed by the body.

500g or 1lb 2oz sauerkraut

2 tsp caraway seeds

2 tbsp safflower oil

1 tbsp cider vinegar

2 large old carrots, peeled and finely grated

1 tbsp chopped fresh parsley

Drain the sauerkraut. Mix in the caraway seeds.

Mix together the oil and vinegar and add to the carrots.

Put the carrots into the middle of a serving dish, arrange the sauerkraut around the outside and sprinkle with the parsley.

Serves 4

Restores digestive balance and increases nutritional uptake. Adding carrots provides a huge boost of **betacarotene**, while caraway seeds aid the digestion of sauerkraut and counteract its well-known flatulence factor.

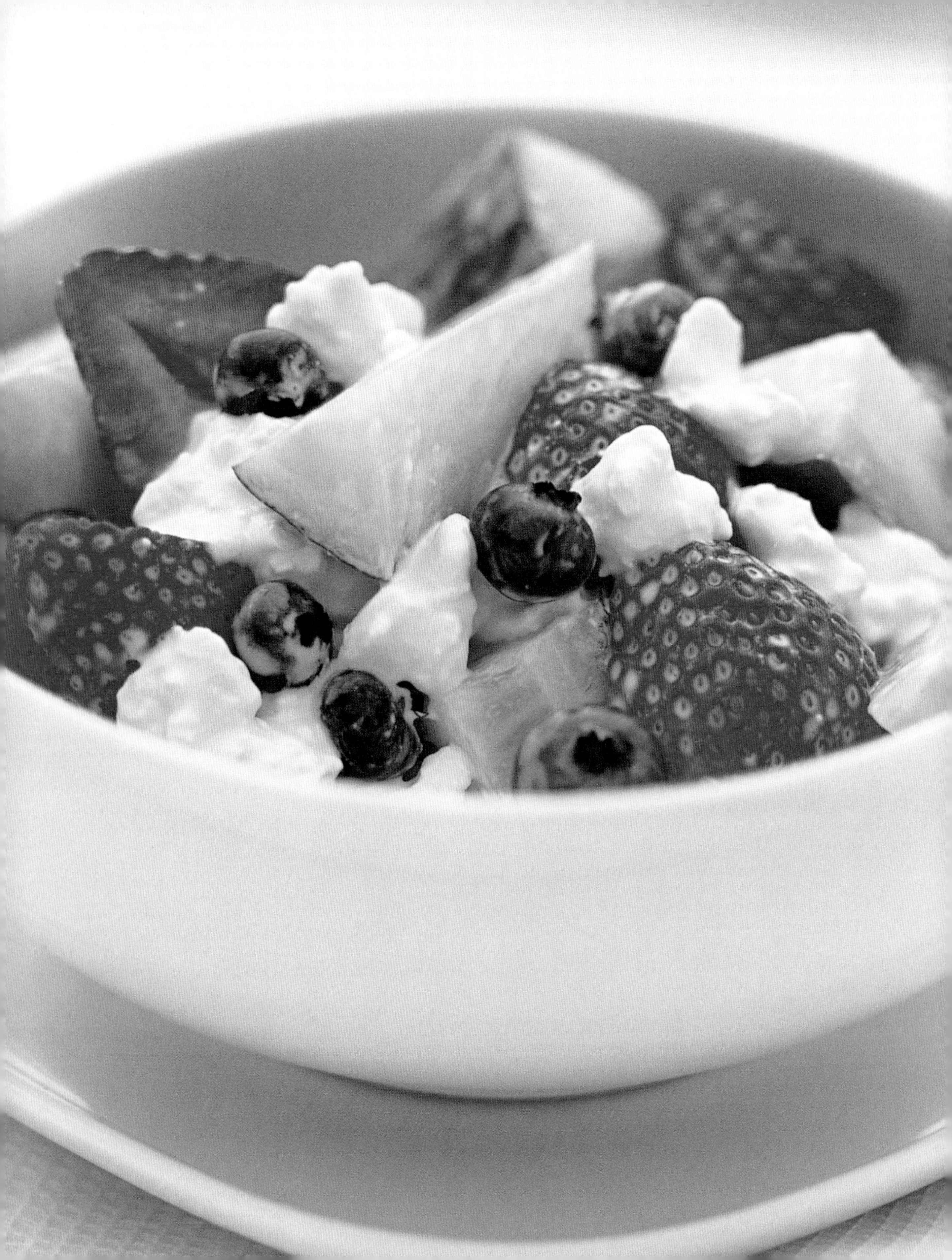

strawberry fare

An antioxidant cocktail for a quick **recovery**. Restoring your **immune system** is the key to quick recovery after any period of excessive stress or illness – and this is just the salad to give you a kick-start.

½ large cucumber, peeled, deseeded and diced

12 large ripe strawberries, quartered

300g or 10½oz blueberries

1 x 150g carton cottage cheese

juice 1 lime

1 tbsp extra-virgin olive oil

2 tsp balsamic vinegar

6 fresh mint leaves

Combine the cottage cheese, lime juice, oil and vinegar.

Wash and dry the mint. Arrange the cucumber in a serving bowl and scatter with the strawberries and blueberries. Add a large dollop of the cottage cheese dressing and mix lightly together.

Sprinkle with mint leaves, and serve.

Serves 4

Not only is this full of **vitamin C**, but the natural substances that give strawberries and blueberries their colour are among the most powerful of the immunity-boosting **antioxidants**. Add the easily absorbed **protein** from the cottage cheese, and you have a dish that appeals to the eye as well as the taste buds.

blueberry hill

An **extremely protective** drink that, thanks to the cranberries, is great for anyone with cystitis. For those with recurrent **urinary infections**, it is preventative as well as therapeutic. The natural pigments provided in every glass supply essential nutrients and protective phytochemicals.

115g or 4oz frozen cranberries

115g or 4oz fresh or frozen raspberries

100g or 3½oz fresh blueberries

200ml or 7 fl oz chilled sparkling mineral water

Defrost the frozen fruit.

Put all the ingredients through a juicer, or whizz in a blender or food processor until smooth.

Add the mineral water to taste.

Serves 1–2

Cranberries contain a natural form of vegetable mucilage that lines the walls of the urinary tract and bladder, preventing bacterial growth. As well as large quantities of **vitamin C** and **antioxidant** plant chemicals, you'll get **potassium** for the heart, and carotenoids for healthy skin and eyes, together with a powerful boost to your immune system.

a passion for fruit

Not only does this juice taste wonderful, it's a real morning eye-opener. It contains enough nutrients to fuel your body and provide nutritional **protection** for hours. Vitamins, minerals, and a vast array of plant-chemical protectors build your defences, nourish your tissues and protect every cell from potential damage.

6 medium strawberries

2 kiwi fruits, unpeeled

2 passion fruits, flesh scooped out

2 peaches, unpeeled and stones removed

1 pomegranate, flesh and seeds scooped out

175g or 6oz seedless grapes

Put all the ingredients through a juicer. Mix thoroughly and serve.

Serves 1–2

A glass of this juice will provide four times the daily requirement of **vitamin C**. **Betacarotene** and other carotenoids protect skin, vision and immune system. Kiwi fruit is rich in **potassium** and **bioflavonoids**, which protect the heart and blood vessels. Grapes provide antioxidants and natural fruit sugars.

liquorice and cinnamon booster

This healing drink combines some of the most ancient remedies known to man: soothing honey, lemon, cinnamon and the amazing properties of liquorice. For **fatigue**, **coughs**, **colds**, **flu**, **sore throats** and even **acid indigestion** and **heartburn**, this is the first choice in the sickroom.

1 piece liquorice about 1cm or ½in long

½ lemon, juiced

1 piece cinnamon about 1cm or ½in long

1 heaped tsp honey

Put the liquorice in a large mug. Cover with boiling water and leave until dissolved.

Add the cinnamon and lemon juice to the mug.

Stir in the honey.

Drink while still warm.

Serves 1

Liquorice extract is used in medicines and confectionery. **Essential chemicals** in the root are antibacterial, expectorant and healing to the mucous membranes of the mouth and throat. In the stomach it creates a protective gel that prevents acid damage and relaxes the digestive muscles.

the luck of the irish

Carrageen, a wonderful Irish moss, has an ancient history of both culinary and medicinal use. It is excellent as a vegetarian substitute for gelatine. This pleasant and satisfying drink is ideal for all **stomach** and **bowel** problems, and is an excellent remedy for heartburn and acid indigestion.

2 heaped tbsp carrageen moss (available from most health stores)

500ml or 18 fl oz boiling water

2 tbsp runny honey

½ unwaxed lemon

Rinse the moss well and put it in a heatproof bowl. Cover with cold water and leave for ten minutes.

Pour over the boiling water. Put into an oven preheated to its lowest setting at 110°C (225°F/gas mark ¼) for about two hours, topping up with boiling water if necessary.

Strain and stir in the honey. Juice the lemon, cut the rind into thin strips and stir the juice and rind into the moss mixture. Serve in mugs or heatproof glasses.

Serves 2

The **vitamin C** and antiseptic properties of lemon and the soothing, healing value of honey are well known. Carrageen is rich in healing **chlorophyll**, betacarotene and **trace minerals**. It's a wonderful restorative during or after any illness.

winter berry punch

Berries come top of the class in the health-promotion tables. They're the richest sources of the protective antioxidants, which **guard every cell** in the body, warding off damage and disease, especially cancer. Adding ginger and cinnamon gives a boost to the circulation, as well as a lift to the spirits.

350g or 12oz frozen or washed fresh mixed berries

600ml or 20 fl oz water

2.5cm or 1in fresh root ginger

4 cinnamon sticks

Put the berries in a saucepan. Add the water. Peel and bruise the ginger, but leave it in one piece and add to the pan. Bring slowly to a simmer and continue simmering for ten minutes.

Remove the ginger and strain the liquid through a sieve, pressing the fruit to extract all the juices. Warm through if necessary.

Serve with cinnamon sticks as stirrers.

Serves 4

This punch overflows with **vitamin C**, carotenoids and cancer-fighting phytochemicals. The **natural pigments** that give the berries their deep-red, -blue and -purple skins are some of the most powerful of all cancer-fighting substances.

blueberry and raspberry crush

One serving provides **more protection** from the ravages of free radicals than most people get in three days. Free radicals attack the body's individual cells, and this dangerous chemical activity is frequently the trigger for heart disease, joint problems, diminishing eyesight and cancer.

200g or 7oz blueberries
200g or 7oz raspberries
crushed ice

Put the fruit into a blender and whizz until smooth.

Serve in long glasses over the crushed ice.

Note: A dash of a spirit such as vodka could make this into a more adult drink.

Serves 1–2

A vitamin C-rich recipe, this crush is much more important for its exceptionally **high ORAC score**. ORAC stands for Oxygen Radical Absorption Capacity: a measure of food's ability to neutralize free radicals. The optimum ORAC score for a day is 5,000. A large glass of this provides almost 6,000 ORACs.

dandelion coffee

If we don't dig them up, mow them down or poison them, we let our pets loose all over them. What a tragic fate for the fabulous dandelion, one of the most valuable of all garden herbs and the easiest to grow! Note that dandelion root is an even stronger **diuretic** than the leaves.

dandelion coffee
(available at good health-food shops)
milk or cream, to taste

Following the packet instructions, add the appropriate amount of coffee and boiling water to a cafetière.

Leave to stand for at least ten minutes; dandelion coffee takes longer to brew than regular coffee.

Pour into mugs and add milk or cream to taste.

Serves 2

Dandelion leaves are a very rich source of **vitamins A, B** and **C**, as well as **potassium**. Dandelion coffee is traditionally made by grinding the dried roots; it is probably the most acceptable of all coffee substitutes. For swollen ankles and general fluid retention, this is one of the safest and most effective remedies.

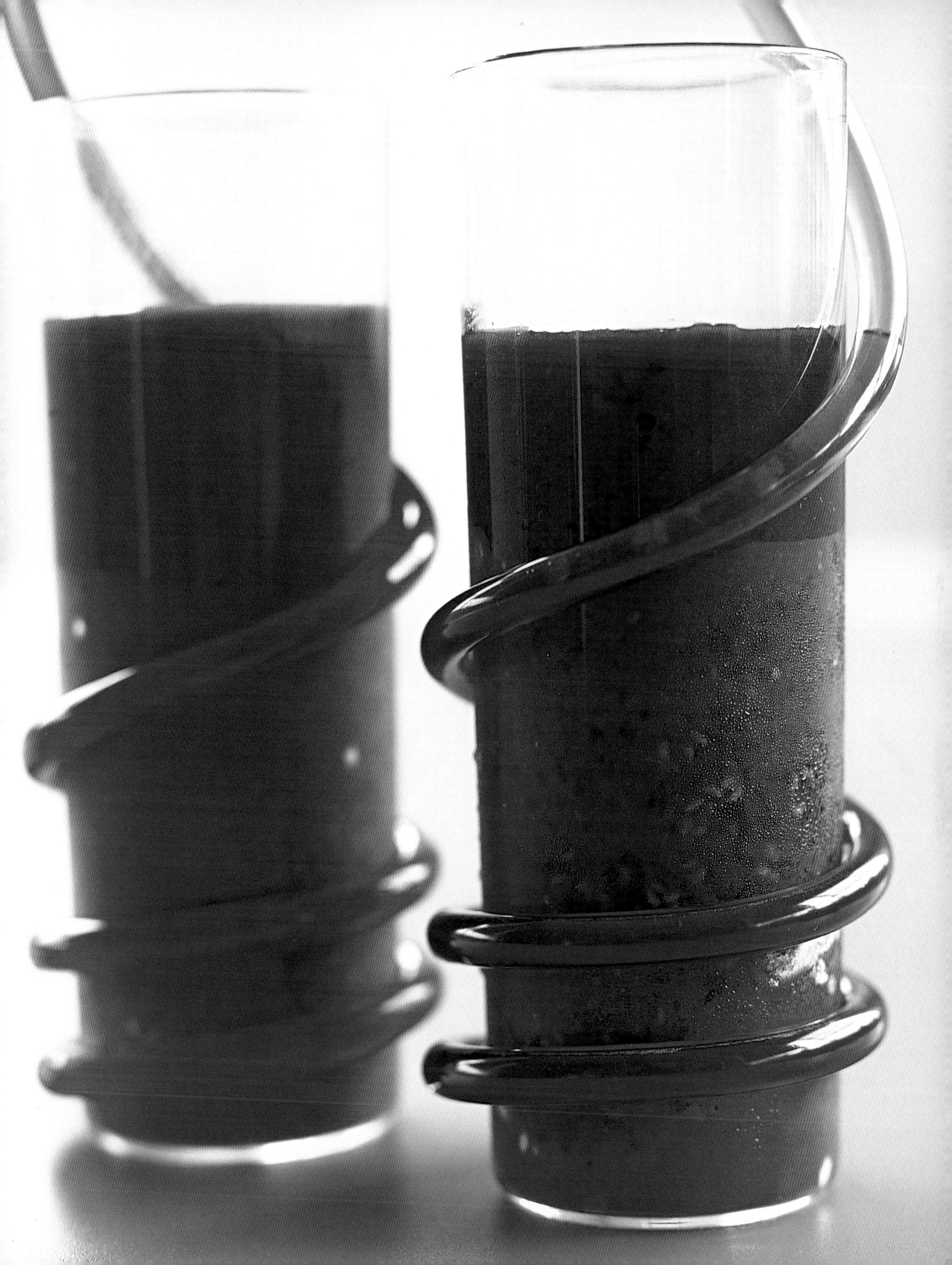

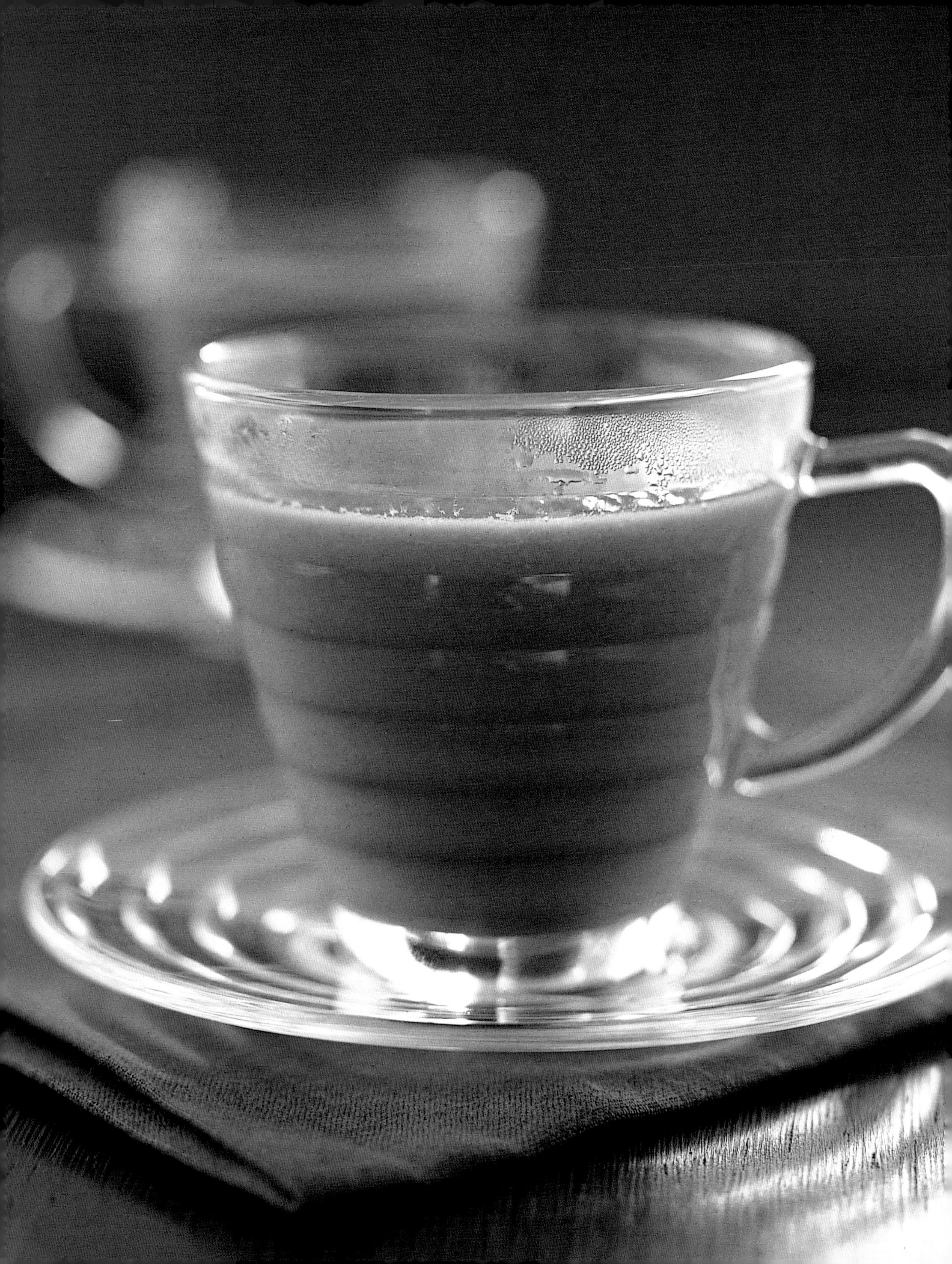

peas, please

This is a sort of instant pea soup – and just what's needed for anyone feeling a bit under the weather, miserable, depressed, anxious or suffering from **seasonal affective disorder** (SAD). The spring onions and the mint add extra essential oils to **boost resistance** and **energy levels**.

2 large spring onions, washed and trimmed

350g or 12oz frozen peas

1 large sprig mint

850ml or 30 fl oz vegetable stock (page 252)

Mix the onions with the other ingredients and warm gently in a saucepan until the peas are tender.

Reserving two tablespoons of peas, liquidize the stock mixture, adding boiling water if necessary.

Serve with the reserved peas floating on top.

Serves 4-6

Extended stress, anxiety or depression drain the body's vitamin B stores, and fresh or frozen peas are an excellent source of **vitamin B_1** and folic acid. They also provide useful quantities of **vitamins A** and **C**, and fatigue-fighting **zinc** and **iron**. Antibacterial and antiviral compounds in the onions help fight infection, making this valuable for infections like flu.

rum-rum, chilli-chilli, rum-rum

I suppose you could say that a generous tot of white rum has some **anaesthetic** effect, but that's not what provides the real benefits in this delicious, tropical-tasting hot drink. Surprisingly, the chilli is the key ingredient, even though it's the coconut that provides the smell of the Spice Islands.

1 small red chilli

300ml or 10 fl oz coconut milk

4 tbsp white rum

Bruise the chilli gently.

Put into a saucepan with the coconut milk.

Bring slowly to a boil.

Strain into two heatproof glasses to remove any chilli seeds, add the rum and serve.

Serves 2

Chillies contain **capsaicin**, a very powerful circulatory stimulant and an effective analgesic. It is used now as a prescription medicine by doctors, and can bring great relief to arthritic joints and injured muscles. It's also one of the few treatments that help relieve the pain of chilblains and Raynaud's syndrome.

starry, starry peach

Peach juice is extremely good to drink, but watch out for cartons or bottles labelled "peach nectar", as these will have large amounts of added sugar. Peaches are an excellent source of carotenoids, but it's the star anise that helps overcome the discomfort of **abdominal distension** and **flatulence**.

4 star anise

500ml or 18 fl oz peach juice

Put the star anise into a small bowl, cover with boiling water and leave for five minutes.

Gently heat the peach juice. Add the star anise and its liquid and simmer gently for five more minutes. Pour into two heatproof glasses, leaving the star anise on top as a decoration.

Serves 2

Peaches aren't hugely nutritious to start with, but the fresher the juice, the more **vitamin C** and **betacarotene** you'll get. **Essential oils** from star anise help disperse wind in the stomach and colon, reducing distension and pain; this juice is also good for the relief of dry, painful coughs.

austrian chocolate

Even if it had no **pain-relieving** properties, this heavenly drink, a variation on the favourite hot chocolate of Viennese coffee shops, would imbue you with sensations of peace, calm and happiness. What could be more self-indulgent than chocolate, cream and spices? All this, and pain-relief, too!

1 organic satsuma

85g or 3oz good organic milk chocolate, like Green & Black's

½ tsp ground cinnamon

425ml or 15 fl oz milk

125ml or 4 fl oz whipping cream

2 pinches freshly ground nutmeg

2 cinnamon sticks

Finely grate the zest off the satsuma (eat the flesh while you're making the drink). Break the chocolate into small pieces.

Put both ingredients into a saucepan, along with the ground cinnamon and two tablespoons of milk, and heat very gently, stirring continuously, until the chocolate melts. Add the rest of the milk, continue heating gently until just boiling and pour into mugs.

Whip the cream until stiff and add a heaped tablespoon to each mug. Serve immediately sprinkled with nutmeg and with the cinnamon sticks stuck into the cream.

Serves 2

This drink isn't an analgesic in the pharmaceutical sense, but it is a major bringer of the feel-good factor. It is this sensation that overrides the pain impulse and makes you feel positive and relaxed. **Theobromine** in chocolate and the gently hallucinogenic **myristicin** in nutmeg generate these feelings – but the rest is pure enjoyment.

lavender barley water

Lavender is a **great relaxant**. Although you may be more used to using it as an oil for aches and pains, a remedy for headaches or a luxurious bath additive, this herb is delicious in food and drink. Combined with wonderfully soothing honey and relaxing barley, it makes the ultimate relaxing drink.

As the preparation time is so long, double or triple the quantities, keep in the refrigerator and warm as required

20g or ¾oz pot barley

2 heaped tbsp finely chopped lavender leaves

425ml or 15 fl oz boiled water

2 tbsp lavender honey

Put the barley and lavender into a saucepan.

Add the water and simmer for ninety minutes.

Strain through muslin or a very fine sieve.

Reheat if necessary.

Stir in the honey before serving.

Serves 2

Natural **carbohydrates** in barley and sugars in honey make this an effective stimulant that encourages the brain to release soothing **tryptophan**. You'll also benefit from the large quantities of healing and relaxing **volatile essential oils** in lavender.

orange and camomile cup

Throughout the Mediterranean, most mothers know how quickly camomile can calm the most irritable, agitated and fractious child. But it works just as well for adults – especially when combined with the **soothing** benefits of honey and the calming fragrance of orange blossom.

1 tsp dried camomile or one camomile tea bag

125ml or 4 fl oz boiling water

1 small or 2 large oranges

1 tbsp orange-blossom honey

Put the herb or tea bag into a saucepan. Pour over the boiling water, cover and leave for five minutes. Meanwhile, juice the orange(s).

Strain out the herb, reserving the liquid, or remove the tea bag.

Pour in the orange juice and warm through.

Pour into a mug or heatproof glass and stir in the honey to serve.

Serves 1

One of the most striking characteristics of camomile is its wonderful fragrance: inhaling the **essential oils** has a direct and calming effect on the brain, which in turn is beneficial to healing the body.

parsley tea

European flat-leaf parsley may be slightly more chewable and palatable than the curly variety, but both are delicious and deserve more than their usual ignominious place as an uneaten garnish. If you're suffering the discomfort of **fluid retention**, this is definitely the herb for you.

2 heaped tsp fresh chopped parsley or 1 tsp dried parsley

1 heaped tsp runny honey (preferably organic)

Put the parsley into an infuser or large mug and fill with boiling water.

Leave for eight minutes before straining.

Add the honey and stir vigorously.

Serve immediately.

Serves 1–2

Apart from significant quantities of **vitamins A** and **C**, iron, **potassium** and **calcium**, parsley has a specific medicinal property: it is a gentle yet effective diuretic and a real boon to women whose periods are preceded by painful swollen feet, ankles, fingers, hands and breasts.

marmalade and ginger tea

Ginger marmalade is a great British tradition; the ginger is added for its piquant flavour. But using ginger in food dates back to the kitchen medicine of the early Christian monks, who knew the **healing** and **pain-relieving** properties of this wonderful spice.

1cm or ½in fresh root ginger (dried ginger doesn't work)

1 tbsp organic thin-cut orange marmalade

Peel and grate the ginger.

Put into a mug or infuser and fill with boiling water.

Leave for five minutes and strain.

Add the marmalade and stir until dissolved.

Serves 1

Even after bitter oranges are turned into marmalade, the peel retains some healing **bioflavonoids**. Adding ginger to this tea releases all the essential oils and other **phytochemicals** from the fresh root. These directly stimulate the circulation and at the same time have a warming effect on the whole body.

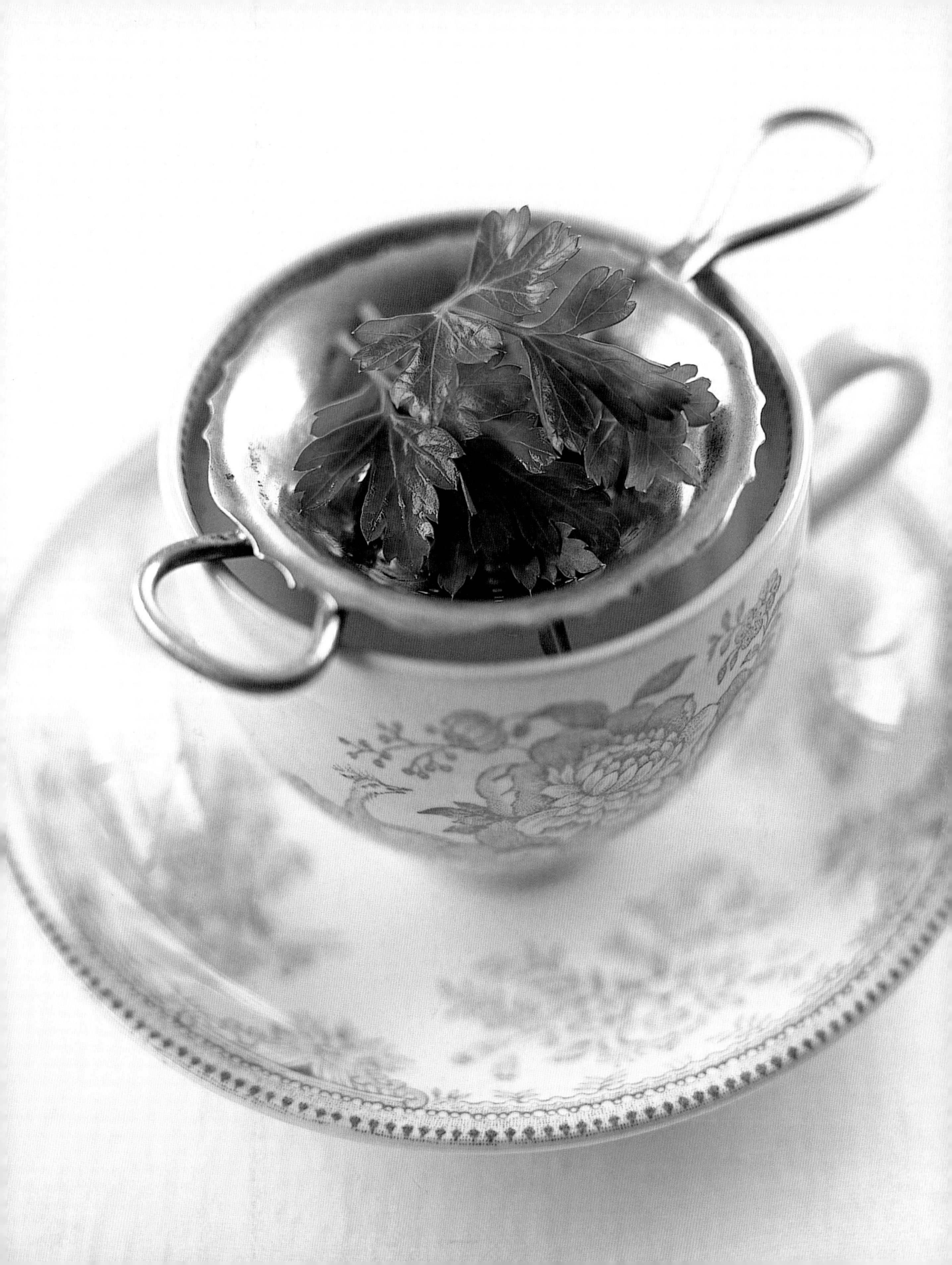

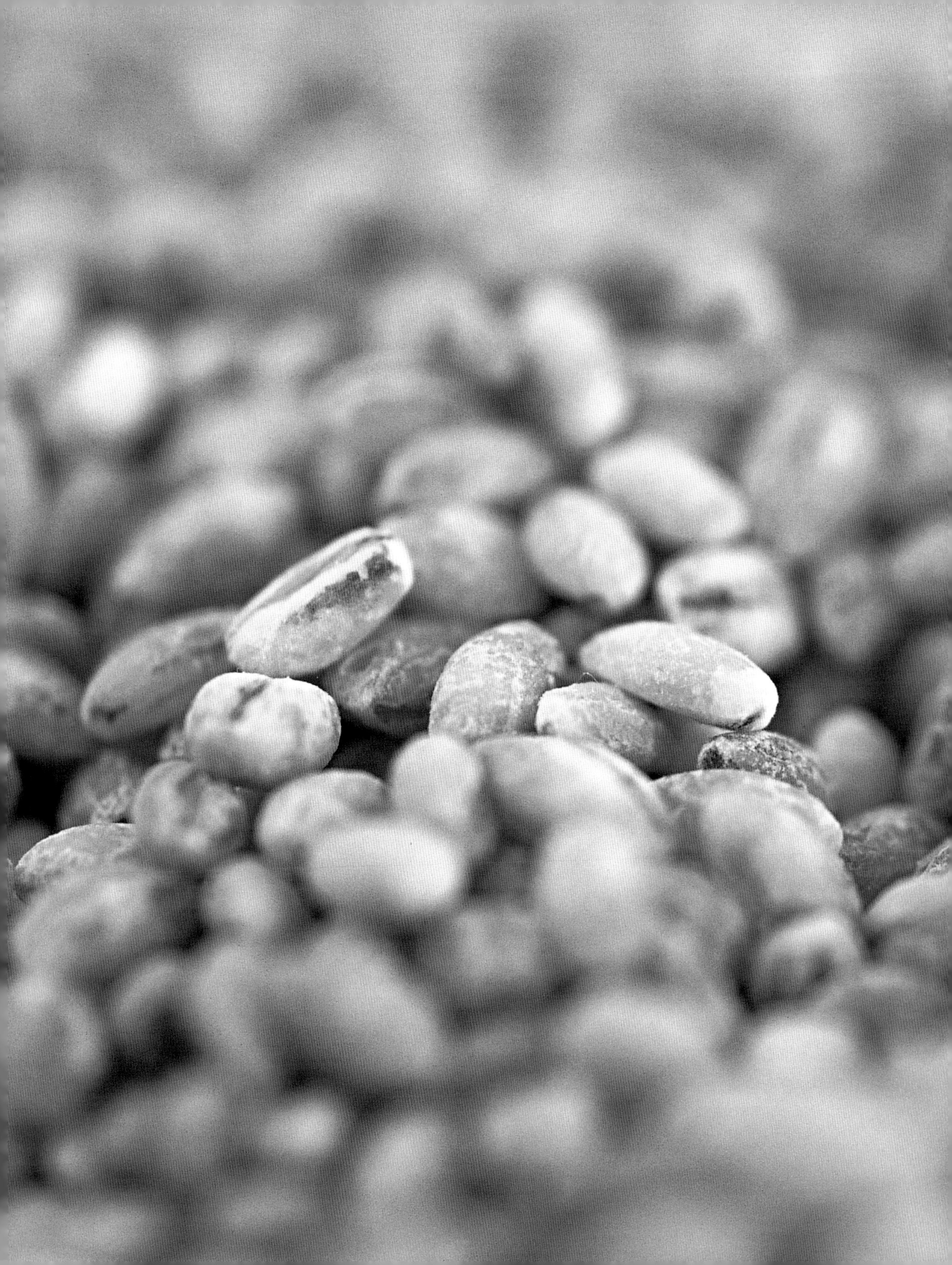

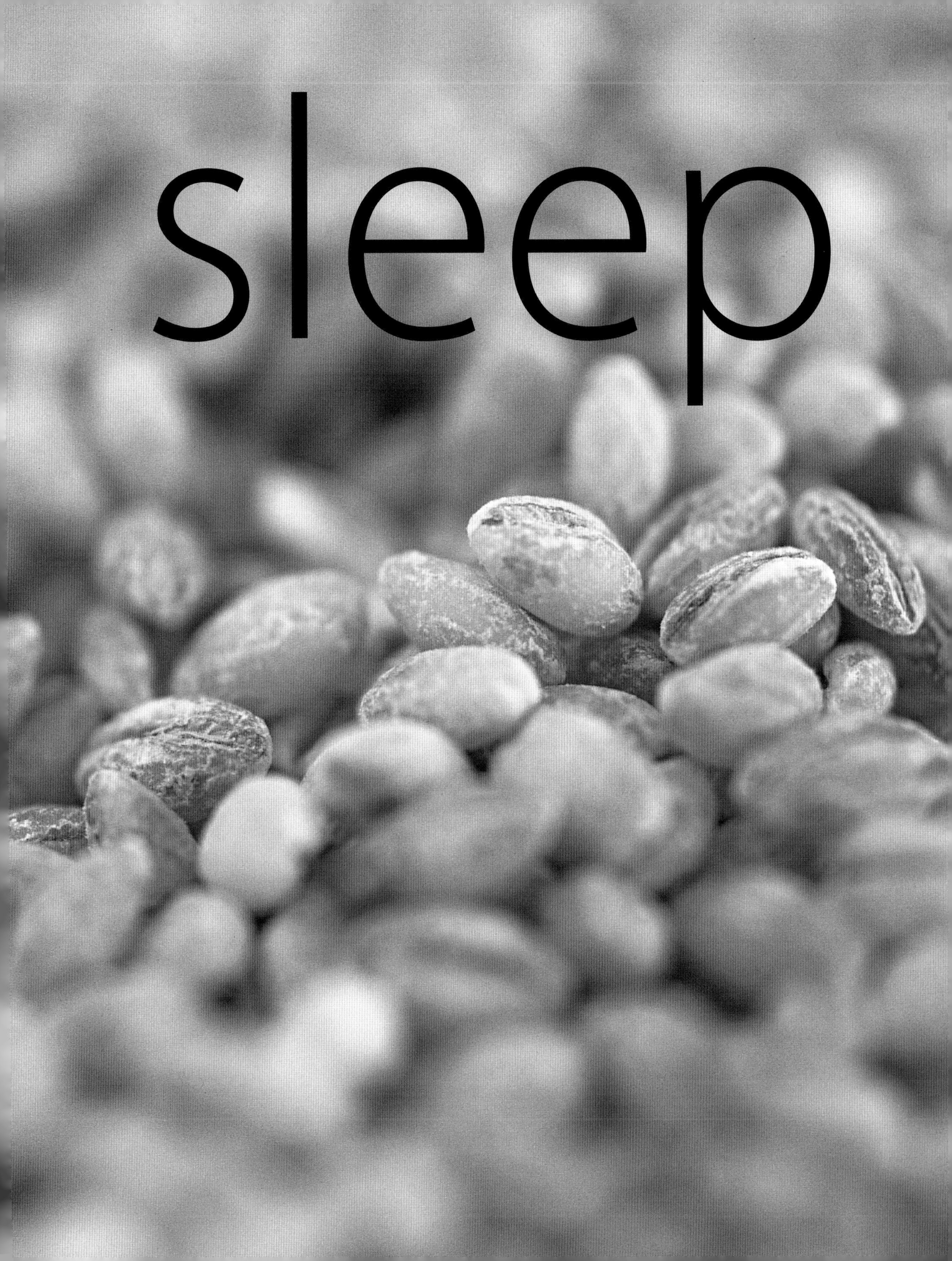

sleep

Few people get through life without the occasional sleepless night due to excitement, anxiety, indigestion, strange dreams, an uncomfortable bed, toothache or noisy neighbours. The occasional loss of beauty sleep isn't a problem. But sadly, there's a huge army of people whose lives are plagued by chronic insomnia – and although this is hardly a terminal disease, it can become an obsessive problem and often destroys people's quality of life.

There are many underlying causes of poor sleep, and habitual insomnia needs to be thoroughly investigated and treated appropriately. Limping through life on the crutch of sleeping pills isn't the answer. However, there's no doubt that food can be a major factor both in the cause and relief of this miserable condition.

Nobody will sleep peacefully two hours after a huge bowl of chicken vindaloo, naan bread, rice and three pints of lager. Nor will you drift into the land of Nod if you go to bed hungry. So the first step is to eat appropriate amounts of food at the right time. Secondly, it's vital to make use of all the herbs, spices and specific foods that help encourage calmness, relaxation and somnolence.

Herbal teas are a simple and effective starting point – and some are equally appropriate for children and adults. In southern Europe, every mother knows that weak camomile tea sweetened with honey is the perfect remedy for fractious children, especially if they're a bit headachey, restless and with a raised temperature.

Lime blossom is an excellent calmative for adults and makes a delicious tea, which is as nice to drink as it is effective. Valerian, hops, passion flower and lavender are also valuable aids to sleep and can be used as fresh or dried herbs, essential oils, liquid extracts or tablets. They can be used in cooking or as massage oils or added to the bath or in a room fragrancer. *Note* Culinary herbs are all fine during pregnancy and breast-feeding, but check with a pharmacist, herbalist or qualified aromatherapist before using them as essential oils or medicines, as some are best avoided at these times.

In this chapter you'll find a selection of dishes that are not only great to eat and not in the least "medicinal", but will dispatch you into the arms of Morpheus without having to count a single sheep.

wholemeal flour

raisins?

cranberry?

- mint + garlic + oregano
- 15g leek + lentil soup

pears

bananas

bulgur

cranberry

Milk features in a number of these recipes as it's one of the traditional foods that trigger the release of brain-calming tryptophans (as do most of the starchy foods), which is why many commercial bedtime drinks that combine milk with malted barley and other cereals are so effective.

The ancient Greeks made much use of the sticky sap extracted from wild lettuce; it contains chemicals similar to morphine and is a powerful sleep-inducer. All modern lettuces are descended from the wild lettuce and, although they contain much smaller amounts of this active ingredient, they're fabulous sleep-inducers and crop up in a number of recipes. A bedtime lettuce sandwich is a perfect combination of natural sleep-inducing substances and starch; it will get you to sleep, it's not addictive like sleeping pills and you won't wake up feeling hungover.

Turkey, oily fish, green vegetables, bananas and nutmeg are all ingredients that will help you achieve a better night's sleep. Any recipe that includes a couple of these should be on your regular menu.

A really traditional nightcap for the insomniac is a cup of hot cocoa. The good news is that chocolate in any form is great for the sleepless. Although chocolate does contain caffeine, it's in very small amounts, so as long as you don't overindulge, the mood-changing and soporific effect of its other main ingredient, theobromine, far outweighs the stimulating action of the caffeine.

Lime-blossom tea is one of the really great bedtime drinks. Not only is it a natural non-addictive sedative, but it also helps prevent panic attacks, soothes headaches and saves you counting sheep. Nutmeg is another super-snooze food that contains a mild hallucinogen called myristicine. It's no accident that Victorian nannies were fond of it and its mildly soporific effect. A generous sprinkle in a bowl of rice pudding might mean their young charges would settle down to sleep easily.

sleepytime checklist

- Eat more lettuce for its sleep-inducing phytochemicals; milk, cheese and bread, which aid the brain's release of calming tryptophans; turkey, bananas, oily fish, green vegetables, nutmeg, cocoa and lime-blossom tea, which all contain some of the calming or sleep-inducing plant chemicals.
- Eat less of the other animal proteins, which generally stimulate the release of the activity hormones.
- Eat less of the wake-up herbs and spices like ginger, turmeric, chilli and most curry mixtures.
- Eat less altogether, as going to bed on a full stomach is uncomfortable and sleep-disrupting.

sorrel soup

Sorrel isn't used nearly as much as it deserves to be. In addition to its mood-enhancing qualities, this delicious herb also works as an effective **detoxifier**. This recipe is helpful for those suffering from **anxiety**, especially when it is associated with insomnia – another common cause of mood swings.

2 large handfuls sorrel, stripped from the stems

55g or 2oz unsalted butter

4 shallots, peeled and finely sliced

200g or 7oz potatoes, peeled and cubed

1.2 litres or 40 fl oz vegetable stock (page 252)

400ml or 14 fl oz set natural, live yogurt

Reserve eight leaves of sorrel and blend the rest briefly in a food processor.

In a small saucepan, melt the butter over low heat – don't allow it to smoke or burn. Combine the processed sorrel into the melted butter and leave in the fridge.

Simmer the shallots and potatoes in the stock for about fifteen minutes until tender. Liquidize or blend the stock mixture until very smooth.

Just before serving, stir in the sorrel and butter mixture and the yogurt. Heat gently.

Serves 4

Sorrel is an excellent source of mood-enhancing **phytochemicals** to soothe and alleviate stressed nerves. Yogurt supplies brain-soothing **tryptophan**.

lavender blue

Mixed here with orange-blossom honey and orange flower water, lavender makes the most delicately flavoured, lightly perfumed and **soothing** bedtime drink.

5 tbsp fresh lavender leaves

200ml or 7 fl oz water

2 tbsp orange-blossom honey

100ml or 3½ fl oz orange-flower water

Put the lavender leaves into a saucepan. Add the water and the honey. Heat gently, stirring continuously, until the honey is completed dissolved. Simmer for one minute.

Strain into cups or heatproof glasses.

Stir in the orange-flower water to serve.

Serves 2

Lavender has one of the longest histories of medicinal herbs. It gets its name from the Latin word lavare, meaning to wash; the Romans used it to perfume bath water. Its **volatile oils** have a gentle, soothing sedative influence. The soporific effects of this drink are enhanced by **essential oils** in the orange flowers and the sleep promoting action of the honey.

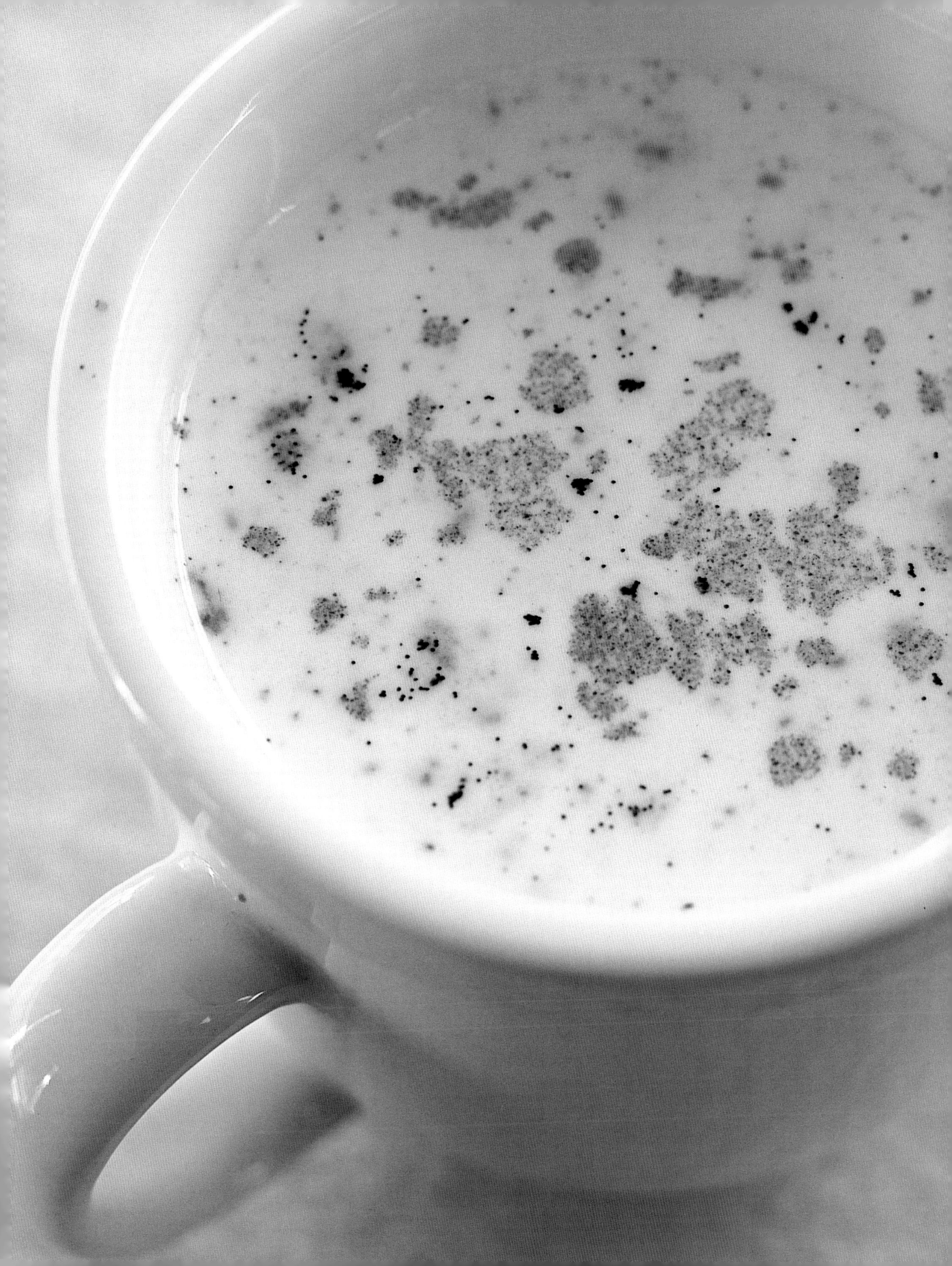

good night, sleep tight

Valerian was much revered by the ancient Romans for its powerful medicinal properties, and it has been used by herbalists since the earliest days of medicine as a **calming** herb. Adding maple syrup imparts an interesting flavour and supplies **brain-soothing** carbohydrates from the natural sugars.

1 tsp dried valerian herb
250ml or 9 fl oz boiling water
1 tsp maple syrup
1 dash peppermint essence

Put the valerian into a mug or infuser. Pour over the boiling water, cover and leave for five minutes.

Strain the liquid into a clean mug.

Stir in the maple syrup and peppermint essence to serve.

Serves 1

The **phytochemicals** in valerian are antispasmodic, calmative and sedative, making this tea an excellent sleeping draught and remedy for stress, anxiety and insomnia. Peppermint is a bonus, as it's antispasmodic and calming in addition to its main medicinal use, which is for the relief of sleep-disturbing indigestion and heartburn.

sultana tea

The fibre in bran helps prevent **constipation** and speed up the passage of food through the intestinal tract. This also helps avoid **indigestion**, wind and uncomfortable spasms of the bowel – common reasons for **disturbed sleep**. Natural sugars, iron and potassium in sultanas relieve stress and anxiety.

115g or 4oz sultanas
40g or 1½oz bran
600ml or 20 fl oz boiling water

Chop the sultanas. Put them into a jug along with the bran.

Pour over the boiling water.

Cover and leave to stand for about eight hours.

Strain, reheat and serve.

Serves 2

Soaking sultanas in hot water helps extract the sugars and other nutrients that make this such a sleep-friendly drink. Additional **B vitamins** and fibre from the bran increase the calming effect and the brain's production of feel-good **tryptophan**.

hops with honey

You're probably aware of how beer can be used to ward off the evils of **insomnia**; this recipe is made with hops. To extract enough of the **soporific** natural chemicals from the dried flowers, you must leave them to infuse for at least ten minutes. Also, make sure you keep the drink covered.

1 tsp dried hops
250ml or 9 fl oz boiling water
1 tsp heather honey

Put the hops into a mug or infuser.

Pour over the boiling water, cover and leave for ten minutes.

Strain into a clean mug. Sweeten with the honey to serve.

Serves 1

Hops, which give beer its sedative effects as well as some **vitamin B_6**, have a long and honourable tradition as a medicinal plant. The only problem is that they don't taste very good, which is why we've added the honey.

sweet dreams

What could be sweeter than this heavenly mixture of flavours and aromas? You only have to smell it to know how **soothing** this drink is – and it takes just a sip or two to realize how effective it will be at helping even the most dedicated **insomniac** have a decent night's sleep.

250ml or 9 fl oz buttermilk
2 tbsp lavender honey
3 pinches freshly grated nutmeg

Heat the buttermilk until just warm.

Add the honey and continue heating, stirring continuously, until the honey is dissolved.

Froth the mixture using a whisk or cappuccino wand. Sprinkle with the nutmeg to serve.

Serves 1

Buttermilk is an excellent source of **calcium**, **beneficial bacteria** and some **protein**. Like all milk products, it's a good sleep-inducer. Flavoured with soothing lavender honey and the extraordinary feel-good, mildly hallucinogenic effects of nutmeg, one mug of this drink will help you look forward to wonderful dreams.

barley broth

A longtime sickroom favourite for **urinary infections** such as cystitis, this is also a great aid to a **good night's sleep** – and doubly valuable because, as well as helping you gently into the land of Nod, it prevents the frequent night-time trips to the bathroom if you have cystitis.

850ml or 30 fl oz water
55g or 2oz pot barley
1 large unwaxed lemon
1 large tbsp honey

Add the water to the barley and put both ingredients into a saucepan.

Cut the lemon into thin slices and add to the pot.

Simmer for ninety minutes.

Strain, stir in the honey and pour into cups to serve.

Serves 4

Barley is a good source of **calcium**, **potassium** and **B vitamins**. This most ancient of all cultivated cereals also has valuable amounts of **fibre** and, like all starches, helps trigger the release of the natural sleep-inducing chemical **tryptophan** in the brain. Honey is used in folk medicine as a sleep promoter.

vanilla soother

It's no accident that milk-based bedtime drinks are popular throughout the world. Milk is one of the classic bringers of Morpheus, the Greek god of **sleep**. The unique flavours of vanilla and allspice come largely from their volatile essential oils, and their fragrance alone is **soothing** and **soporific**.

150ml or 5 fl oz milk
140g or 5oz fromage frais
5cm or 2in length of vanilla pod
1 pinch allspice

Stir the milk and fromage frais together until they are well blended. Pour into a saucepan, along with the vanilla pod. Simmer for ten minutes.

Remove the vanilla pod.

Serve with the allspice scattered on top.

Serves 1

Calcium is one of the most effective nutrients for overcoming sleep problems; thanks to milk and fromage frais, it's abundant here. Milk also triggers the release of sleep-inducing **tryptophan** in the brain. The process begins when you inhale the **volatile oils** and their delicious aromas, released by heating the vanilla and allspice.

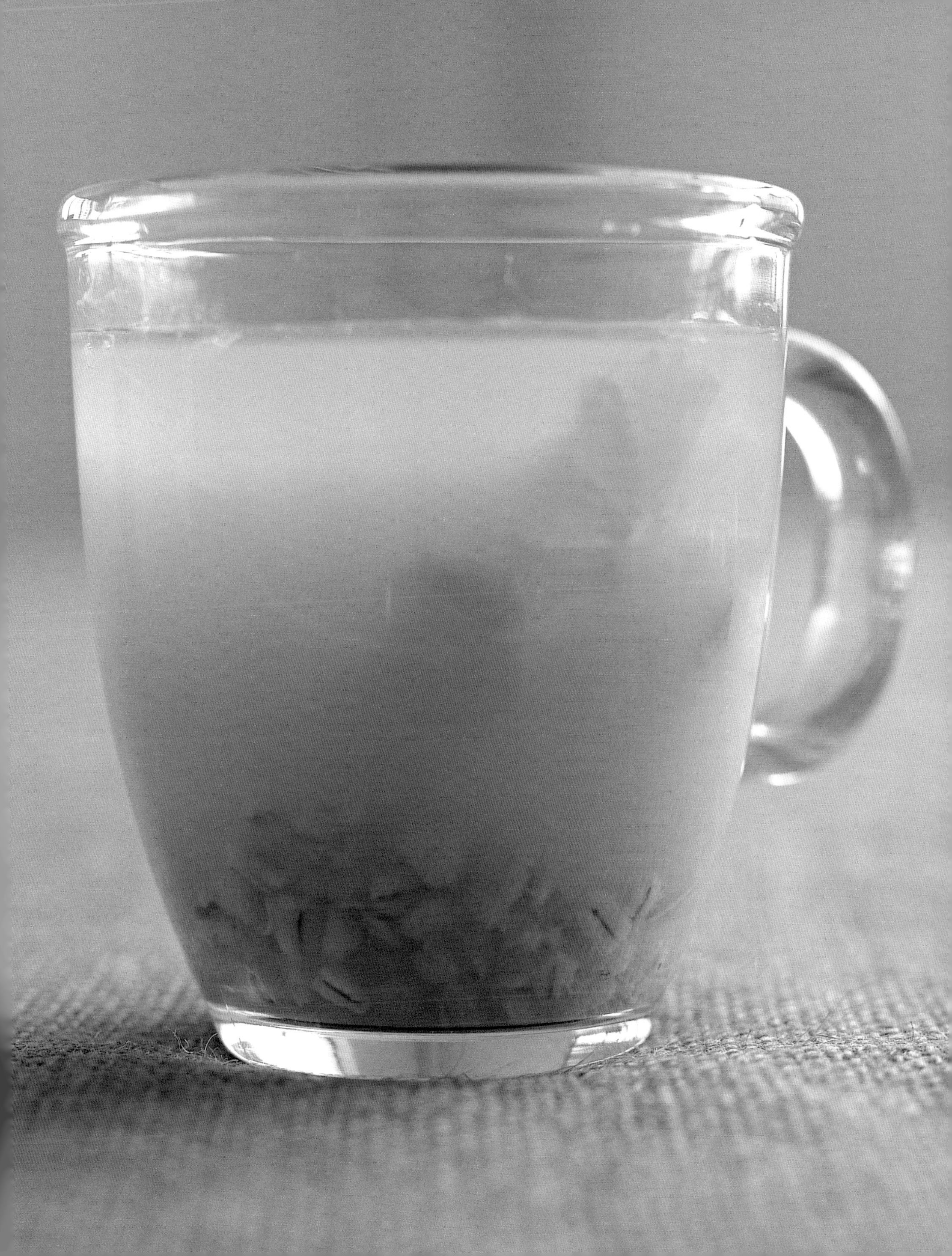

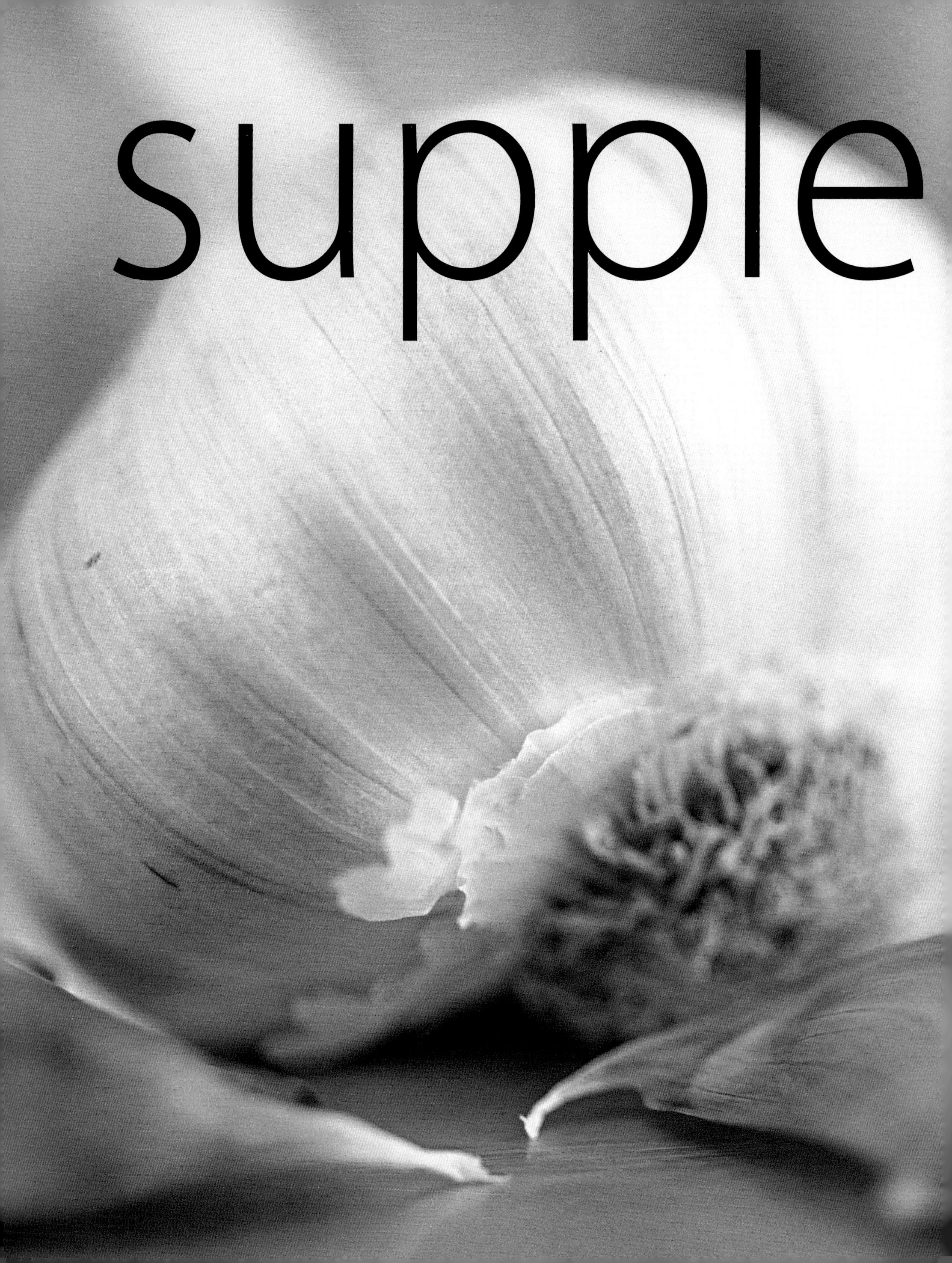
supple

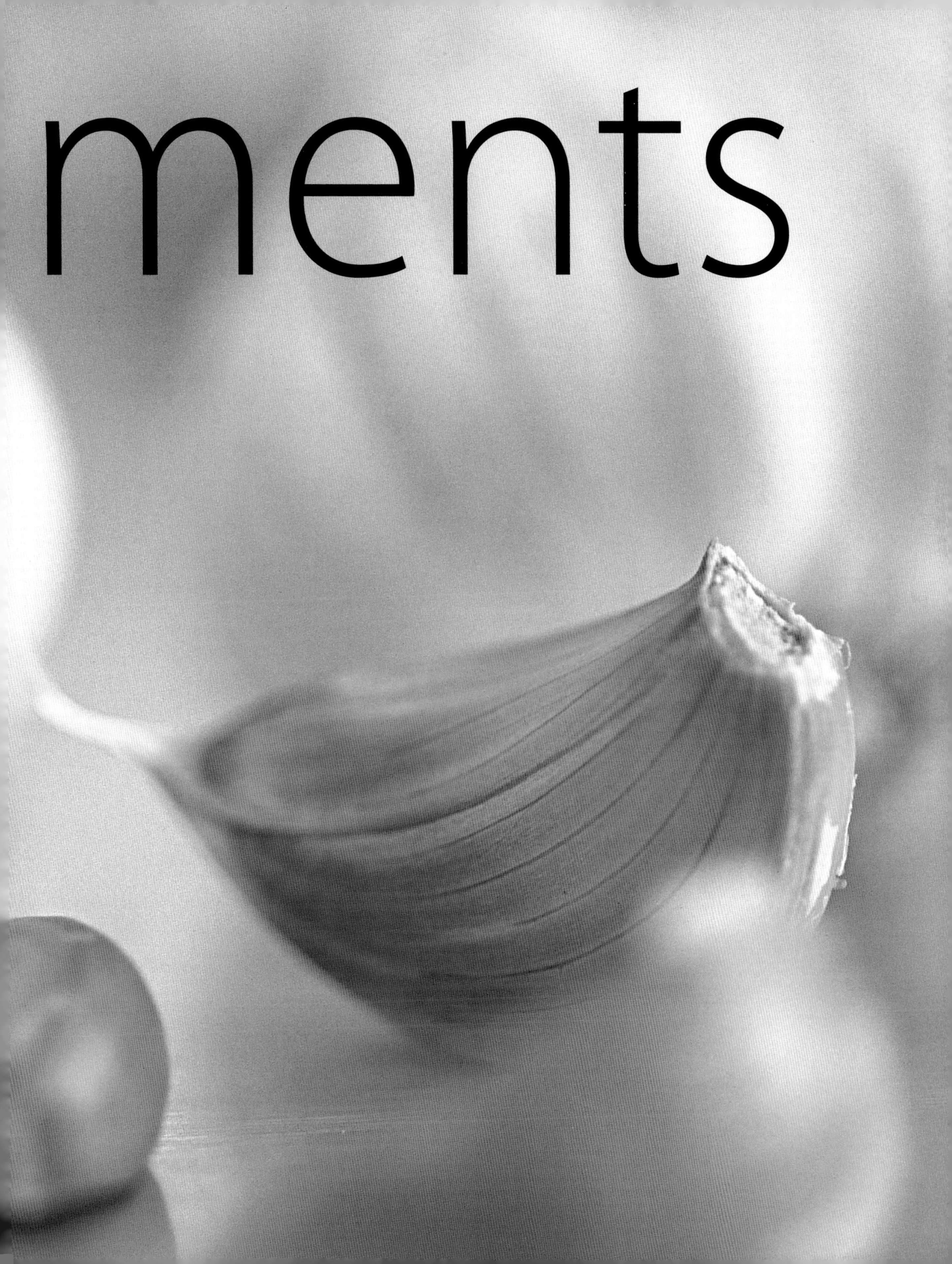
ments

The question most people ask is, "do I need to take extra vitamins?" The theoretical answer is no, not if you are eating a well-balanced diet and using a wide variety of foods. However, few people manage to do this, and even fewer persuade their partners or children to do it. Pressures of time, working couples, no school meals and the relentless march of the fast-food industry all make it more difficult.

There are obvious times when both adults and children need more vitamins and minerals: pregnancy, breastfeeding, illness, before and after operations, or when digestive problems or dental trouble prevent proper eating. The very young and the very old usually need to boost their intake, as do those under extra stress or with physically demanding jobs and high levels of sporting activity. But even the rest of us who are otherwise healthy may be missing out because we eat foods that have been processed, badly stored, are stale or were intensively grown on soils that are themselves deficient in nutrients. Even when buying fresh fruit, salads and vegetables, how they are stored at home can make a difference to their nutritional value. Keeping fresh produce on a rack next to the cooker or anywhere in a warm kitchen speeds up their loss of vitamins, so make sure yours are in a cool place or even in the fridge.

Whenever you do opt for supplements, however, choosing the right one is not an easy task. You dash to the chemist or health store to pick up a bottle of pills, and by the time you've read the umpteenth label, you're more muddled than ever. Do you choose a multivitamin; six individual bottles; mega-dose, slow-release, vegetarian capsules; tablets made without gluten, yeast, colourings or sugars; a brand with seventy different ingredients; one with five – or, like so many shoppers, do you leave empty-handed?

Even worse, you may waste a lot of your hard-earned cash on supplements you don't need and some that may do more harm than good. Single vitamins and minerals certainly have a place, but as a general rule, they are best taken on the advice of your practitioner – especially any high-dose ones. If you mix and match yourself, you may find that the products overlap and you get more of some nutrients than you bargained for.

The official UK government policy is that nobody needs extra vitamins or minerals because we all eat well enough to get all the essential nutrients from our food. Sadly, this is far from the truth; millions of people's intake of vital vitamins and minerals falls way below the lowest amount essential to prevent illness. Which is why natural health insurance in the form of an inexpensive, well-formulated multivitamin and mineral pill *can* be a good idea. It will make up for the missed meal, the extra demands of a stressful life and the vitamin losses during storage, transport and cooking. It will also help after illness.

Apart from vitamins and minerals, other supplements can be extremely useful. Fish and fish-liver oils are anti-inflammatory and may help behavioural problems in children; antioxidant combinations containing lycopene are useful for cancer prevention; lutein or zeaxanthin protect the eyes; seaweed extracts improve thyroid function. Many other valuable supplements may be appropriate from time to time, but anyone who believes they can live on a diet of junk food, takeaways and bags of crisps, and simply pop a few vitamin pills and be healthy had better think again.

Supplements are just that – supplemental. They are not alternatives to proper eating.

supplements checklist

- Read labels carefully. Avoid pills with artificial colours, flavours and preservatives. Watch out for added sugar. Many children with asthma, eczema or other allergies react badly to some food chemicals.
- Don't waste money on expensive products that are gluten-, yeast-, egg-, milk- and everything else-free. Unless you know that you're allergic to these (and comparatively few people are), there is no need to go to these lengths.
- Choose products with substantial levels of the main nutrients, rather than huge lists of things you've never heard of.
- Adult formulations are not normally suitable for children; the latter need specific children's products. Under-twos should only get vitamins on professional advice.
- Vitamins may interfere with prescribed medicines, so check with your doctor before dosing yourself.
- It's simply daft to try to gain some essentials from pills. Fibre is one of these, and it can cost around £5 for 28 days' supply.

vitality

bio-strath elixir

available as

Liquid tonic

what it is

BIO-STRATH elixir is the only proprietary product listed in this book, and it is here for two reasons. First, it is available in most parts of the world. Second, it is unique.

BIO-STRATH is made by feeding a complex mixture of many medicinal herbs to a very special and nutritious variety of yeast. During the process, the yeast cells digest and absorb all the beneficial contents of the herbs. A fermentation process follows that ruptures the cell walls of the yeast, releasing the contents, which now include beneficial enzymes from the yeast. Organic honey and orange juice are added, resulting in an easily absorbed and amazingly versatile natural food supplement. For many years, this booster has been a favourite of some of the world's great elite athletes and leading show-business personalities – all people whose livelihoods and success depend on having that "it" factor, which means unflagging vitality.

what it does

The Pestalozzi family who make BIO-STRATH on the edge of Lake Zurich in Switzerland have been involved in serious scientific research for more than thirty years. These studies have shown that the product has the effect of boosting natural immunity, increasing physical endurance and performance, enhancing mental ability and even helping to protect cancer patients against the side effects of radiation treatment. In short, BIO-STRATH is vitality in a bottle. It is suitable for children, adults and the elderly, and because of its unique manufacturing process, it is very quickly absorbed into the body, where it can start its work.

how to use it

This is one of the very few natural supplements that should be taken on a long-term and regular basis, because it protects against infection and enhances performance. It is best taken before meals for optimum absorption.

precautions

There are no reported adverse reactions or interactions with other medications. BIO-STRATH is suitable – and, in fact, advisable – to take throughout pregnancy and during breast-feeding. It is safe for children of all ages.

dosage

Take 5ml three times daily, doubled if necessary.

evening primrose oil

what it is

Evening primrose oil is a rich source of gamma linolenic acid (GLA). This is what is known as a fatty acid, and it has a valuable property of being converted by the body into a substance known as prostaglandin. Prostaglandins are some of the most powerful natural anti-inflammatories, and they also improve blood flow through the smallest of capillaries. Prostaglandins also have a role in helping to reduce the stickiness of blood, thus lessening the risk of clots and thrombosis. The much more easily obtained linoleic acid is widespread in vegetable oils, seeds and nuts; in optimum circumstances this, too, may be converted into prostaglandins. Unfortunately, a variety of situations can interfere with the process, which is why gamma linolenic acid is such a sought-after and widely used natural booster. Borage oil and blackcurrant-seed oil are also good sources of GLA, although the vast majority of research work has used evening primrose oil.

what it does

Evening primrose oil is valuable in a wide range of inflammatory conditions such as eczema, arthritis, tendonitis and cyclic breast lumps. But from a vitality-boosting point of view, its greatest benefit is in the relief of premenstrual syndrome. There is nothing more draining of vitality than this wretched condition, which frequently deprives huge numbers of women of two weeks of their normal lives in every month. The benefits of GLA are much enhanced by the addition of vitamin B_6, zinc, magnesium and vitamin C, so it is always useful to combine capsules of evening primrose oil with these nutrients.

how to use it

For severe PMS, take 1g three times a days for the ten days before your next period is due. PMS in particular responds best if a concurrent daily supplement of vitamin B_6, zinc, magnesium and vitamin C is taken throughout the month.

precautions

There are no reported adverse side effects or interactions with prescribed medications. Evening primrose oil is safe and advisable during pregnancy and breast-feeding. It is suitable in smaller doses for children over the age of twelve, particularly for the treatment of eczema.

dosage

Up to 3g daily.

available as

Capsules

Oil

guarana *(paulinia cupana)*

available as

Capsules

Chewing gum

Liquid extract

what it is

Of all the medicinal plants of the Brazilian rainforest, the best known is guarana. Rainforest Indians have used this plant for many thousands of years as a tonic, stimulant and aid to vitality. Traditionally, the seeds are turned into hard sticks, which are then grated into boiling water to make guarana tea. First discovered by the Maues-Sateres Indians, guarana was so valuable that they traded it as a form of money with neighbouring tribes. When the seventeenth-century missionary Bettendorf came across this group of Indians, he described them as the sturdiest and healthiest of all the tribes he found during his travels.

what it does

Studies show that guarana increases energy, reduces stress and improves mood and performance. There are claims that the benefits of guarana are due to its caffeine content; the truth is that the prepared extracts act in a totally different way from caffeine and produce none of the side effects of coffee, the world's most widely used stimulant drug. The amount of caffeine in a daily dose of guarana is, at 35mg, far less than that in a cola drink, less than half that found in a cup of tea and only about fifteen per cent of the amount found in a cup of real coffee. The reason guarana works as a highly effective, slow-release energy and vitality booster is that it is absorbed extremely slowly into the body.

Because it is a member of the soapwood family, guarana is also rich in natural fats – which accounts for this beneficial slow absorption. Guarana is not an instant high, does not raise blood pressure, nor is it addictive. In fact, it has none of the side effects of caffeine and is of enormous help in the treatment of ME, chronic fatigue and Tired All the Time syndrome. On a day-to-day basis, it provides the vitality to cope with long hours of work, sporting endurance and even a night on the town.

how to use it

Guarana can be taken as capsules, liquid extracts, chewing gum or made into tea.

precautions

Although its caffeine content is very small, guarana should be avoided during pregnancy and breast-feeding. Do not take it if you have high blood pressure or are caffeine-sensitive. Anyone with sleeping problems should avoid guarana late in the day.

dosage

Take 2g of guarana powder or 1 grated stick in a cup of hot water; either will provide approximately 50mg of the active substance known as guaranine.

red clover *(trifolium pratense)*

what it is

This perennial herb with its dark-pink flowers is a native of Europe and Asia but has become naturalized in Australia, New Zealand, and the US. Agriculturally, red clover is an effective crop; like other clovers, its roots fix nitrogen into the soil, so it is often used as one of the regenerating plants in fallow fields. Traditionally used in both Chinese and European herbal medicine as an expectorant for bad coughs and skin problems, and as an external application for breast cancer, its most valuable properties were discovered by accident.

A sheep farmer in New Zealand found that the fertility of his flock seemed to be in decline for no apparent reason. The sheep all looked healthy, were well nourished and had not been fed on anything but what grew in the fields they grazed. The mystery was solved when the vet realized they were in a field full of red clover. Analysis revealed that the flowers of red clover are rich in plant hormones called isoflavones, particularly genistein, which is known to have oestrogenic properties. The sheep were moved to another field without red clover and fertility returned to normal.

what it does

Because of its gentle oestrogenic effect, red clover certainly has some of the traditional properties that have been ascribed to it. As an anti-inflammatory in skin disease, an anti-cancer agent and a heart-protector, this is a valuable plant. By far its most popular everyday use, however, is in the relief of menopausal symptoms.

Red clover is second to none as a vitality booster during difficult phases of menopause, helping to control mood swings, hot flushes, depression and irritability. It also helps reduce the increased risk of heart disease in postmenopausal women.

how to use it

Take as a tea made from the dried flowers. For precise doses, extracts of red clover are available as tablets and capsules.

precautions

There are no reported side effects or interactions with prescribed medications. Because of its oestrogenic properties, avoid during pregnancy or breast-feeding. Not suitable for children.

dosage

Take 2-3g of the dried flowers in tablet form daily; three cups of tea, made with dried flowers; or 3ml of tincture in warm water three times daily.

available as

Capsules
Dried flowers
Tablets
Tincture

schisandra *(schisandra chinensis)*

available as

Dried berries

what it is

Growing to more than 6m (20ft) in length, this fragrant vine has pink flowers, red berries and an ancient history of use as a tonic in traditional Chinese medicine. The Chinese name *wu-wei-zi* translates as "five-flavoured plant", and the berries do indeed have a very complex sweet, sour and salty flavour.

Schisandra is native to China and is widely cultivated for medicinal use. The plant is also found in nearby regions of Korea and Russia. As with many other traditional Chinese medicines, schisandra has become increasingly popular in the West and is available from Chinese herbalists as well as traditional health-food stores.

what it does

Schisandra berries contain a complex mixture of natural substances, including essential oils, lignans such as schizandrin and gomisin, phytosterols and a number of natural acids. Ancient Chinese texts maintain that schisandra is invaluable for the relief of stress and restoring zest for life. Some modern research has also shown that this herb can be valuable in the treatment of liver disease and can help in the treatment of hepatitis. Modern herbalists describe schisandra as an adaptogenic, which means it helps the body adapt to a whole range of stressful situations, thereby improving concentration and mental and physical strength. Folklore also ascribes powerful aphrodisiac effects to this extraordinary berry.

how to use it

The dried berries can be chewed, or the active constituent can be obtained from using a tincture.

precautions

There are no reported interactions with other medications and virtually no adverse reactions. Rarely, some gastric disturbance or loss of appetite may occur. Avoid during pregnancy and breast-feeding.

dosage

Up to 5g a day of the fruit or 2ml of tincture three times a day.

immunity

cat's claw *(uncaria tomentosa)*

what it is

Cat's claw is a vine that grows high in the canopy roof of the Amazonian rainforest and gets its name from the claw-like thorns that protrude from its woody stems. Besides its native Amazon, it is also found in tropical regions of Peru, Colombia, Ecuador and other parts of South America.

Cat's claw is popular with many Peruvian tribes, which are known to have used it for at least 2,000 years, yet it was virtually unheard of in the rest of the world until the 1970s. At that time, stories began appearing in the press about its use as a cancer medicine, and the fame of this traditional remedy spread worldwide almost overnight. Traditionally, the plant has been used as an anti-inflammatory, for wound-healing, and as a treatment for rheumatism, ulcers and dysentery; in addition, early research into its cancer-fighting properties has shown promise. In 1993, however, scientists found that cat's claw could also boost the immune system of patients with HIV.

what it does

Cat's claw is one of nature's great immunity-boosters. It contains some very important chemicals called oxyindole alkaloids, which have a specific effect of stimulating the immune system. Only small amounts of these alkaloids are necessary to boost immunity by around fifty per cent; other studies have shown tumour- and leukaemia-fighting benefits, too. The overall immunity-boosting benefits of cat's claw make this rainforest plant an excellent choice as a protector and general helpmate for the body's natural defence mechanisms. As yet, there is no definitive evidence of its benefits in the treatment of HIV, AIDS or cancer, but it is certainly worth trying as an adjunct to conventional therapy.

how to use it

Make a tea by boiling 1g of root bark in a cup of water for ten minutes; cool, strain and drink a cup three times daily. Alternatively, certified tea bags deliver an infusion equal to 1,500mg to 1,800mg of plant extract. The herb is also available in capsules of 500mg or 1,000mg.

precautions

There are no reported interactions with other medications, and no serious adverse effects have been noted. However, avoid during pregnancy and breast-feeding.

dosage

Up to 60mg of standardized extract daily or 1,000mg whole dried plant.

available as

Capsules

Dried bark

Tea bags

cranberry *(vaccinium macrocarpon)*

available as

Capsules

Fresh berries

Juice

Tablets

what it is

Cranberries are native to North America. For centuries, Native Americans used these extraordinary berries as both food and medicine. They bathed their wounds in cranberry juice, and their medicine men made cranberry poultices to draw out the poison from arrow injuries. Ever since the North American Indians discovered the health-giving benefits of cranberries, they have become a favourite medicinal fruit of traditional herbalists and naturopaths. In recent years, science has unravelled some of the mysteries of this extraordinary bog plant and confirmed its traditional value. Most women know about cranberry juice and cystitis, but the latest research shows that the berries may protect against breast cancer, too.

what it does

Traditionally, it was thought that the acidity of cranberry juice produced its antibacterial effect. However, between 1984 and 1986, when Dr Anthony Sobota, Professor of Microbiology at Youngstown State University, Ohio, published the results of his research, the true explanation began to emerge. Cranberries contain a component that covers the walls of the bladder, kidneys and interconnecting tubing; this substance prevents bacteria from attaching to these sensitive tissues, where they would normally live and multiply. Sobota found that a glass of supermarket cranberry juice each day was ten times as effective at killing urinary bacteria as conventional antibiotics.

A follow-up study, published in March 1994 by doctors Gerry Avorn, Mark Monane, Gerry Gurwitz and others of the Harvard University Medical School, reported the findings of the first placebo-controlled, large-scale clinical trial to test the effects of cranberry juice. Within a month of beginning the trial, positive results appeared in the majority of patients drinking the real cranberry juice. Other research has shown that the most chronic sufferers stay infection-free as long as they drink their one glass of cranberry juice a day.

how to use it

Drink at least one pint a day of a 50/50 dilution of cranberry juice with water, both as a treatment during an attack of cystitis and for long-term protection against it. Cranberry extract is also available in tablet and capsule form.

precautions

There are no known interactions with other medications and no reported side effects. Cranberries and cranberry juice are safe to take during pregnancy and breast-feeding.

dosage

Take 100-300mg of standardized cranberry extract per day.

echinacea *(echinacea angustifolia)*

what it is

Another Native American herbal remedy, echinacea has become an important natural medicine throughout the world. Although it is still often harvested from the wild, most commercial preparations come from farmed crops of the plant. Both the leaf and root have medicinal properties. American Indians traditionally used it on cuts, burns and other injuries to prevent infection, and the Sioux and Comanche tribes revered the plant for its healing properties. Historically, it has been used for a wide range of conditions, including allergies, asthma and chilblains, but most modern research has studied its value as a natural, safe immunity-booster.

what it does

A century and a half ago, echinacea first appeared in the United States Dispensatory and was listed as a medicine that increased resistance to infection. Physiologically, it stimulates the production of white blood cells for protection against bacteria and helps the body produce more interferon for increased protection against viruses. Its main constituents are polysaccharides, betaine, alkalides and echinolone. The combination of these natural chemicals is the key to the plant's immunity-boosting success, which also extends to protection against fungal infections. Echinacea is a great gargle for sore throats and can be extremely helpful in the treatment of chronic viral conditions such as ME.

how to use it

Take standardized extract, capsules or tinctures at the first sign of any infectious illness. If colleagues or family catch colds, then take echinacea before you get sick – but not for more than two or three weeks.

precautions

There are no reported adverse reactions with other medications. Echinacea appears safe to take during pregnancy and breast-feeding. However, do not take continuously for ongoing protection, since this may reduce the strength of your natural immunity.

dosage

Half a teaspoon of tincture in water three times a day. Capsules of 300mg powdered root and leaf, plus 125mg standardized extract: one, three times daily.

available as

Capsules

Tablets

Tincture

lapacho *(tabebuia impestiginosa,* pau d'arco)

available as

Capsules

Dried bark

what it is

Of all the herbs used by the ancient Incas, lapacho was one of the mainstays. In the four centuries since the Spanish Conquest, the herb has cropped up from time to time in Europe. Tsar Nicholas II and Gandhi are both known to have done what millions of Brazilians do: start their day with a cup of lapacho tea. Also called pau d'arco, ipe roxo or taheebo, lapacho is a rainforest medicine made from the inner bark of the large native South American tree known as tabebuia. Throughout South America, indigenous tribes have drunk tea made from the shredded inner bark to boost the effectiveness of the body's own immune defence mechanisms. They have also used this traditional remedy for centuries in the treatment of asthma, bronchitis, infection and also some forms of cancer. As far back as 1882, one of lapacho's constituents was isolated and identified as lapachol, an antimicrobial and potentially tumour-fighting chemical. Today, scientific evidence shows that crude extracts of lapachol – more potent than refined versions – offer effective protection against a wide range of bacterial and fungal organisms, including *Candida albicans*, which causes thrush.

what it does

Rainforest Indians have always valued lapacho as a powerful medicine for strengthening immunity and protecting them against gut parasites. Research at São Paulo, Harvard, the University of Munich, the University of Rio de Janeiro and the American National Cancer Institute has increased awareness of this amazing natural medicine. In many parts of the world, physicians are recognizing it as an aid to patients with immune-deficiency illnesses. For ME, chronic fatigue syndrome, Epstein-Barr, and Tired All the Time syndrome, lapacho can be a great aid to recovery, due to its positive effects on the immune system.

how to use it

As capsules of finely ground bark powder, usually 500mg in each. These should be taken at a dose of two to three capsules three times daily.

precautions

Using whole bark has no known serious side effects, nor are there reported interactions with other medicines. However, this herb is not suitable during pregnancy or lactation. Care should be taken if using concentrated extracts, since overdosing can cause vomiting, nausea and bleeding.

dosage

Take 2-5g of powdered bark daily.

lemon balm *(melissa officinalis)*

what it is

Lemon balm is a perennial herb growing up to 1.5m (5ft) in height, with a mass of tiny white flowers. Although it originated in the Mediterranean and central Europe, it is now common throughout America and has escaped from English gardens to spread throughout the countryside. The ancient Greeks dedicated this herb to the goddess Diana and named it *melissa* – meaning "bee". More than 2,000 years ago, they observed that bees adored the fragrant white flowers and were attracted by the pollen. To this day, clever gardeners plant lemon balm around their orchards to encourage pollination, and beekeepers use it to keep their swarms close to home. The main constituents of lemon balm are volatile oils, flavonoids and polyphenols, which endow the plant with such an extraordinary range of benefits.

what it does

The ancient Greeks used lemon balm to improve the memory, relieve headaches and overcome depression. From the Middle Ages onwards, it has been a popular remedy for tension, headaches, toothache, skin conditions and depression. While these effects are a factual matter of observation, the most exciting modern use of lemon balm is as an antiviral. Local applications of essential oil can shorten the duration of an attack of *Herpes simplex* (the cold-sore virus) by several days. At the very first sign of prickling and tingling in the lips, apply the oil several times daily and drink two to three cups of lemon-balm tea. Regular use of this delicious aromatic herb in salads and cooking will certainly strengthen the immune system and protect specifically against viral infections. It can also be valuable in the treatment of neuralgic pain and indigestion.

how to use it

Use as tea (with one heaped tablespoon of fresh leaves to a cup of boiling water), tincture or essential oil. Use fresh leaves in salads and cooking.

precautions

There are no reports of serious adverse reactions or of interaction with other medications. Lemon balm is safe to take when driving, as well as with modest amounts of alcohol. Lemon-balm tea and tincture are safe when pregnant or breast-feeding. Some reports indicate that lemon-balm essential oil may have an adverse effect on anyone suffering from glaucoma, since it has been shown to increase the pressure in the eye.

dosage

Tea: two to three cups daily. Tincture: half a teaspoon in water three times a day. Essential oil: five drops to a teaspoon of grapeseed oil for local application.

available as

Essential oil

Fresh leaves

Tea bags

Tincture

tea tree *(melaleuca alternifolia)*

available as

Essential oil

Dried leaves

what it is

Tea tree, a relative of the myrtle, is a modest evergreen tree that grows to about 7.3m (24ft). Native to Australia, it is one of the most important local medicines used by the Aborigines. Their knowledge of its powerful healing properties has been passed from generation to generation for thousands of years. They used it by pounding the leaves and placing them on the affected area like a poultice or by bathing in pools over which tea trees grew. It was Captain Cook who gave the tree its name, because he and his crew used the leaves as a substitute for Indian or China tea.

what it does

Tea tree is powerfully antiseptic, antifungal and antibacterial, and it has the effect of giving your immune system a shot in the arm. The action of the plant's natural terpenoids accounts for these properties; the most important of them is terpinen-4-ol. This potent substance is a very important antiseptic that is also non-irritating to most skin types. Scientific evidence of tea tree's remarkable powers has abounded in Australia since the 1920s, and products made from it have proliferated during the past ten years. Good-quality organic tea-tree oil is a pure, safe substance that deserves a place in every home's medicine chest. It is now available commercially in shampoos, lotions, creams, talcum powder and even as a foot spray for the treatment of athlete's foot.

how to use it

A few drops of essential oil in a bowl of hot water releases decongestant steam for the nose and throat. Six or seven drops in the bath helps prevent thrush and other fungal diseases. Two or three cups of tea-tree tea, made from a teaspoon of dried leaves or half a teaspoon of tincture to a cup of warm water, increase resistance to bacterial, viral and fungal attacks.

precautions

Do not apply tea-tree oil to broken skin or to rashes, or near the eyes, nose, mouth or genital regions. When using tea-tree oil for the first time, test on a small sensitive area of skin, such as the inside of the forearm, and wait twenty-four hours before using it on larger areas. There are no reports of adverse reactions with other medications. Tea-tree oil is safe for external use during pregnancy and breast-feeding, but avoid internal mixtures.

dosage

For topical application: five drops of essential oil to 15ml of grapeseed oil or any other available pure vegetable oil; or add five drops to one teaspoon of any moisturizing cream. For internal use: half a teaspoon of infusion to a cup of warm water twice daily.

turmeric *(curcuma longa)*

what it is

Turmeric is a member of the ginger family and is native to India and China. It grows to a height of approximately 1m (3ft) and is cultivated for the medicinal value of its root, which is most commonly used as a flavouring and yellow colorant in Chinese and other Far Eastern cooking. Turmeric is available in both fresh and dried forms. This essential ingredient of curry powder is also widely used in southern Asian cooking. It is a key to successful Asian vegetarian food and is thought particularly important in the preparation of lentils. The most valuable of the plant's chemicals are its volatile oils, particularly curcumin, which is extracted and sold as a specific medicinal substance.

what it does

Prescribed for centuries by Ayurvedic practitioners in India, turmeric was used in the treatment of bad eyesight, rheumatism, arthritis and liver problems. As well as confirming the traditional activities of turmeric, scientists are now fascinated by its powerful antioxidant and protective properties, which appear to work in a similar way to the latest non-steroidal anti-inflammatories, the Cox-2 inhibitors. But turmeric has one huge advantage: there are no side effects.

how to use it

Incorporate turmeric in cooking to make it a regular part of your daily diet. For emergency situations, when your resistance is low or bacterial and viral infections are rampant, take capsules of curcumin for a two- to three-week period.

precautions

There are no reports of adverse reactions or interactions with other drugs. Using turmeric as a culinary spice is safe during pregnancy and breast-feeding. However, there is no data available on large doses of curcumin in respect of pregnancy, so it is probably best avoided.

dosage

Up to 1.5g a day of curcumin extracted from turmeric, or one teaspoon of dried turmeric powder to a cup of water three times daily.

available as

Capsules

Dried powder (for cooking)

Fresh plant

cleansing

artichoke, globe *(cynara scolymus)*

available as

Fresh plant

Capsules

what it is

Every French housewife knows that the globe artichoke is a boon to the digestion and a powerful stimulant of the gall bladder and liver. The globe artichoke is a type of thistle that originates from the Mediterranean part of Europe. It is not to be confused with the Jerusalem artichoke, a North American plant that found its way to France during the 1600s. The latter, a knobbly little tuber related to the sunflower, is rich in potassium but not much else.

what it does

Rich in a bitter chemical called cynarine, artichokes traditionally form the first course of any over-rich meal. Because they stimulate the production of bile, this makes the digestion of fats much easier. Bile works in the same way as dishwashing detergent on greasy dishes: it breaks fat down into minute globules, dramatically increasing the surface area that is exposed to the stomach's digestive juices. Herbalists have traditionally used extracts of artichoke to treat high blood pressure, and it is also known to help the body get rid of cholesterol. Together with its diuretic properties, artichoke is a cleanser and detoxifier – which makes it useful for people suffering from gout, arthritis or rheumatism. Both types of artichoke also contain a plant chemical called inulin; like fibre, inulin is not broken down during digestion, but is fermented in the colon (large bowel). It has a similar action to fibre, but can be a source of embarrassing flatulence.

how to use it

Eat fresh baby globe artichokes raw with a little olive oil, or sauté lightly and mix with pasta. You can also cook the leaves together with the peeled, chopped stalks for additional cynarine. Standardized extracts are available as capsules and can be taken as a liver-protector before and after rich food or a night on the town. Jerusalem artichokes are best eaten as soup.

precautions

There are no reported side effects or interactions with other medications.

dosage

Take 300-600mg of standardized extract or 10-20g of fresh leaf daily.

dandelion *(taraxacum officinale)*

what it is

It is no surprise that the French call this plant *pis en lit* and that the English country name for it is "wet the bed". *Pis en lit salade* is available in street markets throughout France. The dandelion is a common plant that grows throughout the world. It is related to endive, and its leaves have a similarly bitter taste. The name comes from the French *dent-de-lion* – a reference to the shape of the leaves, which some say resemble lion's teeth. For all gardeners seeking a perfect lawn, dandelions are a bane, but the leaves are delicious in salads and, apart from their medicinal value, are a rich source of iron. They are also valuable for their roots, which, when dried and ground, can be used as a coffee substitute.

what it does

Dandelions contain carotenoids (including lutein), potassium, vitamin C, taraxacoside, taraxerol and iron. This cleansing herb is a strong diuretic, tonic and anti-inflammatory; there is even some evidence of anti-tumour benefits. Useful for kidney and liver problems, it also reduces fluid retention – especially around period time. Thanks to their eliminative properties, dandelions are also helpful for those with rheumatism.

how to use it

As long as dogs, cats and spray-on chemicals are kept away from your lawn, you, too, can enjoy the unique flavour and all the health-giving benefits of young, bright-green dandelion leaves added to a salad. Eat the leaves raw or use a prepared alcoholic extract or dried-root herbal extract. Commercial products are available as liquid or tablets.

precautions

No known side effects or interactions.

dosage

Take 3-5g of dried root, 5ml of alcoholic tincture or 200mg standardized extract, all taken up to three times a day.

available as

Capsules
Dried root
Fresh plant
Liquid extract
Tablets

flax *(linum usitatissimum)*

available as

Capsules

Oil

Seeds

what it is

Flax is one of the most ancient of all cultivated plants and is known to have been used by man since 5,000BC. Egyptian mummies were wrapped in cloth made from the stems of flax, and this extraordinary plant is mentioned in the ancient writings of Greece, Rome and Egypt, as well as in the Old Testament. Both the seeds and seed oil have medicinal value. Linoleic and linolenic essential fatty acids are both present in the oil – essential precursors to the anti-inflamatory prostaglandins. Just like evening primrose oil, this is what makes flaxseed (linseed) oil such a valuable remedy for inflammatory skin and joint disorders.

what it does

Flax seeds are an excellent laxative and have a cleansing effect on the entire digestive system. They are also useful for the reduction of inflammation of the stomach, as well as of the small and large intestines. They can be an effective remedy for irritable bowel syndrome (IBS) and diverticulitis, and help to repair damage done by laxative abuse. The oil is a rich source of essential fatty acids and can be used for the treatment of inflammatory joint problems, eczema and psoriasis. Crushed flax seeds make an effective poultice for the cleansing of boils and other skin infections. Flax seeds are a useful aid to cholesterol reduction. Some studies have shown them to have cancer-fighting properties as well.

how to use it

As a laxative, soak one teaspoon of seeds in cold water overnight; eat them in the morning. For inflammatory problems, use crushed (but not powdered) seeds and take one teaspoon with a large glass of water daily for maximum oil release. For severe inflammatory problems, use capsules of oil, usually 1,250mg per capsule, taken one to three times daily.

precautions

Taking excessive amounts of seeds and too little water may cause bowel obstruction. Take seeds separately from other medications, since they may slow drug absorption.

dosage

One teaspoon of seeds or 1-3g of oil daily.

milk thistle *(silybum marianum)*

what it is

Milk thistle belongs to the same family as the artichoke. It grows wild on roadside embankments, derelict sites and in most gardens. The plant's vivid purple flower heads are a favourite with florists, but the seeds of the dried flowers are used medicinally. The plant has been employed as a medicine since the birth of Christ, and the great English herbalist Nicholas Culpeper recommended it as a treatment for liver disorders during the 1700s. The seeds contain a complicated bioflavonoid called silymarin, and it is this that has the liver-protective and liver-stimulating activity.

what it does

In traditional herbal medicine, milk thistle was used to kick-start and increase the flow of milk for nursing mothers. Like many other bitter herbs, it also has a long history of use as a digestion and appetite stimulant. Milk thistle's silymarin content protects the liver from poisonous toxins and has even been used against poisoning by the death-cap mushroom. Its other important action is to stimulate the regrowth of liver cells to replace those damaged by disease or toxic substances. Like the artichoke, milk thistle stimulates the gall bladder and helps the digestion of fatty foods, as well as cleansing the liver after excessive consumption of alcohol or rich dishes.

how to use it

Take up to 420mg of standardized silymarin per day as capsules. Use 5g of ground seeds to a cup of boiling water and drink up to three cups of tea daily.

precautions

There are no reported side effects, and this herb is safe to use during pregnancy and breast-feeding. There are no reports of interactions with other medications.

dosage

Take 15g of ground seeds made into tea or 420mg of standardized silymarin daily.

available as

Capsules

Ground seeds

circulation

folic acid *(folate)*

available as

Capsules

Tablets

what it is

Folic acid, also known as folate, is part of the vitamin B complex, and it is essential in the formation of DNA: the genetic "skeleton" of every single cell. A lack of folic acid causes anaemia, and deficiency during the early stages of pregnancy causes genetic abnormalities, specifically spina bifida. Folic acid is found in dark-green vegetables such as broccoli and spinach; in wholewheat bread and wholegrain cereals; and in liver, kidneys and nuts. Unfortunately, it is very easily destroyed by overcooking or exposure to bright sunlight.

what it does

In addition to being essential during pregnancy, latest research has shown that low levels of folic acid in the diet lead to increased levels of homocysteine, which is a strong predictor of heart disease. Some European countries have already legislated to add folic acid to all flour so that their national consumption of this substance is increased. The same legislation is imminent in the UK and should do much to redress the generally low intake of this vital nutrient.

how to use it

In the UK, 200 micrograms daily is advised. Take as a single supplement, as part of a B-complex formula or in a general multivitamin and mineral formula. Increase consumption of folate-rich foods. Regular use of antacids or digestive enzyme supplements can interfere with the absorption of folic acid. If using either, an extra dose of 600 micrograms daily is advised.

precautions

Long-term high dosage of folic acid can mask the symptoms of pernicious anaemia. There are no known adverse reactions with other medications. It is safe during pregnancy and lactation, but only in the recommended doses. Prolonged use of 1,500 micrograms or more a day can lead to abdominal discomfort, appetite loss and the formation of crystals inside the kidney.

dosage

In the UK, the recommended daily requirement of folate is 200 micrograms for men and women, plus an extra 100 during pregnancy and an extra 400 for women planning pregnancy. In America, the levels are 400 micrograms per day for all adults, plus an extra 400 during pregnancy and another 100 when breast-feeding.

garlic *(allium sativum)*

what it is

Garlic is the single most versatile, powerful and widely used medicinal plant in the world. A relative of onions, spring onions, leeks and chives, it has an historic use as an antifungal and antibacterial, especially effective for the treatment of chest infections.

This herb was much loved by the physicians of the ancient world. Slaves building the pyramids were paid in garlic, as were Roman soldiers, who brought the bulb to England, wedged between their toes to ward off athlete's foot. Great Classical healers such as Hippocrates, Pliny and Diascorides all wrote about garlic and used it for many illnesses. You'll find it in the Bible and ancient Hebrew writings, and the Chinese have used it for 2,500 years. Louis Pasteur also studied it and proved that it was a powerful antibacterial in the mid-nineteenth century.

what it does

In the 1980s, research began to demonstrate the amazing value of garlic in the protection of the heart and circulatory system. Several hundred published research papers show that garlic can lower cholesterol, reduce blood pressure and make the blood less sticky, thus reducing the risk of clots. A regular intake of garlic not only protects the heart and circulation and boosts their function, but also protects against food poisoning, other bacterial and fungal infections, and even has some cancer-fighting properties. Sulphur-rich compounds released when garlic is crushed produce not only its characteristic smell but also most of its therapeutic benefits. For this reason, supplements that are deodorized or made solely of extracted garlic oil are not as effective as either the whole bulb or the standardized whole extract.

how to use it

If you can't bear the taste, take garlic as tablets, but everyone would benefit from one fresh clove a day (or standardized tablets providing an equivalent dose).

precautions

There are no known interactions with other medications. Skin reactions may occur from handling large quantities of garlic. Mild digestive discomfort has been reported in a few cases. Because it thins the blood, do not take garlic supplements two or three weeks before undergoing surgery; tell your doctor if you have been using them. Garlic is considered safe to take during pregnancy or breast-feeding.

dosage

One medium-sized fresh raw clove per day, or coated tablets of 300mg dried garlic, standardized to produce 1,800 micrograms of allicin; take two daily.

available as

Dried powder (for cooking)

Fresh cloves

Tablets

ginkgo biloba *(the maidenhair tree)*

available as

Capsules

Tablets

Tea bags

what it is

Ginkgo biloba, also known as the maidenhair tree, is the most ancient and one of the longest-surviving plants on earth. Individual trees can live up to 1,000 years, and its medicinal use is recorded 5,000 years ago in traditional Chinese medicine. The tree's leaves are used medicinally. Gentle drying ensures that only the water is removed, then the whole leaf is crushed and made into tablets, which are standardized to ensure an accurate daily intake of its active ingredients.

what it does

The potent natural chemicals in ginkgo extract have the unique ability to improve circulation to the brain, at the same time reducing the stickiness of the blood. Research shows that ginkgo is highly effective in improving short-term memory loss in the elderly. Even people in the early stages of Alzheimer's disease can benefit from ginkgo biloba. There is no evidence that the plant is in any way a treatment for Alzheimer's, but given in the early stages of the illness it appears to delay the worsening of symptoms by many months. Research conducted by Professor Ian Hindmarch, of the Human Psychopharmacology Research Unit at the University of Surrey, UK, surveyed the impact of ginkgo on a group of volunteers who were young, healthy and had no memory problems. The results demonstrated that ginkgo improved concentration, psycho-motor skills and memory in the group taking 120mg of extract daily. As a general circulatory stimulant, ginkgo is helpful in the treatment of Raynaud's disease, chilblains and tinnitus.

how to use it

Take as standardized-extract, high-dose 120mg tablets – two together with breakfast. Alternatively, take three tablets daily containing 50mg ginkgo extract at meal times.

precautions

There are no reports of interactions with other medications, and no contraindications for use during pregnancy or breast-feeding. Very rarely, people have reported mild headaches or stomach upsets for the first day or two of taking the tablets. These symptoms then fade.

dosage

Up to 220mg daily of standardized ginkgo biloba extract, providing 60mg active ginkgo flavonglycosides and 14.4mg ginkgolides and bilobalide.

horse chestnut *(aesculus hippocastanum)*

what it is

The horse chestnut is a large, deciduous tree boasting "candles" of beautiful pink-and-white flowers and rough-covered seeds – the horse chestnuts themselves. Left to their own devices, the trees can grow to a huge 24.4m (8ft+), with a massive canopy that provides a cooling haven on hot summer days.

Originating in eastern Europe and Asia, the horse chestnut now grows in most temperate climatic zones. It has been known as a medicinal plant since Roman times, and extracts of the seeds were more commonly used throughout Europe than in the UK. In the past, the bark, chestnuts and leaves have all been used, but modern preparations consist of standardized extracts taken from the seeds, which have the richest concentration of active substances.

what it does

Although traditionally horse chestnut was used for its cleansing and anti-inflammatory properties, its most important use is in the treatment of peripheral circulatory disorders. Aescin, the most powerful of its constituents, acts specifically as a tonic to vein walls, making this an excellent remedy for the relief of varicose veins, fluid retention and haemorrhoids. Local application is excellent for reducing swelling after an injury.

how to use it

As a standardized extract of dried seeds. Use as a gel applied to painful regions morning and evening.

precautions

Use only standardized extracts with known aescin content; do not exceed recommended doses. Do not take or use topically if suffering from kidney or liver disease, or if pregnant or breast-feeding, and do not use for children under fourteen. Rarely, horse chestnut may cause local allergic reactions when applied topically. There are no reports of interactions with other medications.

dosage

Take 0.5-1g of dried seed. Standardized extract: take fifteen to twenty per cent aescin content, providing 50-100mg of aescin daily, reducing to 25-50mg for maintenance.

available as

Dried seed

Gel

Tablets

selenium

available as

Brazil nuts

Tablets

what it is

Selenium is an essential mineral that is worryingly deficient in the average person's diet. The minimum daily requirement for adult males is 75 micrograms per day; for females, 60 micrograms per day. The daily amount provided by food has declined by fifty per cent over the past twenty years to an average of 35 micrograms per day for men and women. Americans get most of their selenium from bread made with North American and Canadian wheat. The wheat grows on selenium-rich soil; consequently, it contains substantial amounts. In Britain, however, such grains are no longer imported, and European wheats containing much less selenium are used instead. Other good food sources are brazil nuts, wholegrain foods, onions, garlic, sesame seeds and shellfish. Selenium first came to international prominence through American involvement with China and "Keshan disease". This condition produced a vast rate of heart disease in young men in the Keshan province, where the soil is almost devoid of selenium. An American drug company provided selenium supplements; halfway through a double-blind trial, it was so obvious which group was getting the real pill that the study was abandoned, and selenium supplements were given to all participants.

what it does

Selenium is the essential link in the activation of an antioxidant enzyme called glutathione peroxidase. Without sufficient selenium, the enzyme cannot do its job as a heart-protector and cancer-preventer. Selenium is also essential for normal thyroid function. A large number of studies show that an abundant intake of selenium reduces the risk of fatty deposits in the arteries and damage to the heart muscle, as well as the risk of breast and prostate cancers.

how to use it

A daily supplement is one of the most important superboosters to add to your normal regime. Selenium is normally combined with yeast for better absorption. For all-around heart and circulatory benefits, it is best taken in combination with vitamins A, C and E.

precautions

There are no reports of interactions with other medicines. It is safe to take selenium during pregnancy and breast-feeding, but only at the recommended dose. Long-term use of 1,000 micrograms a day or more can have serious side effects, such as rashes or damage to the nervous system.

dosage

Up to 200 micrograms daily.

vitamin e

what it is

Vitamin E is one of the most essential of all the protective antioxidants. It is vital for the good health and proper functioning of the heart and circulatory system. Although vitamin E was discovered almost sixty years ago, new research continues to produce exciting results. In the US, scientists studied a group of 87,000 female nurses and 40,000 male health workers for eight years; those taking a daily supplement of vitamin E – at least 100 international units (IU) – showed a forty per cent reduction in the risk of heart disease. In the UK, the Cambridge Heart Antioxidant Study (CHAOS), a European multicentre study in which volunteers were given between 400 and 800 IU of vitamin E each day, showed a resulting reduction of seventy-five per cent in the occurrence of non-fatal heart attacks.

what it does

Vitamin E protects the actual membrane of every individual cell in the body, and that includes protecting fat-soluble tissues such as LDL, the dangerous type of cholesterol. It is generally believed that only damaged LDL cells have the ability to cause arterial and heart problems; by protecting the cholesterol cells, vitamin E also protects the heart and blood vessels. The list of benefits covers virtually all inflammatory conditions, but the certain advantages of consuming extra vitamin E come from its cardiovascular activity. It is also useful in the treatment of osteo- and rheumatoid arthritis, eczema, infertility and menopause.

how to use it

Take in capsules, but also ensure a good dietary intake from wheat germ and olive oils, nuts, seeds, eggs, dark-green leafy vegetables and avocados.

precautions

There are no reported interactions with other medications, and no evidence of contraindication during pregnancy or breast-feeding. If your diet contains large amounts of polyunsaturated fats, you'll need to increase your intake of vitamin E.

dosage

Take 200-400 IU daily. Up to 10,000 IU with professional advice.

available as

Capsules

Tablets

mood

black cohosh *(cimicifuga racemosa)*

available as

Dried root

Powdered extract

Tablets

Tincture

what it is

Black cohosh is yet another of the Native American medicines that started life in the eastern regions of America and Canada. It now grows wild in Europe, too, as a garden escapee. An herbaceous perennial, black cohosh is a relative of the buttercup and grows to about 2.4m (8ft) in height, with attractive spikes of cream flowers. The plant was named cohosh by the Algonquin Indians; the word means "rough", which is an apt description of its dark, twisted root. Fortunately, those natives weren't put off by the unpleasant smell and bitter flavour of this herb, which they used to great effect in the relief of rheumatic pain and joint disorders, as well as more traditionally in problems of the menstrual cycle.

The key constituents are triterpene glycosides and a group of isoflavones, which are hormone-like substances. Salicylic acid and isoferulic acid are also present, and the combined pain-reducing and oestrogen-like effects are the result of the herb's complex chemical construction.

what it does

The traditional use of black cohosh is for the relief of the physical and psychological symptoms of the menstrual cycle and, later, menopause. It is particularly effective in the relief of hot flushes and general malaise of menopause, and it helps lift the low mood that often accompanies unpleasant menopausal symptoms. Black cohosh is also a valuable anti-inflammatory and inhibits the production of progesterone from the ovaries by decreasing the levels of stimulated hormones. The general sedative effects of the plant may also be helpful in the relief of tinnitus.

how to use it

The most convenient way to take black cohosh is in tablet form as a standardized concentrated extract. Tablets are usually equivalent to 40-50mg of the fresh herb. Up to 2g a day of the dried root or 500mg of powdered extract or half a teaspoon of tincture are normal daily doses.

precautions

There are no reported interactions with other medications, but it is not suitable for pregnant or breast-feeding women. Women should seek medical advice if using oestrogen-based medication. Large doses can cause headaches, nausea and dizziness, among other side effects. Not advised for children or in large doses for the elderly. Avoid long-term use.

dosage

Standardized extracts as tincture or tablets, 250mg providing 40-50mg of extract or up to 2g a day of dried root.

feverfew *(tanacetum parthenium)*

what it is

Feverfew is an attractive member of the chrysanthemum family, and it was originally native to parts of southern Europe. Today, however, it has spread all over Europe, the UK and North America. This useful perennial grows to a height of about 0.6m (2ft) and has masses of attractive yellow and white flowers that resemble daisies. Gardeners beware: it is highly invasive.

Although feverfew was used traditionally in the treatment of all types of fevers, it was the seventeenth-century English herbalist Nicholas Culpeper who first recommended it for headaches; he also maintained that it was one of the best of all herbs for women. In modern times, this herb has become synonymous with the relief of migraines, an action attributed to the phytochemical (plant chemical) parthenolide. The plant also contains valuable volatile oils and camphor. While a wide range of manufactured feverfew products are on the market, it is easy to grow and use, and it deserves a place in everyone's garden – migraine sufferer or not.

what it does

Feverfew appears to have a powerful anti-inflammatory action, which would explain its historical use in the treatment of rheumatism and arthritis. Roman physicians found it valuable in treating menstrual problems and used it as an aid to stimulate the start of periods. Although feverfew had been used as an effective treatment for migraine and headaches for more than 300 years, it wasn't until the 1970s that any serious clinical evaluation was undertaken. The results confirmed the wisdom of the herbalists and showed that around seventy per cent of migraine sufferers could benefit to a greater or lesser degree from this simple, safe and very inexpensive remedy. Exactly how feverfew works is still something of a mystery, yet it appears that the parthenolide reduces the amount of the hormone serotonin. Serotonin, which is produced by the body, is thought to be a likely trigger of migraine attacks.

how to use it

Eat two to three leaves a day; for many migraine sufferers, this is enough to prevent recurrent attacks. It is important to put the leaves into a sandwich, since eaten alone they can cause severe and unpleasant mouth ulcers. Feverfew is also available as standardized tablets and as capsules of dried powdered leaf.

precautions

Eating the fresh leaf may cause mouth ulcers. Not advised during pregnancy or breast-feeding; not for children under twelve. Do not take feverfew if you have been prescribed aspirin, warfarin or other blood-thinning drugs, because it may reduce the effectiveness of your medication. Rarely, some people may develop skin sensitivity to the leaves.

dosage

Two to three fresh leaves daily. Up to 1.5g of dried-leaf powder daily. As a tincture: add five drops to a glass of water and take three times daily.

available as

Capsules
Fresh plant
Tablets

kava kava *(piper methysticum)*

available as

Capsules

what it is

This large climbing shrub is a native Polynesian vine that is found all over the Pacific Islands. It has been used since the earliest times to make a mind-altering liquid that played an essential part in both social and religious ceremonies. The root of kava kava is transformed into a non-alcoholic drink by the Pacific Islanders. Its use as a modern herbal remedy is based on its traditional mood-enhancing benefits, including a long-standing and justified reputation as an aphrodisiac. This valuable member of the pepper family contains a unique resin made up of kava lactones, as well as the alkaloid pipermethysticine.

what it does

In modest doses, kava kava is best known as a safe treatment for stress and anxiety. Unlike many prescribed tranquillizers, the herb does not cause drowsiness or interfere with the ability to drive or operate dangerous machinery in safety. It is a remarkable remedy for overcoming the problems of extended periods of stress and anxiety, and it also helps relieve the muscle tension and subsequent pain that often accompanies unrelieved emotional stress. Some scientific studies have revealed that kava kava is as good a tranquillizer as the benzodiazepines, but without their addictive problems. Kava kava is also helpful in relieving the pain of osteo- and rheumatoid arthritis, as well as other forms of chronic and intractable pain.

how to use it

Best taken as a standardized preparation of root extract, combined with root powder in the form of capsules.

precautions

Do not take continuously for more than three months. Excessive doses lead to euphoria and the appearance of drunkenness. Not suitable during pregnancy or breast-feeding. Do not take with alcohol or prescribed mind-affecting medication. Not suitable in the treatment of severe depression.

dosage

Up to 200mg of kava lactones per day.

passionflower *(passiflora incarnata)*

what it is

This popular climbing vine, adorned with beautiful purple flowers, can grow to around 9m (30ft) in length. Although indigenous to South, Central and North America, varieties of this vigorous plant now grow almost everywhere. Its delicious fruit seldom develops in the UK or northern Europe, though it may do so during a long, hot summer. Passionflower has been popular with European herbalists since the late 1500s, and its virtues as a tranquillizing herb have been praised in herbal textbooks since that time. In North America, the herb has been widely used and studied for at least one hundred and fifty years. A traditional treatment for anxiety and insomnia – and applied locally for headaches and injuries – it has an ancient history among the Aztecs, Amazonian Indians and native North Americans. The plant acquired its name from sixteenth-century Spanish missionaries, who believed the flower represented the crucifixion: the three styles for the nails through Christ's hands and feet, and the five stamens for His wounds.

what it does

The most important constituents are flavonoids, especially apigenin and isovitexin, and the glycosides, including gynocardin. The flowers, leaves and stems are used fresh or dried for their calming effects. Passionflower is extremely valuable for the treatment of insomnia, agitation, irritability and anxiety. Less well researched, though high on the list of traditional uses, are its antispasmodic qualities: it may be safely used for stomach cramps, palpitations, high blood pressure and colic.

how to use it

Passionflower can be taken as a tea, tincture or as commercially available tablets or extracts. It is often found combined with lemon balm, valerian or other mood-enhancing herbs.

precautions

There are no reported side effects or interactions with other medications. Some experts suggest that it should not be taken with the MAOI category of antidepressants. Passionflower is safe for children and there are no known reports of harmful effects during pregnancy or breast-feeding.

dosage

Recommended dosage is 6g of dried herb as an infusion (made as tea) daily.

available as

Capsules

Tablets

Tincture

st john's wort *(hypericum perforatum)*

available as

Tablets

what it is

An upright perennial growing to around 1m (3ft) high with attractive, brilliant-yellow flowers, St John's wort grows wild throughout Europe. It flowers normally around St John's Day, 24 June, which is how it gets its common name. For centuries, St John's wort been used in the treatment of chest infections, bladder problems, for wound healing and as a gentle sedative. Its modern use, however, is mainly for the treatment of mild to moderate depression; more than two million people have tried it for this reason in the UK alone. Even this is not a new treatment; the ancient Greeks called St John's wort the "sunshine herb", because it brought light back into the lives of depressed people.

what it does

St John's wort contains volatile oil, flavonoids and, most importantly, hypericin, which is not only antidepressant but also has powerful antiviral properties. Hypericin is found in all parts of the plant. A recent analysis of twenty-three different clinical trials has shown beyond doubt that St John's wort is extremely effective in the relief of mild to moderate depression. Yet even mild depression can trigger a range of distressing symptoms: insomnia, exhaustion, tiredness, muscle pain, headaches and palpitations – symptoms that can all be helped by St John's wort. Repeated double-blind studies have proved that individuals suffering from mild to moderate depression respond as well to this gentle and non-addictive herb as they do to more powerful chemical sedatives, tranquillizers and antidepressants. Despite some suggestions of interactions with other medications (*see* "precautions"), I believe that St John's wort is infinitely safer than aspirin, paracetamol or other anti-inflammatory drugs. To put it another way, eighty-seven million St John's wort tablets were manufactured by the Kira firm in the past two years; to date, the company hasn't received a single report of an adverse side effect from customers or their doctors.

how to use it

St John's wort is best taken as a tablet with a standardized concentration of hypericin.

precautions

There is evidence of interaction with some prescribed medicines, specifically the blood-thinning drug warfarin. It could also interfere with drugs for HIV, organ transplants and epilepsy, with theophiline for asthma, some antidepressants, triptans for migraine and low-dose contraceptive pills. It is best avoided during pregnancy and breast-feeding.

dosage

Recommended dosage is 400–600mg of dried extract, equivalent to 900 micrograms total hypericin daily.

valerian *(valeriana officinalis)*

what it is

Valerian is an attractive perennial with pretty pink flowers. It grows throughout Europe and is now well established in North America. As far back as the first century AD, the physician Dioscorides used it, as did Hippocrates before him, and Paracelsus after that. In the Middle Ages, valerian was used for many medicinal purposes, though proof of its efficacy in the treatment of epilepsy has never been substantiated. While the ancient Greeks and Romans understood the herb's value as a gentle sedative, it wasn't until the middle of the eighteenth century that it became widely accepted in the treatment of anxiety and insomnia. Valerian contains many active constituents, including volatile oils, iridoids and alkaloids.

what it does

Prolonged periods of stress lead to a state of constant heightened arousal and overproduction of the activity hormone adrenaline. This is the hormone that prepares the body for "fight or flight": the heart rate increases, blood pressure rises and mental faculties are sharpened so that mind and body are prepared for instant action. Valerian can break this vicious circle. Taken in small doses, its action is calming without causing drowsiness. Larger doses become mildly sedative and help to restore regular sleep patterns in those suffering from insomnia. As a bonus, valerian is an effective antispasmodic that helps to relieve colic, stomach cramps and irritable bowel syndrome (IBS).

how to use it

Most commonly taken as tablets, but see "dosage" for alternatives.

precautions

There are no reported side effects or interactions with prescribed medications. Valerian is safe to use during pregnancy or breast-feeding.

dosage

Up to 3g of dried plant, equivalent to 700mg of standardized extract. As tincture: 20 drops in a cup of hot water four times a day for anxiety, or half an hour before bed for insomnia.

available as

Tablets

Tincture

digestion

camomile *(chamomilla recutita)*

available as

Capsules

Dried herb

Fresh herb

Tablets

Tea bags

Tincture

what it is

Camomile, or German chamomile, grows throughout Europe, often wild, but it is cultivated on a large scale for medicinal use. It has been a valuable herb since Roman times and was extremely popular with medieval herbalists. In southern Europe, camomile tea is used extensively as a gentle, safe remedy for children. This attractive member of the daisy family has a deliciously sweet aroma and was often planted for lawns so that its fragrance was released when walked on. Used externally as lotions and creams, camomile makes a soothing application for skin irritation, abrasions, bites and stings, but it is as an aid to digestion that it has earned its reputation.

what it does

Camomile flowers contain volatile oils, the most important of which are proazulenes, alpha-bis-abolol and spiroether, together with bioflavonoids and quercetin. This combination is anti-inflammatory and antispasmodic, which accounts for its 2,000-year history in the treatment of digestion problems. This herb is particularly beneficial in the relief of irritable bowel syndrome (IBS), stomach cramps, bloating and colic. Weak camomile tea with a little honey is excellent for children with a temperature, headache or restlessness.

how to use it

Camomile is most simply taken as a tea: one teaspoon of dried flowers to a cup of boiling water. If using a tincture: one teaspoon to a glass of water.

precautions

Camomile has no known interactions with other medications and is safe to use during pregnancy and breast-feeding. There have been rare reports of allergic reactions, more likely in people allergic to ragweed and chrysanthemums.

dosage

One teaspoon of tincture in a glass of water after each meal. If taking tablets or capsules, use the equivalent of 2g of plant per day. For tea, see "how to use it".

fennel *(foeniculum vulgare)*

what it is

Originally found growing wild throughout Europe, fennel is now widely cultivated around the world and has a history dating back to the ancient Greeks and Romans. Prime among its many medicinal uses are its beneficial effects on the digestive system, but the ancients also used it as an aid to slimming, due to its function as a strong appetite suppressant. Both the seeds and the delicate fronds are used widely in cooking, particularly in stews, soups and with fish dishes. The crushed seeds, together with dill, are a basic ingredient in some colic medicines for babies.

what it does

The most important natural chemicals in fennel are anethole and fenchone, now thought to have oestrogen-like properties and also to have a specific effect on smooth muscle contraction. For this reason, fennel is invaluable in the treatment of constipation, irritable bowel syndrome (IBS), colic and indigestion. Seeds also stimulate the production of bile, thus improving liver function and fat digestion. In India and the Middle East, it is common to chew a few fennel seeds after a meal to improve digestion and prevent flatulence.

how to use it

Fennel seeds may be chewed or used to make tea. The plant can also be made into a tincture. And, of course, you can eat it as a vegetable.

precautions

There are no reports of interactions with other medications, but fennel seeds are toxic if taken in large amounts. They can badly affect the nervous system and cause convulsions, so do not exceed the recommended dose. Though there are no reports of fennel causing problems during pregnancy, it is probably best avoided.

dosage

Half a teaspoon of crushed seeds to a cup of boiling water: drink three cups a day. Tincture: half a teaspoon in water three times a day.

available as

Fresh bulb

Seeds

fenugreek *(trigonella foenum-graecum)*

available as

Seeds

what it is

This strongly aromatic spice is native to the eastern Mediterranean and North Africa. It grows wild on any leftover pieces of waste ground but is widely cultivated for its culinary and medicinal purposes. The ancient Egyptians used it as one of the ingredients of embalming fluid, and prescriptions include fenugreek in the historical Ebers papyrus, which was compiled 3,500 years ago. The seeds are used medicinally, and due to their bitter taste, they are usually available "debittered". In India, *methi* (the dried leaves) are added to root-vegetable dishes for a strong taste and smell.

what it does

Fenugreek is a great remedy for constipation, as well as for the reduction of blood cholesterol. The seeds contain plant steroids, particularly saponins and flavonoids, and vitamins A and C, along with small amounts of minerals. They were traditionally prescribed during convalescence, for the treatment of gastric ulcers and inflammation of the stomach lining. More recent research shows that fenugreek seeds can also help lower blood-sugar levels in diabetics and that they may also slow down the spread of liver tumours.

how to use it

Seeds are usually added to food during cooking and can be used whole, lightly roasted and crushed or finely ground. They can also be sprouted, making a tangy and extremely healthy addition to salads.

precautions

There are no reports of interactions with other medications, and fenugreek is extremely safe to use in cooking. However, the seeds should not be eaten during pregnancy, since they may produce contractions of the uterus. Do not exceed 100g of seeds per day.

dosage

Recommended dosage is 25–75g of seeds per day.

ginger *(zingiber officinale)*

what it is

Ginger is one of the greatest of all natural medicines, used by Chinese doctors since 1,000BC and popular with European herbalists from the Middle Ages. The root of this extraordinary plant is used in both food and medicine, and it is reputed to have been one of God's gifts to man in the Garden of Eden. Ginger grows throughout China and the rest of Asia, in the tropics and South America. Although some inedible varieties make powerful anti-inflammatories, ginger is the only one in common usage.

what it does

Ginger is one of the most potent of digestive remedies and an almost certain cure for various types of nausea. It is particularly effective for the relief of early morning sickness in pregnancy and is safe for both mother and baby. It works equally well for the prevention and treatment of travel sickness and is even used to prevent nausea after anaesthetics. Migraine-sufferers can also benefit – providing they take their ginger before the onset of vomiting. The plant is gaining growing acceptance as an adjunct to radiotherapy and chemotherapy, both of which commonly cause severe nausea. Ginger contains extremely powerful, active volatile oils, which provide both its distinctive taste and smell, as well as medicinal benefits. Zingiberene, zingerone, boreal, bisabolene and shogaols are the most important chemical constituents. These anti-inflammatory compounds are responsible for the other main medicinal value of ginger, which is as an anti-inflammatory for the treatment of rheumatism and arthritis. Although ordinary ginger does help with these conditions and is also an effective circulatory booster, other inedible Chinese varieties are even more potent.

how to use it

Fresh root: slice or grate into food, or grate 2.5cm (half an inch) into a mug, cover for ten minutes and strain for tea. Powder can be more pungent than fresh root, and the volatile oils decline rapidly. Commercial ginger capsules are widely available.

precautions

There are no reports of adverse reactions with other medications. However, some people may initially suffer heartburn after taking ginger. Those with stomach ulcers, hiatus hernia or gastric-reflux problems should start with small doses and always take ginger with food.

dosage

Fresh grated root: 2g three to four times daily.
Dried ginger powder: 1g three times daily.
Capsules of standardized ginger extract: up to 1g daily.

available as

Capsules
Dried powder
Fresh root

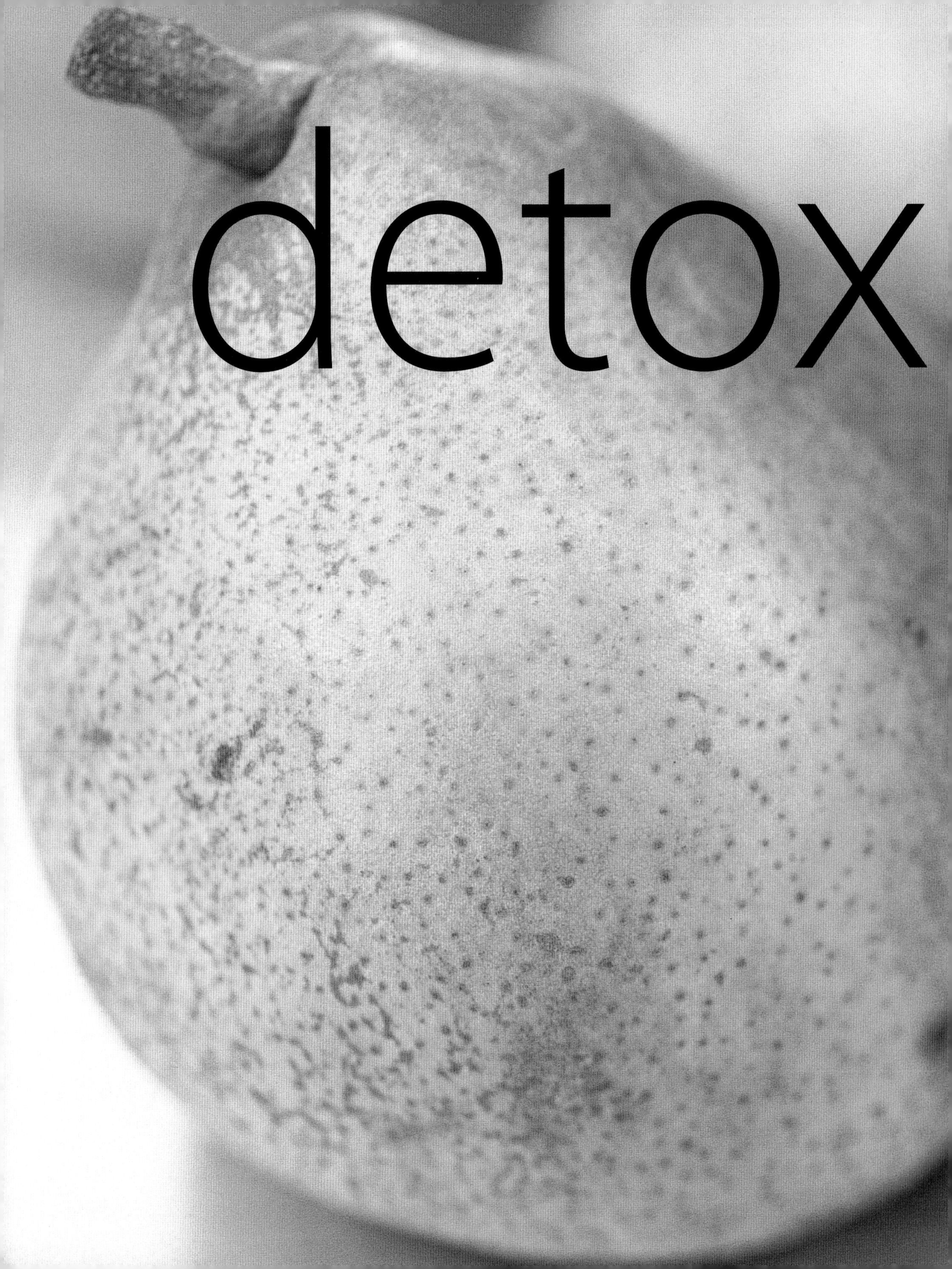

detox

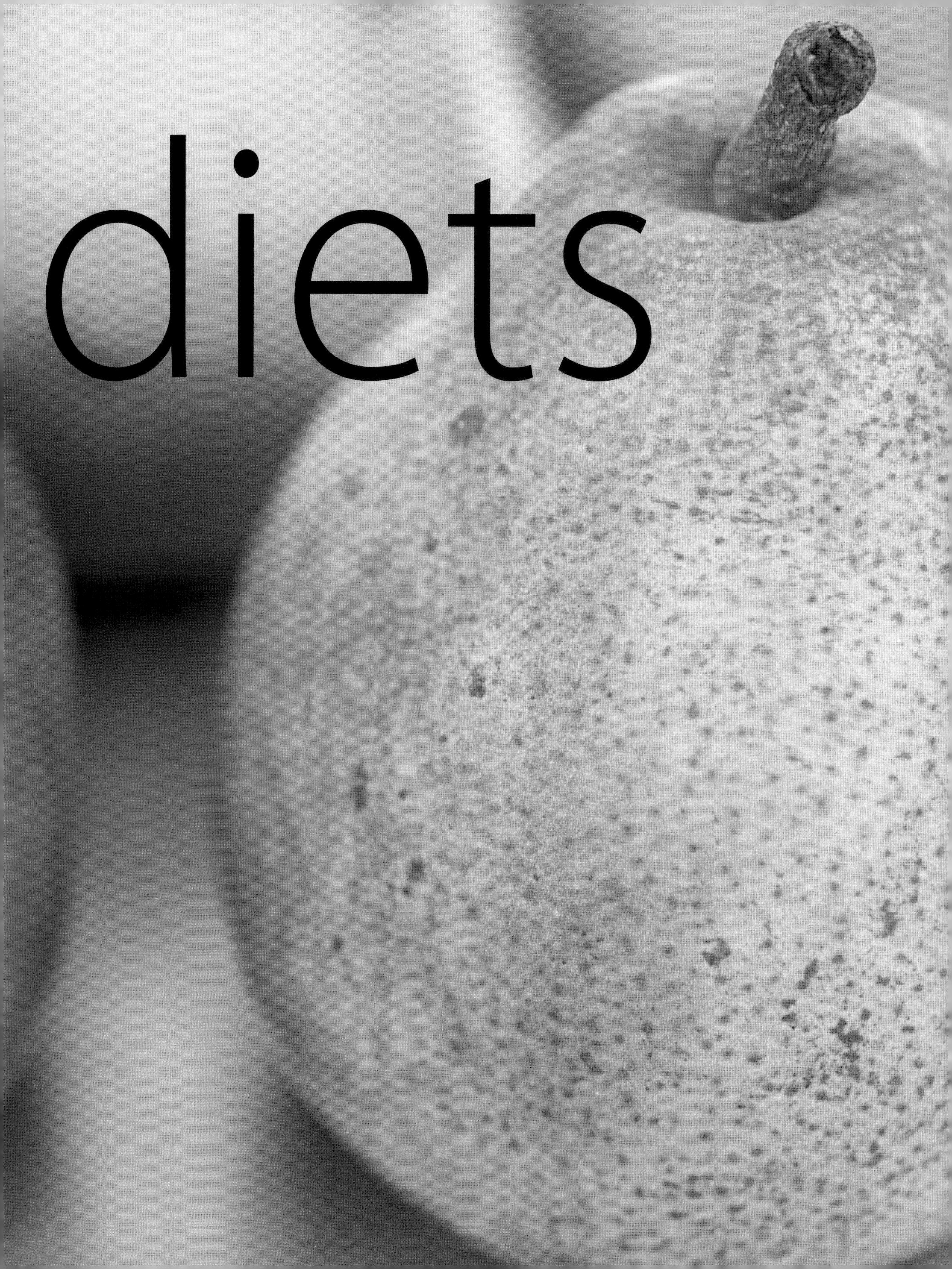
diets

Detox has become a real buzz-word during the last year or so. Unfortunately, it's also become a much-abused word and has been attached to a whole range of pills, potions, lotions and strange diets that do not fulfil the proper functions of a detoxifying regime.

Detoxification, or cleansing, is the traditional platform of naturopathy. It was commonly used in ancient times, often as part of religious ceremonies aimed at purifying body, mind and soul. The modern concept dates from the late nineteenth to early twentieth centuries when the European pioneers of the modern nature cure were developing their techniques, which later spread to America through practitioners like the famous Dr Kellogg and his Battle Creek sanatorium.

Until recently, the medical profession discounted the benefits of fasting, but modern science has shown that short periods without food increase the number of the blood's white cells: nature's policemen, which attack and overcome invading bacteria and viruses. A fast also helps to kill off unwanted bugs that are already living in the body and that may be the cause of chronic illness.

This chapter will guide you through a number of step-by-step regimes. Here, you will find a unique combination of all the traditional attributes of fasting and cleansing diets with the most up-to-date and scientifically proven benefits of herbal medicines, as well as natural food supplements that take you on to the next steps of re-energizing, revitalizing and rebuilding your own vitality. Discover the secrets of sustained natural energy to see you through the demands of work; how to get that extra burst of energy if sport is your thing; how to survive the rigours of an activity holiday, a weekend in the garden or redecorating your home without feeling like a wet rag on Monday morning.

These different detox plans will guide you through the maze of staying healthy after detoxing, providing detailed information on specific foods and supplements to suit your lifestyle and protect you against health problems. Again, there is now scientific evidence to support the value of foods as medicines. Tomatoes, spinach, blueberries, cranberries, strawberries, artichokes, cabbage, watercress, garlic, mustard, chillies, turmeric, parsley, sage, rosemary and thyme... all these and many others are proven protectors and wonderful foods. Trying the different plans that follow will help you understand the lifelong benefits of kitchen medicine, not just for you but for the rest of your family, too.

Skin shows some of the earliest signs that your body may not be functioning at its most efficient, and it also responds more rapidly to appropriate detox regimes than any other part of the body. Your body requires hundreds of nutrients for an unblemished complexion, perfect hair and nails and, of course, the bright eyes that complete the healthy look. With detoxing, you can overcome greasy skin, choose foods that provide the essential vitamin E and carotenoids you need, and learn to make the sensible food choices that will help you keep your perfect complexion and supple, wrinkle-free skin. The skin is the biggest organ of the body, and it's not just your face that matters. What you'll discover from detoxing is how to protect, preserve and improve your skin from your nose to your toes.

Chronic fatigue is one of the most common reasons that people consult their doctors, and when the usual prescription drugs fail, they turn to holistic practitioners of naturopathy like me. Lack of energy, exhaustion and chronic fatigue affect both mind and body. These symptoms are associated with a build-up of environmental pollutants: toxic chemicals from intensive farming, volatile organic compounds, heavy metals like lead and arsenic, and myriad synthetic additives in our food. A detox plan will help.

One really important aspect of detoxing is the way in which it helps beat the scourge of modern affluent society manifested by high blood pressure, strokes, raised cholesterol, heart disease, gallstones, IBS, PMS, osteoporosis, allergies, obesity and diabetes. There are a number of ways in which you could fit detox plans into your normal lifestyle. You may find it easier to follow a detox fast for one day a week like my dear friend and one of the world's greatest footballers, Sir Stanley Matthews, who used to fast on juices and raw fruit and vegetables every Monday. You may prefer a seasonal approach, like the twenty-four-hour summer and winter detox plans.

A three-day fast using a juice or herb detox is a practical monthly exercise, or you may prefer a one-week organic detox every quarter to keep you firing on all cylinders all the time. In this chapter you'll find a special twenty-four-hour detox to prepare you for "the big day"; a three-day immune-boosting programme and the three-day powerhouse energy-boosting diet. Whatever your choice, you'll find these plans easy to follow and really worth the effort you put into them.

Providing you're generally fit and well, anyone can do a short detox fast. Don't undertake any of these plans, however, if you're pregnant, seriously underweight or if you have any acute or chronic underlying illness that might make it imprudent to follow any type of restricted eating scheme.

twenty-four-hour summer detox

Here is a simple plan for a twenty-four-hour detox fast designed for the warmer months. But first, a word of warning: this is not suitable for diabetics, and if you have a serious illness or are currently taking prescribed medication, do check with your doctor before trying it (although it should be suitable for almost everyone). Use this for an occasional short, sharp cleansing process or – better still – do it once a month to keep your body's toxic load to a minimum.

It's best to start this fast on a day when you're not working, and it's much more effective if on the day before, you keep off alcohol, coffee, red meat and dairy products. The day after the detox do the same, then return to your normal but (hopefully healthier) eating patterns.

Drink at least six glasses of water, and as much herb or weak China tea as you like throughout the day. Don't add milk, sugar or sweeteners and avoid fizzy water, canned drinks, squashes, alcohol and coffee.

First thing in the morning, make up a jug of parsley tea. Pour 850ml or 30 fl oz of boiling water over a generous handful of chopped parsley. Cover, leave for ten minutes, strain, refrigerate and drink throughout the day. Parsley tea is a mild diuretic, which eliminates excess fluid and helps the cleansing process. Make sure it's all gone by bedtime.

on waking

1 large glass of hot water with a thick slice of organic, unwaxed lemon.

breakfast

1 large glass of hot water with a thick slice of organic, unwaxed lemon.

1 glass of Ginger and Lemon Zizz (page 125).

mid-morning

1 large glass of hot water with a thick slice of organic, unwaxed lemon.

lunch

Mediterranean Muscle (page 39).

mid-afternoon

1 large glass of hot water with a thick slice of organic, unwaxed lemon.

supper

A Passion for Fruit (page 168).

Camomile tea.

evening

Primary Pepper Punch (page 34).

bedtime

Lime-blossom tea.

twenty-four-hour winter detox

This is another short, sharp twenty-four-hour detox fast designed for the colder months. As with the summer detox, this is not suitable for diabetics, and if you have some other serious illness or are currently taking prescribed medication, do check with your doctor before trying it.

It provides a great lift to your metabolism, and a quick boost to your white-cell count, increasing your natural resistance. Although you may develop a headache by the evening as your blood-sugar levels drop, it will be gone by the morning, and you will wake up feeling refreshed, revitalized and raring to go.

It's best to start this fast on a day when you're not working, and it's much more effective if on the day before, you keep off alcohol, coffee, red meat and dairy products. The day after the detox do the same, then return to your normal but (hopefully healthier) eating patterns. During the afternoon and early evening, be sure to drink at least six large glasses of water.

on waking

1 large glass of hot water with a thick slice of organic, unwaxed lemon.

breakfast

1 large mug of Green Tea with Apples (page 70) and 1 glass of water.

mid-morning

1 large mug of Lemon and Ginger Tea (page 150) and 1 handful of raisins.

lunch

Hot Banana Smoothie (page 127) and 1 large glass of hot water with a thick slice of organic, unwaxed lemon.

mid-afternoon

Hot Tommy (page 137), six dried apricots and 1 large glass of water.

early-evening

Chicken Yum-yum (page 17) and 1 glass of hot water with a large slice of organic, unwaxed lemon.

mid-evening

1 large mug of Sweet Dreams (page 185) and 1 tablespoon each of pumpkin seeds and walnuts.

bedtime

Camomile tea.

three-day juice detox

If you've overindulged and feel a bit sluggish, it's time for the three-day juice detox. Boost immunity; ward off colds; cleanse your liver and colon; rest your kidneys... and, as a bonus, lose four or five pounds.

There are few calories here, so be warned: you'll feel hungry. But don't cheat; you'll thank yourself for it later. There's also no coffee and only weak tea, which means no caffeine, and that's almost certain to cause headaches. Avoid the painkillers, though, and drink plenty of water. The headaches are transient, and you're going to feel great by day four and bursting with protective antioxidants.

I advise you to start the first two days of the diet when your workload is at its lightest.

day 1

breakfast

Pro-Bonus 1 (page 69).

1 orange, ½ grapefruit, 1 large slice of melon. Herb tea with honey.

lunch

Pro-Bonus 2 (page 69).

1 plateful of raw red and yellow peppers, cucumber, tomato, broccoli, cauliflower, celery, carrots, radishes and lots of fresh parsley. Add extra-virgin olive oil and lemon juice as a dressing.

evening meal

Peak Performer (page 33).

1 large mixed salad: lettuce, tomato, watercress, onion, garlic, beetroot, celeriac, fresh mint and any herbs you like. Add extra-virgin olive oil and lemon juice as a dressing.

day 2

breakfast

Hot and Smooth Prune (page 39).

Hot water with a thick slice of lemon.

mid-morning

Punch of Power (page 30).

1 handful each of raisins, dried apricots and fresh nuts.

lunch

Granny's Lemon Barley Water (page 106).

1 large salad of green leaves with radishes, celery, a sprinkle of sunflower seeds, lemon juice and olive oil. Herb or weak Indian tea with honey (no milk).

mid-afternoon

Lemon Express (page 106).

evening meal

Cucumber and Mint Slush (page 100).

1 Large jacket potato drizzled with olive oil and black pepper. Herb tea or weak Indian tea.

during the evening

A mixture of dried fruits and unsalted nuts and as much fresh fruit as you like.

day 3

breakfast

Blueberry Hill (page 167).

1 carton of live yogurt mixed with a tablespoon of unsweetened muesli. Weak tea or herb tea.

mid-morning

Minty Morning (page 109).

6 dried apricots.

lunch

Life Saver (page 149).

1 small bowl of raisins, sultanas, walnuts and almonds. Herb or weak Indian tea.

mid-afternoon

Tango Smoothie (page 72).

evening meal

Waterfall (page 111).

1 bowl of pasta with chopped garlic, olive oil and fresh, chopped tomatoes. 1 large mixed salad. 1 carton of low-fat live yogurt. Herb or weak Indian tea.

Treat your system gently on day four, and don't rush back to normal eating. Avoid red meat, and start with plainly cooked chicken or fish, some starchy foods, plenty of fruit, salads and vegetables. And no dairy products except yogurt, until day five.

three-day herbal detox

This three-day cleansing plan starts with a short, sharp shock specifically designed to detoxify the liver, rest the kidneys and cleanse the colon. As a bonus, it provides a huge boost for the body's natural immunity defences. Take heed, however: this short fast is not a diet for life, nor is it one that should be followed for weeks on end. Based on the traditional principles of fasting, its main objective is to boost the body's protective white-cell count and give it a chance to restore vital functions to their optimum performance.

day 1

The first detox day is designed to kick-start your metabolism by providing lots of potassium, vitamins A, B_1, B_6, C and E, folic acid and niacin. You should drink at least 1½ litres of fluid – water, weak tea or herbal tea – in addition to the menu below.

breakfast

1 orange, ½ grapefruit and a large slice of melon.

1 glass of unsalted vegetable juice.

1 cup of Sorrel Tea (page 128), with honey if desired.

lunch

1 plate of raw red and yellow peppers, cucumber, tomato, broccoli, cauliflower, celery, carrots, radishes, fresh parsley and fennel, with extra-virgin olive oil and lemon juice dressing.

1 large glass of unsweetened fruit juice.

dinner

1 large mixed salad – lettuce, tomato, watercress, onion, garlic, beetroot, celeriac, fresh mint, rocket and thyme – drizzled with extra-virgin olive oil and lemon juice. 1 large glass of unsweetened fruit juice or unsalted vegetable juice.

day 2

The second day of the plan provides an abundance of phosphorus, magnesium, potassium, copper, vitamin A, B_1, B_6, C and E and folic acid, along with protein, calcium, fibre, iron and selenium.

breakfast

1 large glass of hot mint tea with a thick slice of lemon and a tablespoon of honey.

1 small carton of natural low-fat live yogurt.

mid-morning

1 large glass of unsalted vegetable juice.

1 handful each of raisins, dried apricots and fresh nuts.

lunch

1 salad of grated carrot, red cabbage, apple, sliced red pepper, tomato, radishes, celery, marjoram, chicory, basil and a sprinkling of sunflower seeds, lemon juice and olive oil.
1 cup of Dill Tea (page 100).

mid-afternoon

1 glass of fruit juice and a banana.

dinner

Any three cooked vegetables (but not potatoes) sprinkled with thyme and capers and drizzled with olive oil, nutmeg and lemon juice. Fresh mint leaves in 1 cup of boiling water.

evening

A mixture of dried fruits and unsalted nuts and as much fresh fruit as you like.

day 3

The last day of the detox plan provides more than the daily requirement of fibre, phosphorus, magnesium, potassium, copper, vitamins A, B_1, B_2, B_6, C and E, niacin and folic acid, along with some vitamin B_{12}, calcium and iron.

breakfast

1 fresh fruit salad of apple, pear, grapes, mango and pineapple.
1 carton of live yogurt and a tablespoon of unsweetened muesli. Camomile tea (page 180).

mid-morning

6 dried apricots. 1 glass of unsweetened fruit juice or unsalted vegetable juice.

lunch

Lettuce soup: soften ½ a chopped onion in a large pan with a little olive oil; add ½ a shredded iceberg lettuce, stir for a few minutes, add 900ml (32 fl oz) of vegetable stock and lots of black pepper; simmer for twenty minutes, then sprinkle with a large handful of chopped parsley. 1 chunk of crusty wholemeal bread (no butter). Dandelion coffee (page 170).

mid-afternoon

1 apple and 1 pear.

dinner

Pasta with lettuce pesto: use the rest of the iceberg lettuce from lunch, processed with a handful of pine nuts, a little olive oil, 1 clove of garlic and 1 carton of low-fat fromage frais. Tomato, onion and yellow pepper salad. Fresh mint leaves in 1 cup of boiling water.

Well done! If you haven't cheated, you're probably four or five pounds lighter, your eyes are bright, your skin is clear and you feel terrific. Powerful herbs have worked their magic, and the natural chemicals in unadulterated food have lifted you, both physically and mentally.

seven-day organic detox

My patients have used this seven-day detox regime with great success. Be warned: the first day is tough, and you'll probably have a headache, but after that it's plain sailing.

day 1

A real fasting day, so choose a time when you can get plenty of rest.

breakfast, lunch, dinner

1 glass of unsweetened organic fruit juice or unsalted organic vegetable juice. 1 small carton of live low-fat natural yogurt.

Drink at least 3 litres of still mineral water or herbal teas (don't use milk, but you can add half a teaspoon of organic honey).

day 2

standard breakfast (to eat throughout the week)

1 portion of fresh fruit (vary throughout the week): apple, pear, mango, grape, pineapple or grapefruit.

2 slices of wholemeal toast spread with low-fat cottage cheese.

1 small carton of live low-fat yogurt.

1 small glass of skimmed milk. 1 cup of herbal or weak Indian tea without milk or sugar.

lunch

1 kiwi fruit. 200g or 7oz mixed raw vegetable salad: a bed of lettuce filled with grated carrot, celeriac and raw beetroot, with a squeeze of lemon juice and a drizzle of olive oil. 170g or 6oz of any steamed vegetables, sprinkled with a chopped garlic clove and a drizzle of olive oil. Herbal or weak Indian tea.

dinner

60g or 2oz organic berries in 120g or 4oz unsweetened organic muesli mixed with the juice of an orange and a small carton of live low-fat yogurt. Herbal or weak Indian tea.

day 3

standard breakfast

lunch

1 large mango. 170g or 6oz mixed salad (watercress, mint, spring onions, tomato, red/yellow peppers, chicory, baby spinach, bean sprouts) with lemon juice and olive oil dressing.

1 large jacket potato (with skin) with 60g or 2oz low-fat fromage frais, whipped with chopped chives and a clove of garlic. 1 glass of vegetable juice.

dinner

1 small carton of live low-fat yogurt with mixed berries and a teaspoon of honey.
1 crusty wholemeal roll with a matchbox-size piece of soft organic cheese: Brie, Camembert or similar. Herbal or weak Indian tea.

day 4

Your main food today will be organic rice. Make enough for the entire day: 100g or 3½oz dry brown rice cooked in 500ml of water (or half water and half vegetable stock for a more savoury flavour). Drink only water (at least 3 litres) with meals and in between.

breakfast

85g or 3oz rice with 145g or 5oz stewed apple with honey, cinnamon and lemon rind.

lunch

85g or 3oz rice with 200g or7oz steamed vegetables: celery, leek, carrot, tomato, spinach, broccoli and shredded cabbage.

dinner

85g or 3oz rice mixed with soaked dried apricots, raisins, sultanas and the flesh of a pink grapefruit.

day 5

standard breakfast

lunch

1 apple and 1 pear. 170g or 6oz raw vegetable salad (cauliflower and broccoli florets, carrot, spring onion, grated red cabbage, mange tout) tossed in olive oil and cider vinegar dressing, sprinkled with a teaspoon of raisins, and 3 chopped brazil nuts.
1 large jacket potato (with skin) filled with 85g or 3oz steamed spinach, chopped, with 2 teaspoons of olive oil, 1 chopped garlic clove and a generous grating of nutmeg.
Herbal or weak Indian tea.

dinner

85g or 3oz fromage frais mixed with 1 carton of live, low-fat yogurt, poured over a generous bowl of mixed fruit salad, including kiwi, pineapple, orange, grapes, berries and apple.
Herbal or weak Indian tea.

day 6

Standard breakfast

lunch

1 banana. 170g or 6oz mixed salad: mixed shredded lettuce leaves (cos, little gem, lamb's

lettuce, radicchio), tomato, olives, red pepper, carrot, spring onions, cucumber, 1 clove of garlic, fennel and watercress, with a dressing of lemon juice, walnut oil and tarragon. 1 large jacket potato filled with 85g or 3oz steamed French or runner beans sprinkled with a dessertspoon of sunflower oil and finely chopped onions. Herbal or weak Indian tea.

dinner

85g or 3oz muesli mixed with 1 dessertspoon of lemon juice, 1 teaspoon of honey, 1 grated apple and 1 small carton of live low-fat yogurt.

1 slice of wholemeal bread, with a matchbox-sized piece of Brie, Camembert or similar soft organic cheese.

1 slice of wholemeal bread with honey. Herbal or weak Indian tea.

day 7

standard breakfast

lunch

170g or 6oz mixed salad (watercress, baby spinach, mixed lettuce leaves, parsley, celery, garlic, chives, basil, tomato) with a dressing of ⅓ walnut oil, ⅓ olive oil, ⅓ cider vinegar and 1 teaspoon of Dijon mustard (make a large amount and store in bottles), sprinkled with sunflower seeds.

85g or 3oz boiled potatoes in their skins. 1 trout stuffed with finely chopped parsley, onion, tomato and pine nuts, covered in thinly sliced lemon, baked in foil with a little olive oil. Vegetarian alternative: stir-fried tofu with shredded carrot, bean sprouts, mangetout and soy sauce. 1 glass of dry white wine.

dinner

1 whole pink grapefruit. 2 poached eggs on 2 slices of wholemeal toast with a scrape of butter. Herbal or weak Indian tea.

Well done! If you haven't cheated, you're probably four or five pounds lighter, your eyes are bright, your skin is clear, and you feel terrific. The high-fibre content of this week has really got your digestion working and all the super-protective natural chemicals in pure, unadulterated organic food have lifted your spirits. Best of all, you'll finish the week with lower blood pressure, less cholesterol and a rested liver.

Taking some exercise is also vital to a detox regime. No matter what the weather, dress appropriately and get into the fresh air and daylight whenever possible. Even on overcast days, you'll get enough sunlight to help ward off the problems of seasonal affective disorder syndrome (SAD). A brisk, 20-minute walk three times a week will make all the difference.

three-day immune diet

This three-day eating plan is perfect at times of stress, when resistance is lowered and when flu, coughs and colds are rampant. During each day, drink at least 1 litre of water and an equal quantity of other fluids (herbal teas, fruit/vegetable juice, weak Indian or China tea).

day 1

breakfast

½ grapefruit, 1 poached egg and 2 poached tomatoes.

lunch

Avocado, tomato and mushroom salad plus 115g or 4oz of low-fat cottage cheese. 1 large bunch of grapes.

dinner

1 large bowl of thinly sliced cucumber with lots of black pepper, cider vinegar and 1 teaspoon of extra-virgin olive oil. A generous portion of mixed stir-fried vegetables served on a bed of plain boiled rice.

day 2

breakfast

1 large fresh peach and 6 ripe strawberries.

lunch

1 large green salad and a mixture of lots of steamed vegetables – carrots, courgettes, new potatoes, peas, string beans, sweetcorn – tossed in a light teaspoon of butter and sprinkled with fresh chopped mint and parsley.

dinner

1 bowl of vegetable soup. 1 large red or yellow pepper stuffed with rice, and a generous portion of lightly cooked spinach with a drizzle of extra-virgin olive oil and 1 clove of garlic.

day 3

breakfast

1 large bowl of cherries and 1 small carton of live, low-fat natural yogurt.

lunch

1 mixed green salad. A generous portion of pasta topped with olive oil, garlic and parsley.

dinner

1 small carton of live, low-fat natural yogurt with cucumber, fresh mint, garlic, black pepper and olive oil. 1 skinless grilled chicken breast, with grilled tomato, lettuce and boiled potatoes.

twenty-four-hour big-day diet

For maximum concentration and brain power during a stressful time, it's best to reverse some normal eating patterns. The object of this exercise is to be at peak performance during the morning and afternoon, and to unwind, relax and sleep well during the evening and night.

The same eating plan will sharpen your concentration and keep your brain in top gear for important interviews, crucial business meetings or vital social events. Combined with the mood-boosters that suit your needs, you'll have no worries – whatever the occasion.

Nutritionally perfect for extended periods of brain work, the daily diet below provides approximately 2,000 calories, lots of protein, low carbohydrates, low fat, low salt and well over the recommended daily requirement of each essential nutrient. Follow this, and your mind will be fully alert when you need it most.

breakfast

This needs to be high-protein, low-fat, and little carbohydrate, so...

1 large glass of fresh orange or pineapple juice. 1 small carton of live, low-fat natural yogurt with toasted almonds or pistachios. 1 poached egg with baked beans and 1 apple or pear.

mid-morning

1 snack of dried apricots, raisins, dates and plain fresh nuts.

lunch

1 mixed salad with cold meat, fish or low-fat cheese. Add sesame seeds, sunflower seeds and pumpkin seeds to the salad, and include plenty of watercress and tomatoes.

mid-afternoon

1 piece of low-fat cheese (if you haven't had it already today) or 1 hard-boiled egg with 1 apple, pear or bunch of grapes.

evening meal

1 thick, root-vegetable casserole made with potatoes, parsnip, turnip, carrot, onion, celery, shredded cabbage, canned kidney beans and rice or barley, or 1 generous portion of pasta or risotto with your favorite low-fat sauce. Finish with 1 delicious carbohydrate-rich rice pudding – add plenty of nutmeg. During the evening, eat 1 banana and a few dates or dried apricots.

If your mental faculties are needed in the evening, and you want a calm day, stick to cereals and bread for breakfast, then have the starch meal for lunch and the protein meal for dinner.

three-day powerhouse diet

These three days feature mouthwatering recipes that taste good, look good and do you good. Once you've experienced the energy surge provided by these vitality foods, you'll want to use them at least one or two days each week as part of your normal eating plan.

To avoid a lack of energy, make sure you never skip breakfast and don't go more than three hours without food: always have a banana and a bag of unsalted fresh nuts, raisins and dried apricots handy to satisfy hunger pangs. In addition to the menus below, drink at least 1½–2½ litres of fluid a day – herbal tea or water – to flush out your system.

day 1

breakfast

Sliced oranges and pink grapefruit. 1 small carton of live, low-fat natural yogurt, sprinkled with 1 teaspoon of chopped nuts and 1 teaspoon of honey.

lunch

Scrambled eggs with mushrooms on a bed of mixed salad leaves. Dried-fruit compote: add boiling water, a rosehip tea bag, 1 tablespoon of honey and 2 cloves to a bowl of mixed dried fruits – prunes, apricots, figs, apple rings, pears, peaches etc. Cover and leave to stand overnight. Remove the tea bag and serve with a sprinkle of flaked almonds.

dinner

1 red and 1 yellow pepper stuffed with brown rice, raisins, onion, parsley, mint and pine nuts and cooked. Serve with crusty wholewheat bread. Fresh dates and figs.

day 2

breakfast

Dried-fruit compote with 1 small carton of live, low-fat natural yogurt and 1 orange.

lunch

½ an avocado, sliced, with watercress, tomatoes and cucumber, on mixed leaves, sprinkled with 1 generous squeeze of lemon juice. 1 crusty wholewheat roll.

dinner

Mustard-Marinated Salmon Steaks (page 240) served with puréed spinach, seasoned with nutmeg. A selection of vitality-boosting tropical fruits: pineapple, mango, kiwi, pawpaw and passion fruit.

day 3

A meatless day, just to show that vegetarian food doesn't have to be all brown rice and lentils. Vegetarians are less likely to have high blood pressure, heart disease, gallstones, constipation, haemorrhoids and bowel cancer, so why not give it a try?

This is also a heart-friendly day, with little cholesterol or saturated fat, a low dose of salt but plenty of heart-protective monounsaturated fats. Lots of vitality vitamins are guaranteed to put a spring in your step.

breakfast

2 hot wholewheat rolls spread with a little butter and 1 banana.

lunch

Risotto con Salsa Cruda (page 241) with 1 green salad. For dessert, have a mixture of some raisins and nuts.

dinner

Aubergine Caviar with Crudités (page 241).

mustard-marinated salmon steaks

4 salmon steaks

For the marinade:

2 tbsp extra-virgin olive oil
2 tbsp finely chopped onion
4 tbsp dry white wine
salt and pepper, to taste
2 tbsp Dijon mustard

To garnish:

lemon slices
fresh cilantro sprigs

Place the marinade ingredients in a screw-top jar, shake then pour into a large, shallow dish.

Add the salmon steaks to the dish, coat with the marinade and refrigerate for approximately three hours, turning once.

Brush the rack of a grill pan with oil. Lift the salmon out of the marinade with a slotted spoon, place on the rack and brush each steak with some of the marinade. Grill at a high temperature for four minutes on each side.

Serve garnished with lemon and cilantro.

Serves 4

risotto con salsa cruda

250g or 9oz long-grain brown rice
a pinch salt
4 medium tomatoes, chopped
½ medium cucumber, peeled and diced
2 cloves garlic, finely chopped
4 medium spring onions, finely chopped
4 medium carrots, finely chopped
4 medium radishes, finely chopped
3 small courgettes, finely chopped
1 tbsp fresh or frozen peas
125ml or 4 fl oz extra-virgin olive oil
ground sea salt, to taste
freshly ground black pepper, to taste
chopped chives and parsley, to taste

Bring a pan of slightly salted water to the boil – the amount of water should be twice the volume of the rice.

Wash the rice, add to the boiling water, cover and cook gently for about forty minutes. Check it occasionally, but don't stir.

When cooked, remove the rice from heat, drain and leave uncovered for ten minutes, until dry and separated.

In a bowl combine the tomatoes, cucumber, garlic, spring onions, carrots, radishes, courgettes and peas. Add the olive oil and season lightly. Allow to marinate for thirty minutes.

While the rice is still warm, gently stir in the vegetable mixture. Season to taste, and sprinkle with the chopped herbs.

aubergine caviar with crudités

2 large aubergines
juice of 1 large lemon
3 tbsp extra-virgin olive oil
1 clove garlic, crushed
2 tbsp live, low-fat natural yogurt
ground sea salt, to taste
freshly ground black pepper, to taste
½ tsp cilantro seeds, crushed
chopped chives and parsley, to taste

Preheat the oven to 200°C (400°F/gas mark 6). Bake the aubergine until soft (about twenty minutes).

Cut the aubergine open, and scrape the flesh into a bowl. Add the lemon juice to the flesh and beat in the olive oil, drop by drop, to form a smooth cream.

Stir the garlic and yogurt into the aubergine mixture. Season with salt, pepper and the crushed cilantro seeds. Combine well, cover and chill for an hour.

Serve with crudités – strips of carrot, celery, cucumber, fennel and sprigs of cauliflower.

raw ingredients a–z

ingredient	source of
Alfalfa sprouts	Calcium, silicon, vitamins A, B complex, C, E and K
Apples	Carotenes, ellagic acid, pectin, potassium, vitamin C
Apricots	Betacarotene, iron, potassium, soluble fibre
Artichokes, Jerusalem	Inulin, iron, phosphorus
Asparagus	Asparagine, folic acid, potassium, phosphorus, riboflavin, vitamin C
Banana	Energy, fibre, folic acid, magnesium, potassium, vitamin A
Basil	Volatile oils: linalol, limonene, estragole
Beetroot	Betacarotene, calcium, folic acid, iron, potassium, vitamins B_6 and C
Blackcurrants	Anti-inflammatory and cancer-fighting phytochemicals, carotenoids, vitamin C
Blueberries	Antibacterial and cancer-fighting phytochemicals, carotenoids, vitamin C
Brazil nuts	Protein, selenium, vitamins B and E
Brewer's yeast	B vitamins, biotin, folic acid, iron, magnesium, zinc
Broccoli	Cancer-fighting phytochemicals, folic acid, iron, potassium, riboflavin, vitamins A and C
Cabbage family	Cancer-fighting phytochemicals, folic acid, potassium, vitamins A, C and E
Carrots	Carotenoids, folic acid, magnesium, potassium, vitamin A
Celery	Coumarins, potassium, vitamin C
Chard (Swiss)	Calcium, cancer-fighting phytochemicals, carotenes, iron, phosphorus, vitamins A and C
Cherries	Cancer-fighting phytochemicals, flavonoids, magnesium, potassium, vitamin C
Chicory	Bitter, liver-stimulating terpenoids, folic acid, iron, potassium, vitamin A (if unblanched)
Chives	Betacarotene, cancer-fighting phytochemicals, vitamin C
Cinnamon	Coumarins, tannins and volatile oils with mild, sedative/analgesic blood pressure-lowering effects
Cloves	Volatile oil (especially eugenol) with anti-nausea, antiseptic antibacterial and analgesic properties
Coconut milk	Calcium, magnesium, potassium, small quantities of B vitamins

ingredient	source of
Coriander	Coumarins, flavonoids, linalol
Cottage cheese	Calcium, folic acid, magnesium, protein, vitamin A and B
Cranberries	Cancer-fighting phytochemicals, specific urinary antibacterials, vitamin C
Cucumber	Folic acid, potassium, silica, small amounts of betacarotene in the skin
Cumin seeds	Flavonoids that relieve intestinal wind and spasm, volatile oils
Dandelion	Betacarotene, diuretic and liver-stimulating phytochemicals, iron, other carotenoids
Dates	Fibre, folic acid, fruit sugar, iron, potassium
Fennel	Volatile oils: fenchone, anethole and anisic acid, all liver and digestive stimulants
Figs	Betacarotene, cancer-fighting phytochemicals, fibre, ficin (a digestive aid) iron, potassium
Garlic	Antibacterial and antifungal sulphur compounds, cancer and heart disease-fighting phytochemicals
Ginger	Circulation-stimulating zingiberene and gingerols
Grapefruit	Betacarotene, bioflavonoids – especially naringin, which thins the blood and lowers cholesterol, vitamin C
Grapes	Natural sugars, powerful antioxidant flavonoids, vitamin C
Horseradish	Natural antibiotics, protective phytochemicals, vitamin C
Jalapeño pepper	Carotenoids, capsaicin: a circulatory stimulant, flavonoids
Kale	Betacarotene, calcium, cancer-fighting phytochemicals, folic acid, iron, phosphorus, sulphur, vitamin C
Kiwi fruit	Betacarotene, bioflavonoids, fibre, potassium, vitamin C
Kohlrabi	Cancer-fighting phytochemicals, folic acid, potassium, vitamin C
Lamb's lettuce	Folic acid, iron, potassium, vitamins A, C and B_6, zinc. Also contains calming phytochemicals
Lecithin	Phospholipids extracted from soya beans: heart protective and beneficial to nerves
Leeks	Anti-arthritic, anti-inflammatory substances, cancer-fighting phytochemicals, folic acid, potassium, diuretic substances, vitamins A and C
Lemon	Bioflavonoids, limonene, potassium, vitamin C
Lettuce	Calcium, folic acid, phosphorus, potassium, sleep-inducing phytochemicals, vitamins A and C
Lime	Bioflavonoids, limonene, potassium, vitamin C

ingredient	source of
Mango	Betacarotene, flavonoids, potassium, other antioxidants, vitamin C
Mangosteen	Digestion-friendly mucilage, potassium, vitamin C
Melon	Folic acid, potassium, vitamins A and C, small amounts of B vitamins,
Milk	Calcium, protein, riboflavin, zinc
Mint	Antispasmodic volatile oils, flavonoids, menthol
Mixed salad leaves	Calcium, folic acid, phosphorus, potassium, sleep-inducing phytochemicals (the darkest leaves contain the most nutrients), vitamins A and C
Molasses	Calcium, iron, magnesium, phosphorus
Mooli	Iron, magnesium, phytochemicals that stimulate the gall bladder and heal mucous membranes, potassium, vitamin C
Nutmeg	Myristicin: mood enhancing and hallucinogenic in excess; phytochemicals that aid sleep and digestion
Oranges and citrus fruits (including mandarins, satsumas and tangerines)	Bioflavonoids, calcium, folic acid, iron, limonene, potassium, thiamine, vitamin B_6 and C
Pak choi	Betacarotene, vitamin B and C, cancer-fighting phytochemicals, folic acid,
Parsley	Calcium, iron, potassium, vitamins A and C
Parsnip	Folic acid, inulin, potassium, vitamin B and E
Passion-fruit	Betacarotene, phytochemicals that are antiseptic, sedative and mildly laxative, vitamin C
Pawpaw	Betacarotene, flavonoids, magnesium, papain: a digestive enzyme, vitamin C
Peaches	betacarotene, flavonoids, potassium, vitamin C
Peanuts	B vitamins, folic acid, protein, iron, zinc
Pears	Soluble fibre, vitamin C
Peppers	Betacarotene, folic acid, potassium, phytochemicals that prevent blood clots, strokes and heart disease, vitamin C
Pineapple	Enzymes (especially bromelain, helpful for angina, arthritis and physical injury), vitamin C
Plums	Betacarotene, malic acid: an effective aid to digestion, vitamins C and E
Pomegranate	Betacarotene, enzymes with antidiarrhoeal properties, heart-protective phytochemicals, vitamin E
Prunes	Betacarotene, fibre, iron, niacin, potassium, vitamin B_6
Pumpkin	Folic acid, potassium, vitamins A and C, small amounts of B vitamins

ingredient	source of
Purslane	Essential fatty acids and cleansing bitter alkaloids, folic acid, vitamins C and E
Radishes	Iron, magnesium, phytochemicals that stimulate the gall bladder and heal mucous membranes, potassium, vitamin C
Rosemary	Flavonoids, volatile oils: borneol, camphor, limonene
Sage	Phenolic acids, phyto-oestrogens, thujone: an antiseptic
Sauerkraut	Calcium, cancer-fighting phytochemicals, gut-protective lactic acid, potassium, vitamin C
Seaweed	Betacarotene, calcium, iodine, iron, protein, magnesium, potassium, soluble fibre, vitamin B_{12}, zinc
Sesame seeds	Calcium, folic acid, magnesium, niacin, protein, vitamins B and E
Sorrel	Carotenoids, iron, protective phytochemicals, vitamin C
Soya milk	Calcium, phyto-oestrogens, especially genistein (a powerful breast, ovarian and prostate cancer-fighter), protein. If fortied, also vitamin D
Spinach	Betacarotene, cancer-fighting phytochemicals, chlorophyll, folic acid, iron, lutein, xeaxanthine
Spring greens	Betacarotene, cancer-fighting phytochemicals, carotenoids, iron, vitamin C
Spring onion	Cancer-fighting phytochemicals, diuretic, anti-arthritic and anti-inflammatory substances, folic acid, potassium, vitamins A and C
Stinging nettle	Betacarotene, calcium, iron, vitamin C
Strawberries	Anti-arthritic phytochemicals, betacarotene, vitamins C and E
Sweet potato	Betacarotene and other carotenoids, cancer-fighting phytochemicals, protein, vitamins C and E
Tahini	Calcium, folic acid, magnesium, niacin, protein, vitamins B and E
Thyme	Flavonoids, volatile oils: antiseptic thymol and carvol
Tomatoes	Betacarotene, lycopene, potassium, vitamins C and E
Watercress	Antibacterial mustard oils, betacarotene, iron, phenethyl isothiocyanate: specific lung cancer-fighter for smokers, vitamins C and E
Watermelon	Folic acid, potassium, vitamins A and C, small amounts of B vitamins
Wheat germ	Folic acid, iron, magnesium, potassium, vitamins B and E
Yogurt: milk	Beneficial bacteria, calcium, protein, riboflavin, zinc
Yogurt: soya	calcium, phyto-oestrogens, especially genistein: a powerful breast, ovarian and prostate cancer fighter. If fortified, also contains vitamin D

vitamins and minerals a–z

vitamins	essential for	best food sources
A	Growth, skin, colour and night vision, immunity	Butter, cheese, chicken liver, cod liver oil, eggs, herring, lamb's liver, mackerel, salmon
B_1 (Thiamine)	Conversion of starchy foods into energy	Brewer's yeast (dried), peanuts, peanut butter, pork and pork products, sunflower seeds, veggie burger mixes, wheat germ, yeast extract
B_2 (Riboflavin)	Converting fats and proteins into energy; also for mucous membranes and skin	Brewer's yeast, cheese, eggs, green leafy vegetables, liver, meat, soya products, wheat germ, yeast extracts, yogurt
B_3 (Niacin)	Brain and nerve function, healthy skin, tongue and digestive organs	Brewer's yeast (dried), cheese, dried fruits, eggs, nuts, oily fish, pig's liver, poultry, wholegrain cereals, yeast extracts
B_6 (Pyridoxine)	Protein conversion, protection against heart disease, regulation of menstrual cycle, growth, nervous and immune systems	Bananas, beef, brewer's yeast, cod, herring, lentils, poultry, salmon, walnuts, wheat germ
B_{12}	Metabolism, nervous system, prevention of pernicious anaemia, proper formation of blood cells. With B_6, controls levels of homocysteine, which may cause heart disease	Beef, cheese, eggs, lamb, liver, oily fish, pork, seaweed
Betacarotene	Essential in its own right for protection against heart disease, cancer, and as an immune-booster. Not a vitamin in its own right, but listed here as it is also converted by the body into vitamin A (see above)	Apricots, chard, dark green and red leaf lettuce, dark leafy greens, mangoes, old carrots, pumpkin, red and yellow peppers, spinach, squashes, sweet potatoes, tomatoes, watercress, yellow melons
C	Natural immunity, wound healing, iron absorption; extremely powerful antioxidant that protects against heart disease, circulatory problems and cancers	All citrus fruits, all green vegetables, berries, currants, lettuces, peppers, potatoes, tomatoes, tropical fruits: guavas, mangoes, kiwi fruits and pineapple

vitamins	essential for	best food sources
D	Bone formation, protection from osteoporosis and rickets	Canned sardines, cod liver oil, eggs, fresh tuna, herring, kipper, mackerel, salmon, trout
E	Antioxidant protection of the heart and blood vessels, skin, immune-boosting and cancer-fighting	Avocado, broccoli, nuts and seeds, peanut butter, safflower/sunflower/olive and other seed oils, spinach, sweet potatoes, watercress, wheat germ
Folic acid	Blood cells, prevention of birth defects, protects against anaemia	Brewer's yeast (dried), citrus fruits, eggs, dried fruits, fresh nuts, green leafy vegetables, liver, oats, pulses, soya flour, wheat germ
Calcium	Bone formation and prevention of osteoporosis, proper functioning of heart muscles and nerves	Brazil nuts, cheese, chickpeas, dried seaweeds, figs, greens, milk, shellfish, tinned sardines, tofu, whitebait, yogurt
Iodine	Normal functioning of the thyroid gland	Cod, cockles, haddock (fresh or smoked), milk, mussels, seaweed, smoked mackerel, whelks
Iron	Red blood cells	Liver, kidney, dried apricots, wholemeal bread, spinach, raisins, prunes, dates, lentils, sesame and pumpkin seeds, legumes, nuts, dark-green leafy vegetables, beef and other meats
Magnesium	Energy-producing processes, the functions of vitamins B_1 and B_6, growth and repair	Almonds, brazil nuts, brown rice, cashews, peas, pine nuts, sunflower and sesame seeds, soya-based protein, soya beans
Potassium	Normal cell function, nerves, control of blood pressure	Bananas, cheese, dried fruits, eggs, molasses, nuts, fresh fruit, fruit juices, raw vegetables, tea, wholemeal bread
Selenium	Powerful antioxidant: protects against heart disease, prostate cancer and lung cancer	Brazil nuts, dried mushrooms, lamb's kidneys and liver, lentils, sardines, sunflower seeds, tuna, walnuts, white fish, wholemeal bread
Zinc	Growth, hormone function, male fertility, liver function, immunity, taste	Cheese, dried seaweed, eggs, liver, oysters, pumpkin/sesame/sunflower seeds, pine nuts, shellfish, wholemeal bread

health boosters

ailment	booster	effect
Acne	Artichoke, Dandelion	Artichoke improves liver function and fat digestion. Dandelion is both cleansing and diuretic.
Anxiety	Passionflower, Valerian	Both are calming and mild tranquillizers.
Arthritis	Devil's claw, Glucosamine, Pycnogenols	Devil's claw and pycnogenols are both anti-inflammatories, while glucosamine sulphate helps repair damaged cartilage.
Back pain	Chili, Devil's claw	Chili stimulates the circulation and promotes healing of damaged tissues. Devil's claw is a natural anti-inflammatory.
Boils	Garlic, Tea tree	Both are powerful antibacterials (eat one clove of garlic a day or take as tablets; apply tea tree oil directly to the boil).
Bruising	Horse chestnut, Pycnogenols	Horse chestnut improves capillary blood flow. Pycnogenols are natural anti-inflammatories.
Chilblains	Chili, Ginger, Vitamin E	All stimulate and improve circulation to the extremities.
Cholesterol	Evening primrose oil, Folic acid, Garlic	Evening primrose oil is anti-inflammatory and protects the arteries. Folic acid controls levels of heart-damaging homocysteine. Garlic helps reduce blood cholesterol.
Chronic fatigue	BIO-STRATH Elixir, Coenzyme Q10, Ginseng, St John's wort	BIO-STRATH is an immune-booster, protects against infection and improves nutrient uptake. Coenzyme Q10 improves energy release from food. Ginseng boosts energy. St John's wort helps with depression that accompanies chronic fatigue.
Circulation problems	Ginger, Ginkgo biloba, Vitamin E	Ginger stimulates circulation and improves blood flow. Ginkgo biloba helps dilate the tiny capillaries at the end of the circulatory system. Vitamin E strengthens blood vessel walls.
Colds	Devil's claw, Echinacea, Lapacho	Devil's claw lessens aches and pains. Echinacea and lapacho are both immune-boosters.
Cough	Garlic, Liquorice, Valerian	Garlic is antibacterial. Liquorice is an effective expectorant. Valerian improves sleep that is interrupted by coughing.

ailment	booster	effect
Cramps	Chili, Ginger, Vitamin E	All stimulate and improve circulation.
Cystitis	Cranberry, Dandelion	Cranberry protects against urinary bacteria. Dandelion is diuretic.
Depression	Kava kava, Lemon balm, St John's wort	Kava kava eases stress and anxiety. Lemon balm relieves physical tension. St John's wort helps moderate depression.
Fever	Camomile, Feverfew, Tea tree	Camomile helps ease fevers, especially for children. Feverfew helps lower body temperature. Tea tree is antibacterial.
Flatulence	Fennel, Peppermint	Both relieve symptoms.
Fluid retention	Dandelion	Dandelion leaves are powerfully diuretic.
Gallstones	Artichoke, Fenugreek	Artichoke stimulates the gall bladder and improves liver function. Fenugreek protects and stimulates the liver.
Gastritis	Camomile, Fennel, Peppermint	Camomile relieves stomach pain. Fennel seeds relieve gastric discomfort. Peppermint reduces stomach acidity.
Gout	Dandelion, Devil's claw, Lemon balm, Pycnogenols	Dandelion's diuretic action helps remove uric acid, which causes the pain of gout. Devil's claw and pycnogenols are anti-inflammatories. Lemon balm relieves muscle spasms.
Hair problems	Camomile, BIO-STRATH elixir, Red clover	Camomile helps strengthen weak hair (drink as tea or use tea as a rinse after washing). BIO-STRATH improves nutrient absorption to aid hair health. Red clover provides plant hormones that may help reduce hair loss.
Headache	Artichoke, Dong quai, Feverfew	Artichoke cleanses the liver (good for hangover headaches). Dong quai relieves vascular spasm, so may help headaches associated with blood flow. Feverfew eases headaches.
Heart disease	Folic acid, Garlic, Lycopene, Selenium, Vitamin E	Folic acid controls homocysteine levels, a predictor of heart disease. Garlic lowers blood pressure and cholesterol, as well as reducing the stickiness of blood. Lycopene is a protective antioxidant. Selenium is an essential mineral. Vitamin E protects both heart and arteries against oxidative damage.
Hepatitis	Artichoke, Milk thistle	Artichoke stimulates the liver and gall bladder and improves fat digestion. Milk thistle is useful for all liver problems.

ailment	booster	effect
Herpes	Garlic, Lemon balm	Both are specifically antiviral. Dab the cut end of a garlic clove on to affected areas, eat garlic in food or take as tablets. Take lemon balm as tea; use cold tea as a lotion on any areas affected by the herpes virus.
Hypertension	Coenzyme Q10, Flax seeds, Garlic	Coenzyme Q10 may lead to significant reduction in blood pressure. Flax seed oil aids cholesterol and blood-pressure reduction. Garlic lowers blood pressure and cholesterol.
Impotence	Catuaba, Muira puama, Pfaffia	Catuaba stimulates the central nervous system. Muira puama helps improve sexual function. Pfaffia helps combat stress.
Indigestion	Camomile, Fennel seeds, Peppermint	Camomile relieves stomach pain. Fennel seeds relieve flatulence. Peppermint reduces stomach acidity.
Influenza	Cat's claw, Echinacea, Turmeric	Cat's claw is a great immune booster. Echinacea protects against viruses. Turmeric is antibacterial and antiviral.
Insomnia	Passionflower, St John's wort, Valerian	Passionflower is calmative. St John's wort is an antidepressant; insomnia can be a symptom of depression. Valerian encourages deeper sleep and prevents waking in the small hours.
Memory loss	Ginkgo biloba, Phosphatidylserine	Ginkgo biloba stimulates blood flow to the smallest blood vessels of the brain, specifically improving short-term memory loss. Phosphatidylserine is a vital regulator of brain function and helps improve general memory.
Menstrual problems	Black cohosh, Camomile, Dandelion	Black cohosh helps regulate general physical and emotional disruptions of the menstrual cycle. Camomile eases painful breasts before and during periods. Dandelion helps correct fluid retention, that causes menstrual discomfort.
Mouth ulcers	Garlic, Lemon balm, Probiotics	Garlic oil is excellent for healing mouth ulcers (rub the ulcers with the cut, squeezed end of a clove). Lemon balm is antiviral and prevents secondary infections (use lemon balm tea as an antiviral mouthwash). Probiotics replace the friendly bacteria in the mouth and digestive tract which protect against infections.
Prostate problems	Zinc, oyster extract	Zinc is essential for proper functioning of the prostate.
Raynaud's syndrome	Chilli, Ginger, Ginkgo biloba, Vitamin E	All stimulate and improve circulation to the extremities.

ailment	booster	effect
Seasonal Affective Disorder (SAD)	Ginseng, Lemon balm, St John's wort	While none of these is a true treatment for the condition (light therapy is most effective), together they can produce a remarkable improvement. Ginseng provides an energy boost, which at least enables sufferers to be more active. Lemon balm relaxes physical tension and aids well-being. St John's wort helps to overcome the inevitable depression of SAD.
Tired all the time syndrome	BIO-STRATH elixir, Guarana, Kelp, Schisandra	BIO-STRATH promotes well-being. Guarana provides a gentle, slow-release energy boost. Kelp stimulates the thyroid, which is commonly, though subclinically, underactive. Schisandra restores the zest for life and improves mental state.
Varicose veins	Chili, Garlic, Ginger, Horse chestnut, Vitamin E	All stimulate and improve circulation to the extremities. Vitamin E in particular helps to strengthen vein walls.

vegetable stock

If you're serious about an occasional detox session, then this recipe is a must. Apart from its wonderful flavour, it has none of the unwanted chemicals present in most stock cubes. Ideally, you need a giant stockpot for the job, but if you don't have one, simply reduce the quantities. Place a large pasta basket inside the pot to hold all the vegetables; it saves straining the stock. This stock **freezes brilliantly**, especially in ice-cube trays.

2 large onions, unpeeled, cut in half

3 celery sticks with leaves, chopped

5 large carrots, chopped

3 medium turnips, chopped

3 large leeks, chopped (including green part)

1 entire bulb garlic, unpeeled and halved horizontally

3 ripe plum tomatoes, quartered

1 generous bunch flat-leaf parsley

1 generous bunch thyme, rosemary and bay leaves, tied together (or 2 bouquets garnis)

5 whole peppercorns

4 litres or 135 fl oz water

Put all ingredients into the pan, bring to the boil and leave to simmer gently for two hours without a lid.

If using a large basket to hold the vegetables, lift it out and use a wooden spoon to press the vegetables in order to extract the maximum flavour and nutrients. If you haven't got a basket, pour through the biggest sieve you have, again using a wooden spoon to squeeze the cooked vegetables. The stock will keep happily in the fridge for several days or for up to three months in the freezer.

Because none of the vegetables is peeled, you can make this stock safely only by using **organic** produce. Rich in **potassium** and **vitamin A**, with useful quantities of calcium, phosphorus, folic acid and vitamin C. This stock contains beneficial cancer-fighting, **heart-protective** plant nutrients.

fish stock

Home-made fish stock tastes absolutely stunning and will impart a professional flavour to all fish and shellfish soups, sauces and risottos. It is rich in **iodine**, a mineral often deficient in modern diets.

100g or 3½oz fish trimmings and bones, washed and dried

3 carrots, trimmed and peeled if not organic, cubed

2 sweet, white Spanish onions, coarsely chopped

1 large leek, washed and coarsely chopped

1 generous bunch flat-leaf parsley

1 generous bunch rosemary, mint and tarragon, tied together (or 2 bouquets garnis)

1½ litres or 55 fl oz water, or 1 litre or 35 fl oz water and 500 ml or 18 fl oz dry white wine

8 white peppercorns

½ tsp salt

Put all ingredients into the pan, bring to the boil and simmer gently for thirty minutes without a lid, skimming the surface regularly.

Strain through kitchen muslin or a fine sieve.

chicken stock

After vegetable stock, this is probably the most useful stock recipe. Because it's fairly neutral in flavour, good chicken stock can be substituted for beef or ham stock. It is particularly good for making most soups and risottos.

1 chicken carcass

2 litres or 70 fl oz water

6 spring onions, green tips left on

1 large leek, trimmed, washed and coarsely chopped

2 large stalks of celery, chopped

1 generous bunch of rosemary, sage and thyme, tied together (or 2 bouquets garnis)

half a large bunch parsley

3 bay leaves

10 white peppercorns

⅓ tsp salt

Put the chicken carcass in a large saucepan. Cover with the water, bring to the boil and simmer for about thirty minutes.

Add the rest of the ingredients, return to the boil and simmer for an additional forty minutes.

Strain through kitchen muslin or a fine sieve.

index

Entries in **bold** are recipe names